Textbook of
CANCER BIOLOGY

Textbook of CANCER BIOLOGY

C. Vaman Rao
Former Professor and Head
Department of Biotechnology Engineering
Nitte Mahalinga Adyanthaya Memorial Institute of Technology
Nitte, Udupi, Karnataka, India

Jayaprakash Shetty
Vice-Dean/Professor and Head
Department of Pathology
K. S. Hegde Medical Academy
(Nitte – Deemed to be University)
Mangaluru, Karnataka, India

TECHSAR™
NEW DELHI

Published by
I.K. International Pvt. Ltd.
4435-36/7, Ansari Road, Daryaganj
New Delhi-110 002 (India)
E-mail: tech_info@techsarworld.com
Website: www.techsarworld.com

ISBN: 978-93-90620-40-1

Published/Printed by Krishan Makhijani for I.K. International Pvt. Ltd., 4435-36/7, Ansari Road, Daryaganj, New Delhi-110 002

Dedicated to

the lotus feet of my Sadguru

Shri Shirdi Saibaba

Preface

The *Textbook of Cancer Biology* is meant for undergraduate students of biological sciences, biotechnology, and medical sciences. This book is the outcome of the literature survey on cancer research caried out by the authors and many years of teaching the subject to the undergraduate students. We are sure, this book will enthuse and invigorate interest in undergraduate students who are novice to the subject of Cancer Biology. We are confident that this book will help the students in understanding the basic concepts of causative factors and molecular aspects of cancer, which we hope will stimulate research interest in them, who perhaps will take up research in cancer biology in their future career. The book briefly presents the information on various aspects of cancer development and therapies available for cancer treatment, which is presented in five chapters.

C. Vaman Rao
Jayaprakash Shetty

About the Author

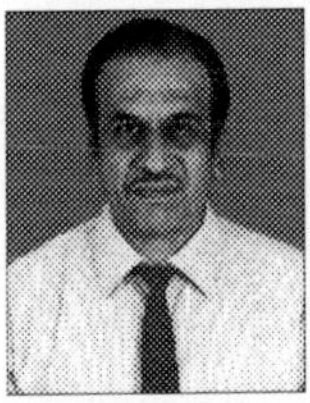

C. Vaman Rao received B. Sc. Degree in Zoology from the University of Mysore in 1977 and postgraduate degree in Zoology with Genetics specialization in 1979 from the same University from Manasagangotri campus. Joined the staff of St. Xavier's College, Mumbai to teach in the Department of Zoology in 1980. In 1988 obtained Ph.D. degree in Biochemistry (Environmental Toxicology) from University of Mumbai (then it was University of Bombay). In 1989 went to USA to pursue postdoctoral studies in Toxicology in the Department of Pharmacology and Toxicology at the University of Mississippi Medical Centre, Jackson, Mississippi, USA as a postdoctoral fellow in Dr. Harihara Mehendale's lab and gained experience in Liver Toxicology and returned to India in 1991 to teach the undergraduate students of B. Sc. Zoology and continued the research in toxicology. He has published *Immunology*, 3rd Ed (2017); *A Textbook of Immunology*, 3rd Ed (2019), and *Biology for Engineers*, 1st Ed (2021). Actively involved environmental toxicology, biofuels research program, has published research papers in reputed Scopus indexed journals. At present carrying out research on plant derived antidote for snake venoms. Has been a life-member of Indian Science Congress, Society of Toxicology-India, Indian Society of Toxicology, Indian Society for Technical Education, and Toxinology Society of India.

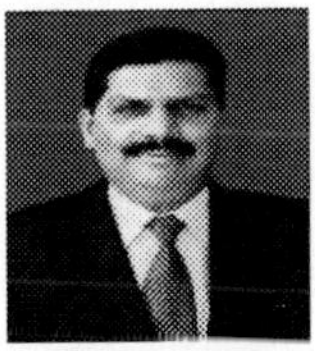

Jayaprakash Shetty, MBBS, MD, FRCP (Glasgow) graduated from Mysore Medical College, Mysore, Karnataka, India, completed his Postgraduation in Pathology at Kasturba Medical College (Manipal University) Karnataka, India and FRCP (Glasgow), [Fellow of Royal College of Physicians - Glasgow, United Kingdom]. Presently, he is Vice-Dean/ Professor and Head – Department of Pathology K. S. Hegde Medical Academy (Nitte – Deemed to be University) Mangaluru, Karnataka, India. He has illustrious teaching carrier of 24 years, apart from publishing over 120 scientific papers in both national and international journals. He is the reviewer of the article for *Journal of Neurosciences and Rural*

Practice, Editorial Board member for *Journal of Pediatric Oncology, and Journal of Evidence Based Medicine* and *Health Care*. He is the recipient of Doctors Day award in 2006 from IMA Headquarters, Delhi. He is the member of foundation steering committee India of the UNESCO Chair Bioethical Unit, Haifa. As a researcher he has completed a Govt. funded project sanctioned by Vision Group of Science and Technology, the project tilted as "Evaluation of prognostic marker for Triple-negative breast cancer" and currently carrying out Govt. funded ICMR Project.

Contents

Abbreviations

Abl	Abelson leukemia virus oncoprotein
ACT	adoptive cell transfer
ACTH	adrenocorticotropic hormone
ADCC	antibody-dependent cellular cytotoxicity
AEV	avian erythroblastosis virus
Ag	antigen
ALL	acute lymphocytic (lymphoblastic) leukemia
ALT	alternative lengthening of telomeres
ALV	avian leukosis virus
AML	acute myelogenous leukemia
AMP	adenosine monophosphate
AMV	avian myelocytomatosis virus
Ang	angiopoietin
AP	(1) apurinic; (2) apyrimidinic
Apaf-1	apoptotic protease-activating factor-1
APC	(1) antigen presenting cell; (2) adenomatous polyposis coli
APL	acute promyelocytic leukemia
ARF	alternative reading frame
AT	ataxia telangiectasia
ATM	mutated in telangiectasia
ATP	adenosine triphosphate
ATR	ATM-related kinase
ATRA	all-*trans*-retinoic acid
BCG	Bacille Calmette-Guerin (mycobacterium)
Bcl-2	B-cell lymphoma gene-2
BCR	B-cell receptor
BER	base excision repair (DNA repair)
BFB	breakage-fusion-bridge
BL	Burkit's lymphoma

BMI	body- mass index
BP	benzo (a) pyrene
bp	base pair
C	constant region of antibody; cytidine; cytosine
CDH1	E-cadherin gene
CDK	cyclin dependent kinase
CdkI	CDK inhibitor
cDNA	complementary DNA
CEA	carcinoembryonic antigen
CML	chronic myelogenous leukemia
CMV	cytomegalovirus
COX-2	cyclooxygenase-2
CSF-1	colony stimulating factor-1
CTL	cytotoxic T lymphocyte
CTLA-4	cytotoxic T lymphocytic antigen-4
DC	dendritic cell
DM	double minute chromosome
DMBA	dimethylbenz(a)anthracene
ds	double stranded DNA or RNA
E2F	transcription factor
EBV	Epstein-Barr virus
ECM	extracellular matrix
EGF	epidermal growth factor
EGF-R	epidermal growth factor receptor
EMT	epithelial-mesenchymal transition
ENU	N-ethylnitrosourea
env	retrovirus envelope glycoprotein
EPC	epithelial precursor cell; endothelial progenitor cell
EpCAM	epithelial cell adhesion molecule
ER	estrogen receptor
ERK	extracellular signal regulated kinase
ES	embryonic stem cell
FasL	ligand of the Fas death receptor
Fc	constant region domain of antibody
FDA	food and drug administration
FGF	fibroblast growth factor
FLIP	flice inhibitory protein
fos	feline osteosarcoma
G	guanine; guanine nucleotide; guanosine
G1	gap 1 phase (cell cycle)

G2	gap 2 phase (cell cycle)
gag	glycosaminoglycan antigen of virus
GF	growth factor
GH	growth hormone
GM-CSF	granulocyte-macrophage-colony-stimulating factor
gp	glycoprotein
GSK-3β	glycogen synthase kinase-3β
Gy	gray (radiationdose unit)
HBV	hepatitis B virus
HCA	heterocyclic amine
HCC	hepatocellular carcinoma
HCMV	human cytomegalovirus
HCV	hepatitis C virus
HDAC	histone deacetylase
HDM2	human homolog of MDM2
HGF	hepatocyte growth factor
HIF	hypoxia inducible factor
HIV	human immunodeficiency virus
HLA	human leukocyte antigen
HNPCC	hereditary non-polyposis colon cancer
HNSCC	head and neck squamous cell carcinoma
HPV	human papillomavirus
IAP	inhibitor of apoptosis
IFN	interferon
IGF	insulin like growth factor
IGF-R	insulin like growth factor receptor
IκB	inhibitor of NF-κB
IL	interleukin
IP3	inositol (1,4,5)-triphosphate
IR	insulin receptor
IRK	insulin receptor kinase
LAK	lymphokine activates killer cell
LOH	loss of heterozygosity
LT	large T antigen of SV40 (or polyomavirus)
LTR	long terminal repeat
M	mitosis
3-MC	3-methylcholanthrene
MDM2	mouse double minute chromosome-2
MDR	multidrug resistance
MMR	mismatch repair

MMTV	mouse mammary tumor virus
MNU	N-methylnitrosourea
myc	myelocytomatosis oncogene
Myc	myelocytomatosis protein
mos	murine osteosarcoma
NER	nucleotide excision repair
NF	neurofibromatosis
NF-κB	nuclear factor-κB
NGF	nerve growth factor
NHEJ	nonhomologous end joining
NK	natural killer cell
NSCLC	non-small-cell lung carcinoma
8-oxo-dG	8-oxo-deoxyguanosine
p	referring to short arm of the chromosome
PAH	polycyclic aromatic hydrocarbon
PDGF	platelet-derived growth factor
PDGF-R	platelet-derived growth factor receptor
PhIP	2-amino-1-methyl-6-phenylimidazo[4,5-b] pyridine
PI	phosphoinositol
PIP	phosphotidylinositol phosphate
PIP2	phosphotidylinositol (4,5) diphosphate
PI3K	phosphotidylinositol 3-kinase
PIP3	phosphotidylinositol (3,4,5) triphosphate
PKB	protein kinase B
PKC	protein kinase C
PML	promyelocytic leukemia
pol	polymerase
pRb	retinoblastoma protein
PTEN	phosphotase and tensin homolog deleted on chromosome 10
q	referring to long arm of the chromosome
R	restriction point
RANK	receptor activator of NF-κB
RAR	retinoic acid receptor
Ras	signal transducer oncoprotein
H-Ras	Harvey Ras oncoprotein
K-Ras	Kirstein Ras oncoprotein
N-Ras	Neural Ras oncoprotein
Rb	retinoblastoma protein
RSV	Rous sarcoma virus

RT	reverse transcriptase
RTK	tyrosine kinase receptor
S	DNA synthesis phase of cell cycle
src	Rous sarcoma oncogene
Src	Rous sarcoma protein
SV	simian virus
T	thymidine; thymine
t	referring to translocation in chromosome
TC	T cytotoxic cell
T_H	T helper cell
TAA	tumor associate antigen
T-ALL	T-cell acute lymphocytic leukemia
TAM	tumor associated macrophage
TERT	telomerase reverse transcriptase
TGF	transforming growth factor
TGF-α	transforming growth factor-α
TGF-β	transforming growth factor-β
TGF-βR	transforming growth factor-β receptor
TIL	tumor infiltrating lymphocyte
TK	tyrosine kinase
TNF	tumor necrosis factor
TNF-α	tumor necrosis factor-α
TPA	12-O-tetradecanoyphorbol-13-acetate (PMA)
TPO	thrombopoietin
TRAIL	TNF-related apoptosis-inducing ligand
Tsp-1	thrombospondin-1
U	uridine; uracil
UV	ultraviolet
V	variable region of antibody
VEGF	vascular endothelial growth factor
VEGF-R	vascular endothelial growth factor receptor
VHL	von Hippel-Lindau
XAF1	XIAP-associated factor 1
XIAP	X-chromosome-linked inhibitor of apoptosis
XP	xeroderma pigmentosum

CHAPTER 1

Fundamentals of Cancers

The term cancer refers to the crab (zodiac sign), which has a unique ability to move backwards and forwards, as well as lateral movement. Based on this character of the crab, the word cancer was coined to the tumor, which shows abnormal growth in all directions. The primary cause of cancer is the mutation of one or more genes leading to misregulation in the cell cycle, which leads to abnormal growth of cells. The mutation in the genes regulating cell cycle may occur in a single cell leading to the development of cancer from that single mutated or abnormal cell; therefore, cancers are clonal in origin. Tumors originating from the genetically altered cell can be either malignant or benign. Malignant tumor is harmful because the cells of malignant tumors are capable of invading neighboring tissue or travelling to any area in the body and initiate tumor development in the area wherever they lodge. The process of malignant tumor progression or migration is called metastasis. The metastasizing cells spread to other parts of the body through lymphatic channels or blood vessels to lymph nodes where they take temporary residence and migrate to other tissues in the body, where they succeed in establishing the colony called micrometastasis, which leads to secondary malignant growths. Benign tumors are not regarded as cancers because they do not spread like malignant tumors since they are encapsulated, and they grow within the encapsulated area; therefore, they do not invade and destroy the surrounding tissue.

Cancerous cells are generally called transformed cells, and the transformation might have been brought about by the RNA or DNA tumor viruses or by chemical carcinogens through mutagenesis or by chromosomal aberrations.

According to the WHO report, there were 1.16 million cancer cases in India in 2018. In the report it was mentioned that 1 in 10 Indian would suffer from cancer and 1 in 15 will die due to the disease. The world cancer report noted that, 7.848 lakh cancer deaths, 2.26 million 5-year prevalent cases in the Indian population of 1.35 billion. Six most common cancer types reported in India are breast cancer, oral cancer, cervical cancer, lung cancer, stomach cancer and colon cancer. Together, these account for 49% of all new cancer cases. Of the 5.70 lakh new cancer cases in men account for 45% of cases, and 5.87 lakh new cancers cases in womJen account for 60% of the cases. (Table 1.1).

Table 1.1. Cancer cases detected in the year 2018

Types of cancers	Men	Women
Oral cancer	92,000	28,000
Lung cancer	49,000	19,000
Stomach cancer	39,000	18,000
Colorectal cancer	37,000	20,000
Esophageal cancer	34,000	20,000
Breast cancer	–	1,62,500
Cervical cancer	–	97,000
Ovarian cancer	–	36,000

In the cancer pattern in India, it is dominated tobacco-related head and neck cancers, particularly oral cancer in men and in women, breast cancer followed by cervical cancer is predominant.

1.1 CHARACTERISTICS OF CANCER CELL

The key characteristics of transformed cells are as follows:

- *Altered morphology (typically round shape in cancer cells):* Cells of normal tissue have particular shape and size, which is lost in cancer cells due to loss of cytoskeletal support to the membrane.
- *Loss of contact inhibition (indicates the ability to grow one over the other)*: This is called density-independent growth or high saturation density (this indicates ability of accumulation of large number of cells in a culture dish without getting attached to the surface) where there is no upper limit for growth of cancer cells in tissue culture. If nutrition is provided, they continue to grow without any inhibition due to crowding in the culture vessel, unlike the normal cells.
- *Anchorage-independent growth (indicates the ability to grow without attaching to solid substrate support*) : It is the unique ability of cancer cells that they do not need any substratum to grow. They grow freely in the culture medium without attaching to the bottom or sides of the culture vessels.
- *Immortalization (ability to proliferate indefinitely)*: Cancer cells attain immortalization by producing their own growth regulatory factors and preventing apoptosis.
- *Reduced requirement for mitogenic growth factors:* Cancer cells do not require any external growth factor to grow in a tissue culture medium. They produce their own growth factors and regulators and grow in an uncontrolled manner in a tissue culture medium.
- *Increased transport of glucose and amino acid across the membrane:* This facilitates the cancer cells to utilize glucose for energy requirement to proliferate and to become immortal.

- *Ability to induce tumors elsewhere on transplantation:* This is a special character of cancer cells. Due to the loss of tissue markers and adhesion molecules, cancer cells in the de-differentiated state, behave like embryonic cells. Therefore, they can lodge themselves anywhere in the body in another tissue of different origin and induce tumor in that tissue. Cancer cells on xenotransplantation (another animal of different genera) or allotransplantation (another animal can survive and induce tumor formation).
- *Altered cell surface and membrane properties:* Increased protein mobility, loss of certain receptors and gain of new receptors.
- *Loss of tissue-specific antigens and markers:* Generally, the cells belonging to a particular tissue have their own specific markers, which are presented on class I MHC. In the cancer cell, class I MHC expression is down-regulated hence, tissue-specific markers are underexpressed.
- *Loss of cell adhesion molecules:* Fibronectin, adherins, cadherins, etc., are lost from the concerned cell surface, due to which cancer cells free themselves from parent tissue and move about freely to show metastasis.
- *Very poor intercellular communication*: Each cancer cell behaves differently within the same tissue of its origin. Therefore, there is no coordinated rhythmic activity, as observed in normal cells.
- *Increased protease activity:* This helps the cancer cell to show metastasis, where the protease induced by the cancerous cells dissolve the barrier walls and facilitate the free movement of cancerous cells to other areas outside the parent tissue origin.
- *Increased transcription, translation, and metabolic activity:* This property helps the cancer cell to produce proteins of their choice for growth and survival.
- Cancer cells obtained from the same tissue origin from two different individuals will not have similar properties. One of the reasons is genes involved in bringing about transformation will be different in different individuals, even though the tissue involved in developing the cancer is the same.

1.2 CLASSIFICATION OF CANCERS

Cancers are classified based on tissue origin. Cancers originating from epithelial cells that protect surfaces like skin, intestinal lining, esophageal lining, and buccal lining are called carcinomas (Figs. 1.3 and 1.4). For example, skin carcinoma, colon carcinoma, hepatocarcinoma, lung carcinoma, etc. About 90% of all malignant tumors are carcinomas, which are the most common type of cancer encountered in humans. Most carcinomas recorded so far belong to two categories: squamous cell carcinomas and adenocarcinomas. Squamous cell carcinomas (Fig. 1.1) originate from the protective epithelial cell layers, for example, skin, nasal cavity, oropharynx, larynx, lung, esophagus, and cervix. The adenocarcinomas (Fig. 1.2) arise from the secretory or glandular epithelia, which is secretory in nature. It secretes substances into the ducts or cavities that are lined by secretory epithelium, for example, lung, colon, breast, pancreas, stomach, esophagus, prostate, endometrium, and ovary.

The malignant cancers arising from nonepithelial tissues found in the body, which are mesodermal or mesenchymal in origin are called sarcomas, constitutes only 1% of the tumors encountered in cancer clinics. Some of the common sarcomas are osteosarcoma (bone cells) (Fig.1.5), liposarcoma (adipocytes-fat cells), leiomyosarcoma (muscle cells), malignant fibrous histiocytoma (macrophages of bone), fibrosarcoma (fibroblast), synovial sarcoma (cells of synovial tissue), angiosarcoma refers to cancer arising from endothelial cells of blood vessels, chondrosarcoma is a cancer arising from cartilage tissue cells.

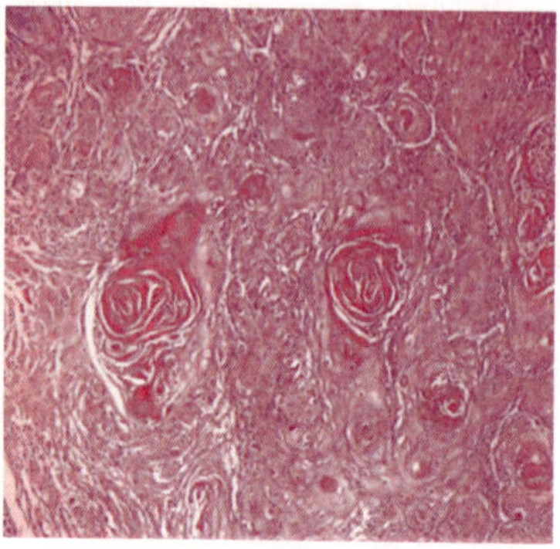

Fig. 1.1. Squamous cell carcinoma

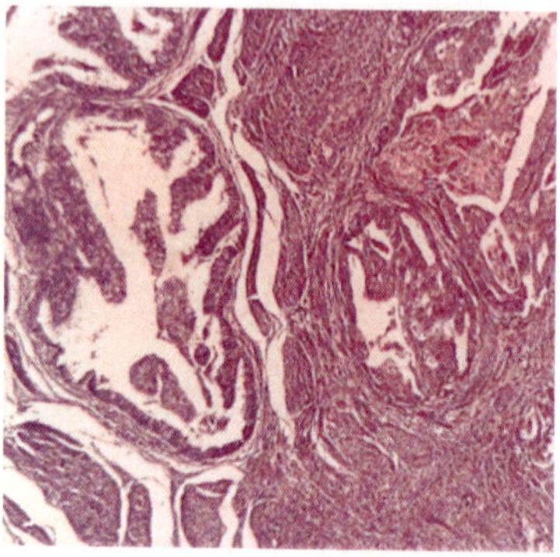

Fig. 1.2. Adenocarcinoma

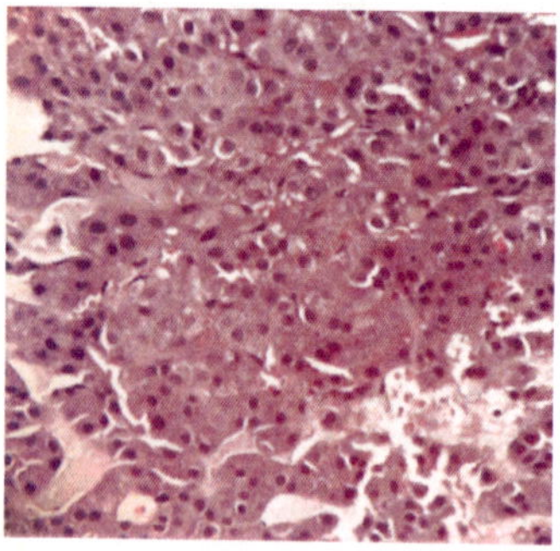

Fig. 1.3. Hepatocellular carcinoma

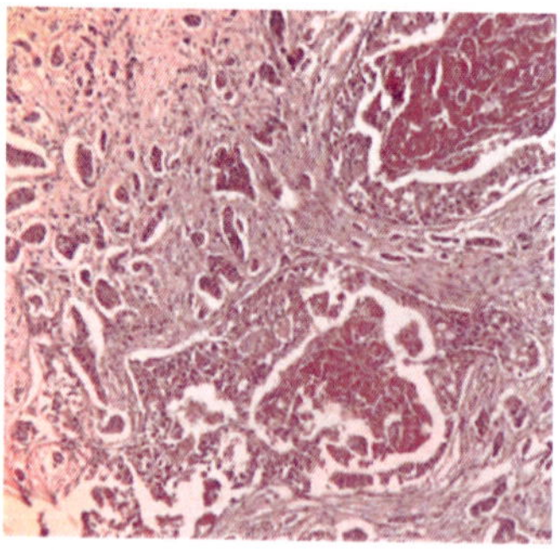

Fig. 1.4. Breast carcinoma

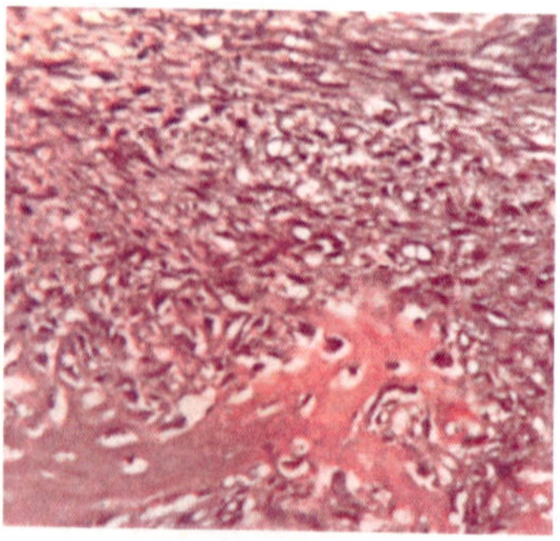

Fig. 1.5. Osteosarcoma

The second group of nonepithelial cancers arises from another category of mesodermal tissue, i.e., blood forming-**hematopoietic tissues**, which includes the immune system cells. The term **leukemia** is used for cancers derived from white blood cells and **lymphomas** (Fig. 1.6) for the tumors originating from the B and T lymphocytes, which are called lymphoid lineage aggregate to form the solid tumor masses in lymph nodes rather than dispersed as single-cell populations of tumor cells as observed in leukemia.

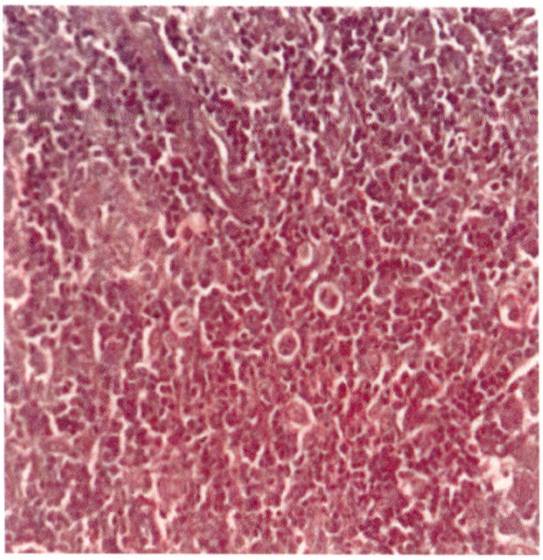

Fig. 1.6 Hodgkin's lymphoma

The third major group of nonepithelial tumors belongs to neuroectodermal tumors that arise from various components of the central and peripheral nervous system. The tumors included under the neuroectodermal category are **gliomas** (Fig. 1.7), **glioblastomas, neuroblastomas** (Fig. 1.8), **schwannomas,** and **medulloblastomas,** which constitute about 1.3% of the cancers diagnosed.

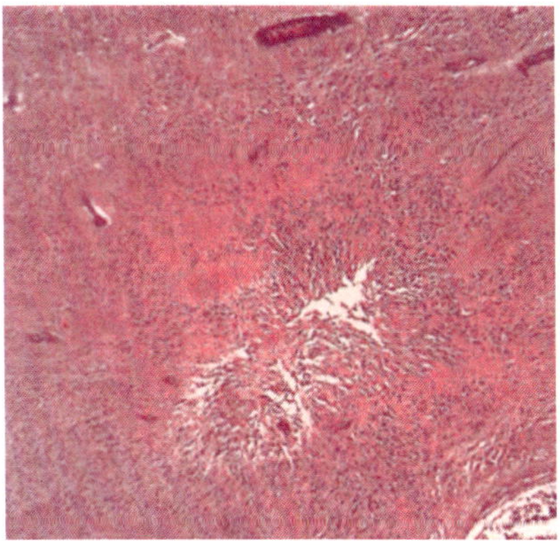

Fig. 1.7. Glioma

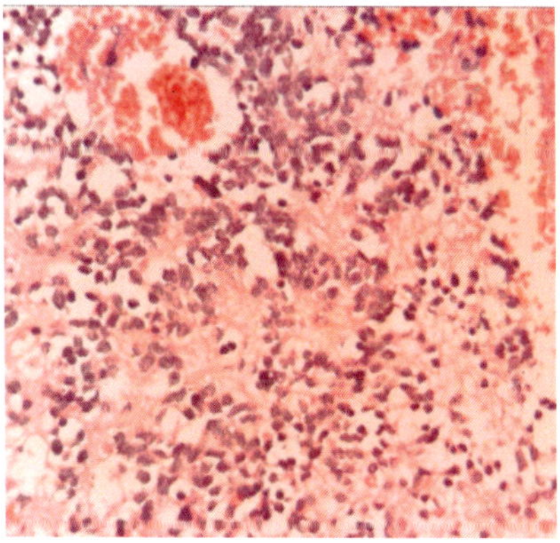

Fig. 1.8. Neuroblastoma

Some tumors cannot be classified into any category, and their origin cannot be traced because of dedifferentiation that they have undergone. Such tumors are said to be **anaplastic.** For example, **melanoma** (Fig. 1.9) is derived from melanocytes, which are pigment-producing cells of the skin and the retina.

The origin of melanocytesis from cells derived from neuroectodermal tissue called neural crest cells and do not retain any connection with the original germ tissue.

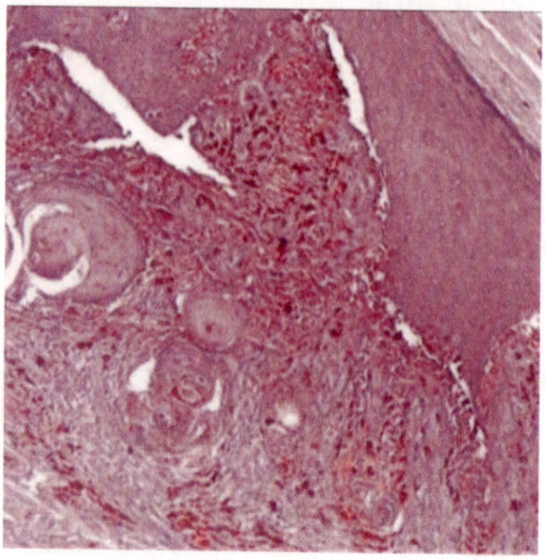

Fig. 1.9. Melanoma

1.3 COMPARISON BETWEEN BENIGN TUMOR AND MALIGNANT TUMOR

Table 1.2. Characteristics of benign and malignant tumors

Benign tumor	Malignant tumor
Generally harmless, localized and grow in a cluster.	Generally harmful, proliferative, and freely moving (spread throughout the body).
The cells resemble normal cells of parent tissue origin.	The cells look different from normal cells and loss of morphology.
Surrounded by connective tissue capsule.	Not surrounded by a capsule, hyperplastic and freely moving, proliferate into neighboring areas.
The tumor grows with time and may block certain passages.	The cells are invasive and spread by crossing the basement membrane.
The rate of cell division is slightly higher than normal.	The rate of cell division is remarkably high.
The cells continue to produce enzymes of parent tissue origin.	The cells produce new enzymes required for metastasis.
The cells are well differentiated and maintain the differentiated status.	The cells undergo dedifferentiation and show morphological alteration.
The cells do not show chromosomal anomalies.	Most of the time show chromosomal anomalies (both ploidy and alteration in chromosome structure).
The cells undergo malignant transformation only on mutagenesis.	The cells readily show malignant transformation.

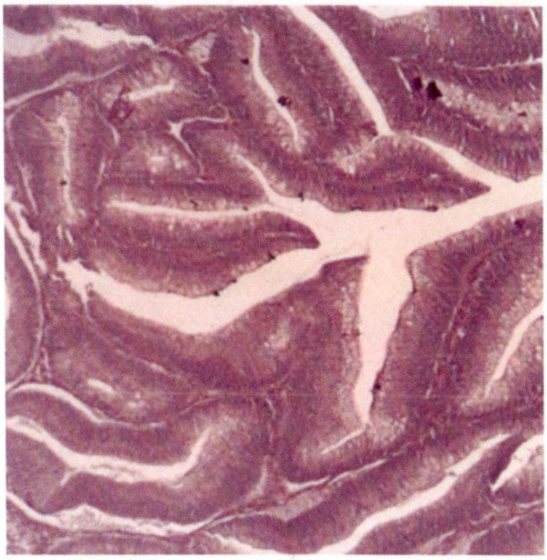

Fig. 1.10. Histology of benign tumor

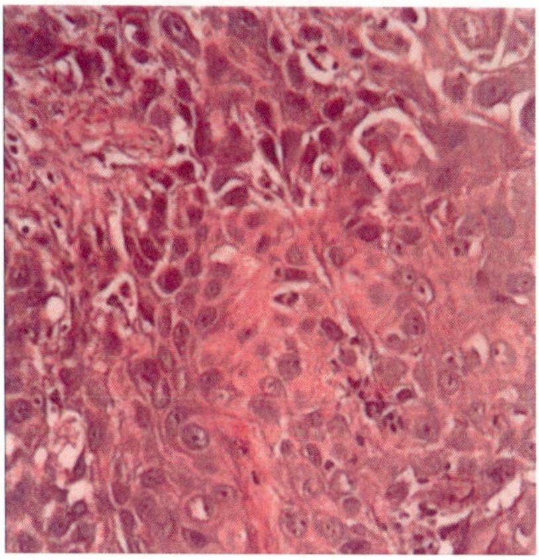

Fig. 1.11. Histology of malignant tumor

The tumor seems to grow excessively without hindrance due to uncontrolled proliferation of cells, which is called **Hyperplasia** Here, excessive number of cells seen in tissue as compared to the normal cell population. **Dysplasia** is a transitional stage found between completely benign and premalignant stage with cells showing abnormal cytology. Benign growths like adenomas, polyps, papillomas, and warts are considered to be dysplastic epithelial tumors, and these tumors are confined within the boundary created by the basement membrane and grow within the boundary.

1.4 STAGES IN THE DEVELOPMENT OF CANCER

By studying different experimental models of carcinogenesis, like liver and skin cancer models, the stages in the development of cancer have been classified into three stages, namely, **initiation, promotion, and progression or proliferation**. For understanding the different stages of carcinogenesis, the Solt-Farber experimental model of liver carcinogenesis is considered here (Fig. 1.12).

Young, healthy mice are injected with 200 mg/kg diethyl nitrosamine (DENA), a potent mutagen as well as a carcinogen. Two weeks later, 0.02% 2-acetaminofluorine (2-AAF) was fed to the animals through diet. One week later, partial hepatectomy (PH) was performed. After 8 to 12 months, animals had developed a metastatic hepatic tumor. To know how cancer developed in the animals, a few animals were sacrificed every week after the treatment with DENA and 2-AAF. Within one month after the treatment with DENA, the liver showed neoplastic foci of different size (0.5 to 2 mm) distributed in the liver, which was confirmed from histological evidence. These foci showed focal proliferation and altered biochemical characteristics. Some cells reverted to the original status of hepatocytes, and some showed apoptosis.

On biochemical analysis of cells of the neoplastic foci, they showed two different characteristics. Some cells showed decreased xenobiotic metabolizing enzymes, which was considered **stage 1 of initiation (I-1)** and some cells showed increased detoxification components and these cells were considered to be in **stage 2 of initiation (I-2).** Decreased xenobiotic metabolizing enzymes were cytochrome p-450, mixed-function oxidase (MFO), sulfotransferases, aldehyde dehydrogenase and enzymes of lipid peroxidation. Increased components of detoxification were glutathione (GSH), glutathione transferase, gamma-glutamyl transpeptidase and multidrug resistance P-glycoprotein. Also, the cells of the hepatocellular foci showed decreased glucose 6-phosphatase and ATPase levels. At this stage of carcinogenesis, if the promoter is made available, the foci will undergo a further change in histology and morphology leading to enlargement in foci with nodular appearance.

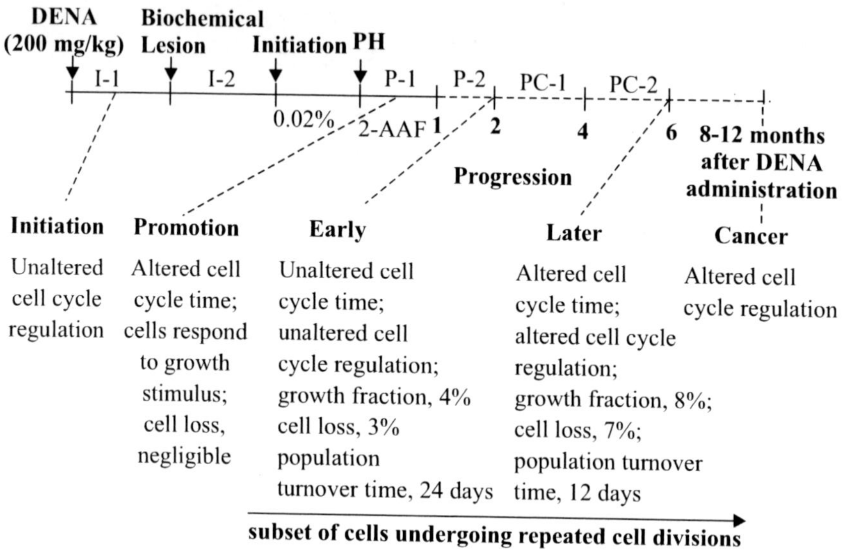

Fig. 1.12. Solt-Farber model of hepatocarcinogenesis

In the Solt-Farber model for liver carcinogenesis, 2-AAF administration leads to the promotion of carcinogenesis. The promoter is referred to as pro-carcinogen or co-carcinogen and could be an inflammatory agent like phorbol ester, or the substance that induces free radical production and membrane injury (Phenobarbital, DDT-dichlorodiphenyltrichloroethane, PCB-polychlorinated biphenyl). Administration of 2-AAF leads to necrotic changes in the liver and promotes further proliferation of neoplastic foci. Promotion of carcinogenesis can also be brought about by choline-deficient diet, which results in 2–5% persistent hepatic nodules, some show spontaneous proliferation, and some undergo remodeling to form normal hepatocytes.

In the Solt-Farber model of liver carcinogenesis, the progression stage begins two months after the initiation, where hepatic foci show a tenfold increase in the proliferation of hepatocytes. There is 4% proliferation of hepatocytes in the nodule and 3% apoptosis, with a net gain of only 1% proliferation leading to slow enlargement of nodules. By six months post-initiation, 8% of hepatocytes in hepatic foci show proliferation. By this time, there is an alteration in the property of hepatocytes in the foci, such as loss of binding ligands, lipoprotein and apoproteins, alkylated and acylated glycoproteins. By 7 to 8 months of post-initiation, the cells of hepatic foci show loss of surface coding property (antigens), acquisition of new antigens and a new pattern of growth. At this stage, they are transplanted into spleen which will develop into hepatocellular carcinoma.

1.5 INFLUENTIAL FACTORS IN HUMAN CARCINOGENESIS

Important role played by different factors in carcinogenesis in an individual are environment, reproductive life, diet, lifestyle (alcohol consumption and use of tobacco in different forms) genetic predisposition, are some of the significant contributors. Detailed epidemiological studies have contributed significantly to understanding these lifestyle factors as contributors to cancer development, which can be altered to prevent cancers in most cases. Some of the factors like accidental or occupational exposure to chemical carcinogens, physiological alterations in hormonal levels influenced by childbirth, birth control measures and viral infections underlie these lifestyle factors. Epidemiological studies of a wide variety of populations have played a significant role in elucidating the contribution of these factors towards development of different cancers.

1.5.1 Environment

Wide range of human-made chemicals released into the environment and recycling through the diet or inhalation are the major causes of increased incidence of cancers. To some extent, occupational exposure to certain chemicals largely contributes to the development of cancer. For example, workers in the azo-dye industry are constantly exposed to the fumes of the dye chemical are prone to bladder cancer. Chimney sweepers exposed to chimney dust containing tar are prone to develop nasal and scrotal cancer. Skin exposed to UV radiation of sun will induce the development of skin cancer, which is predominant in the white race compared to people having skin pigment. Workers exposed to fine dust particles in the cement industry, stone quarrying industry and asbestos industry are prone to develop lung cancer. The incidence of lung cancer will increase if the workers have the habit of smoking tobacco. Coal mine workers and those working in bitumen (coal tar) based industry are prone to various types of cancers. Incidence of liver and lung cancer is very high in these workers if they have the habit of consuming alcohol or are tobacco smokers. Estrogen injection is given to dairy cattle to increase milk yield. Estrogen levels in dairy milk also increase the cancer risk in men and women.

The development of cancer in an individual generally involves multi-step process, which is governed by multiple factors, such as, the genetic constitution of the individual and the surrounding environment in which he or she lives as well as lifestyle. Chances of development of any cancer can be avoided or drastically reduced by changing our surroundings or our lifestyle habits.

From the epidemiological studies it is evident that cancer development can be avoided largely by identifying the specific environmental risk factors and strictly adhering to change of lifestyle to minimize the effect of risk factors. Some of the mutagenic factors operate as tumor initiators that are directly responsible for genetic change. Some other factors presumably serve as tumor promoters that facilitate growth of mutated cells population, which is liable to progress as cancer through further mutation in order to grow as full-blown cancer. The tobacco smoke carcinogens, the aflatoxin found in stored food items act as mutagens and initiate cancer development. The reproductive hormones found in circulation in a woman's body at different stages of her life serve as cancer promoters. There is a significant correlation between a woman's reproductive history and her risk of developing breast cancer and the importance of the role played by the hormones in the development and proliferation in the breast.

1.5.2 Carcinogens

The first example of cancer following the exposure to chemicals was reported in 1775, where scrotal cancer incidence in chimney sweepers was high, which was attributed to exposure to chimney soot. Exposure to chemical carcinogens at the workplace is a common factor for cancers of different types in individuals. For example, individuals exposed to azo dyes are prone to testicular and bladder cancer; similarly, those who work in the chrome plating industry are prone to lung cancer. Individuals working in the asbestos industry are prone to lung and respiratory tract cancer. A systematic epidemiological study of individuals working in different chemical industries had revealed that long-term exposure to certain chemicals leads to cancers. Some examples of such studies are given below.

It is well established that all carcinogens are mutagens, whereas all mutagens are not carcinogens. Most of the chemical carcinogens are electrophiles (electron seeking) and chemically modify DNA by interacting with DNA and form DNA adducts, which leads to mutations. Chemical carcinogens belong to two broad categories, namely, direct-acting and indirect-acting. Direct-acting carcinogens bind to DNA directly without undergoing any further change. For example, propiolactone, ethyl-methyl sulfonate, dimethyl sulfoxide, nitrogen mustard and methyl nitrosourea (MNU), all these are strong electrophiles.

Table 1.3. Most common chemical carcinogens found in the environment and cancers caused by them

Chemical carcinogens	Source and the use	Cancers
Acrylonitrile	Produced by chemical synthesis and used as a polymer for household goods	Colon and lungs
Aflatoxin B1	Fungus that infects stored food, *Aspergillus niger*	Hepatocellular carcinomas
4-aminobiphenyl	Produced by chemical synthesis and used as source for dye production and antioxidant in rubber	Bladder cancer

Aniline derivatives	Produced by chemical synthesis and used as source for dye production	Bladder cancer
α and β naphthylamine	Produced by chemical synthesis and used as source for dye production	Bladder cancer
Arsenic	Arsenic is used as a doping agent in semiconductors and these compounds are used in making special glasses	Skin carcinoma
Asbestos	Artificially produced and used as fire retardant in building construction, roofing, etc.	Lung mesothelium
Benzene	Petroleum derivative, used an industrial solvent	Leukemia
Cadmium salts	Used in cadmium batteries	Prostate and lung
Chromium and chromates	Used for electroplating	Lung and nasal sinus
Carbon tetrachloride	Used as cleansing liquid in industries	Liver
Dimethylbenzanthracene	Found in coal tar and tobacco smoke	Liver
Benzo (a) pyrene	Found in coal tar and tobacco smoke, produced when food is smoked and charred	Liver and other organs
Organochlorines	Produced by chemical synthesis and used as pesticides	Liver
Soot and tar	Produced when food is roasted on charcoal	Skin, lung, bladder, and scrotum
Vinyl chloride	Produced by chemical synthesis and used as a polymer for household goods	liver, lung, and brain
Tobacco and tobacco smoke (60 different carcinogens)	Agricultural crop used in cigarettes, bidis, cigars, cheroots, etc.	Lung, oral cavity, larynx, esophagus, stomach, and pancreas

Indirect acting carcinogens require metabolic activation to become carcinogens or electrophiles, which generally occurs in the liver in the presence of drug-metabolizing enzymes or mixed-function oxidases (MFOs). These enzymes convert hydrophobic substances to hydrophilic to excrete them from the body. In this process, they become electrophilic and react with DNA to form DNA adducts. Some chemicals are converted into epoxides, which are highly reactive compared to any other metabolites and form a strong association with DNA leading to mutations.

1.5.2.1 Metabolism of carcinogen

Metabolism of carcinogen can occur in four different ways, namely, **oxidation at carbon, oxidation at nitrogen, reduction at nitrogen, and conjugation.**

I. **Oxidation at carbon:** Organic chemicals like alkanes, alkenes and aromatics that undergo oxidation at carbon produce alkylating and aralkylating agents.

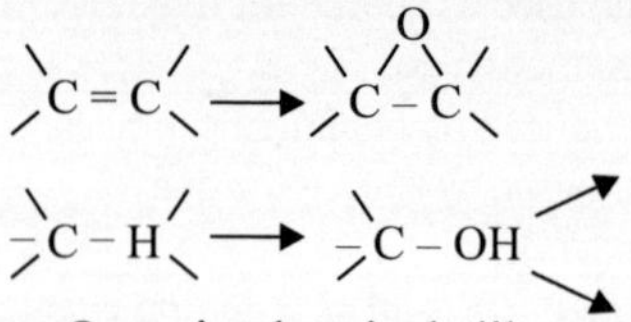

II. **Oxidation at nitrogen:** Organic chemicals like aromatic amines or aromatic amides, oxidized at nitrogen atom can give rise to **arylaminating** agents.

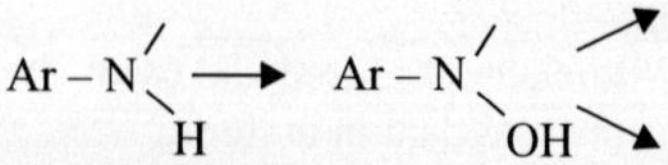

III. **Reduction at nitrogen:** Aromatic nitrates, when reduced at nitrogen, will give rise to **arylaminating** agents.

$$Ar - NO_2 \longrightarrow Ar - NHOH$$

IV. **Conjugation (for hydroxy compounds)**

Ar — C — OH ⟶ Ar — C — X **(Aralkylating)**

Ar — N — OH ⟶ Ar — N — X **(Arylaminating)**

C — X ⟶ C — SG (Glutathione) **Alkylating**

1.5.2.2 Alkylation

Transfer alkyl residues to DNA is called alkylation, and the carcinogens that bring about alkylation of DNA are aliphatic epoxides, aliphatic amines (Diethyl nitrosamine, dimethyl nitrosamine, methyl nitrosourea, haloalkanes, lactones, alkyl triazines, methyl-methane sulfonate and ethyl methane sulfonate. The sites of adduct formation with nitrogenous bases are shown below (Fig. 1.13) with AK and an arrow.

Features observed with alkylating agents are:

- The targets of alkylation are mostly **ring nitrogen** and **exocyclic oxygen** atoms.
- Most frequently alkylated nitrogenous base is **guanine in 7th position.**
- Non-ionic alkylating agents target nitrogen atoms.
- Ionic alkylating agents target oxygen atom.
- Ring nitrogen alkylated complexes are unstable, and thus the biological effect brought about is after secondary chemical transformation.

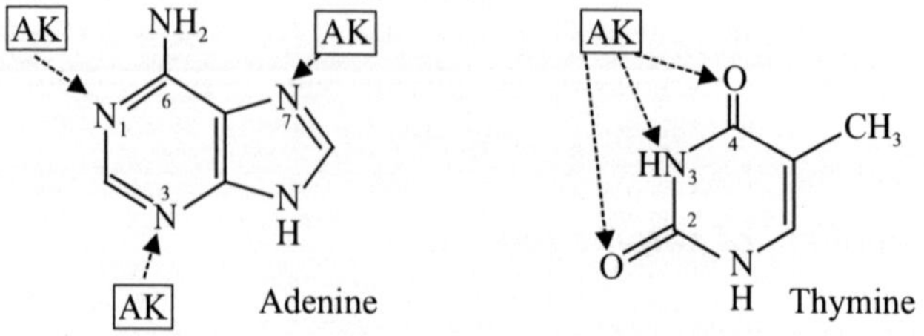

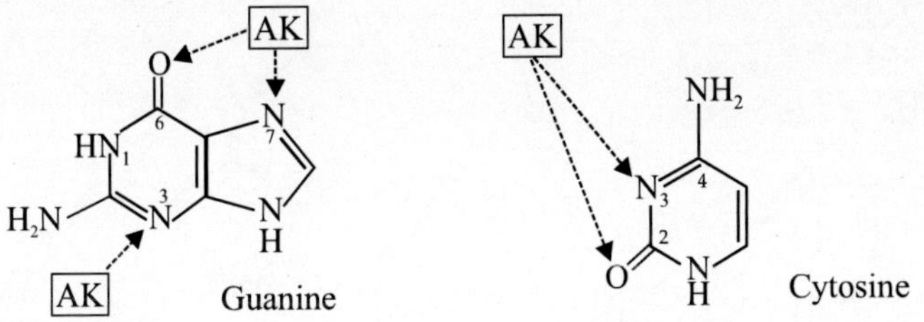

Fig. 1.13. Most frequently alkylated (AK) regions of the nitrogenous bases of DNA

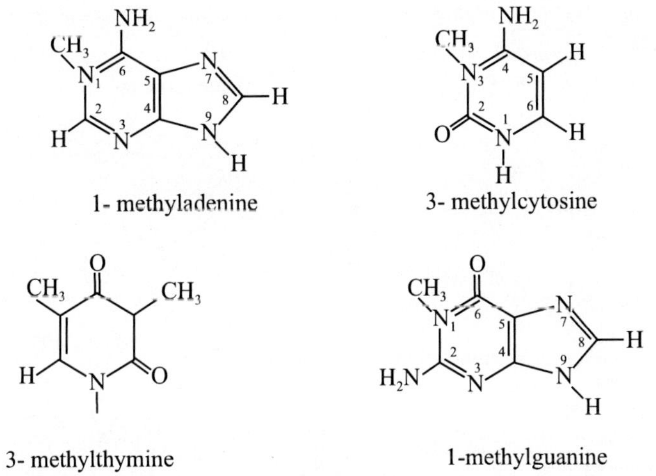

Fig. 1.14. Most frequently observed methylation (alkylation) of nitrogenous bases of DNA

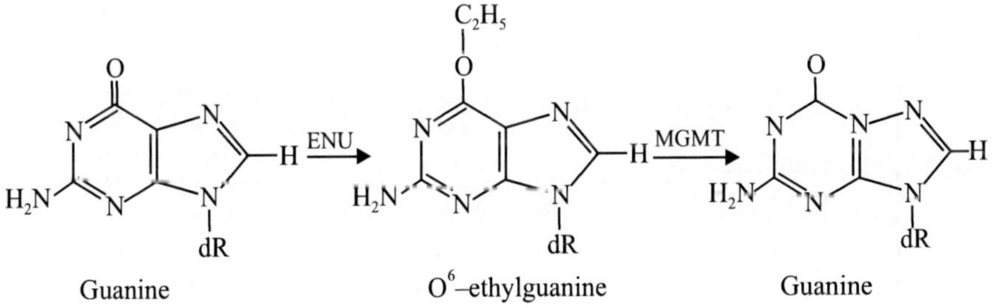

Fig. 1.15. Ethyl nitrosourea (ENU) induced ethylation (alkylation) of guanine residue and further de-ethylation (de-alkylation) by methyl-guanine methyl transferase (MGMT) enzyme

1.5.2.3 Arylamination

They are chemical carcinogens consisting of heterogeneous group that transfer an arylamine group to DNA. For example, aromatic amines and amides, amino azo dyes, nitro-aromatics and heterocyclic aromatic amines (present in deep-fried meat and fish). Features of arylamination are as follows: (Shown with an arrow and AM) (Fig. 1.16)

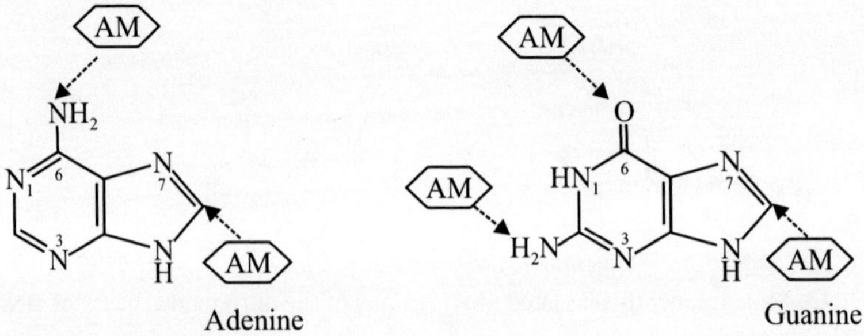

Fig. 1.16. Most frequently arylaminated (AM) regions of the nitrogenous bases of DNA

The arylaminating agents target majorly the **C-8 carbon atom,** and the **amino groups** of deoxy guanosines and the products of arylamination are more stable than alkylation products.

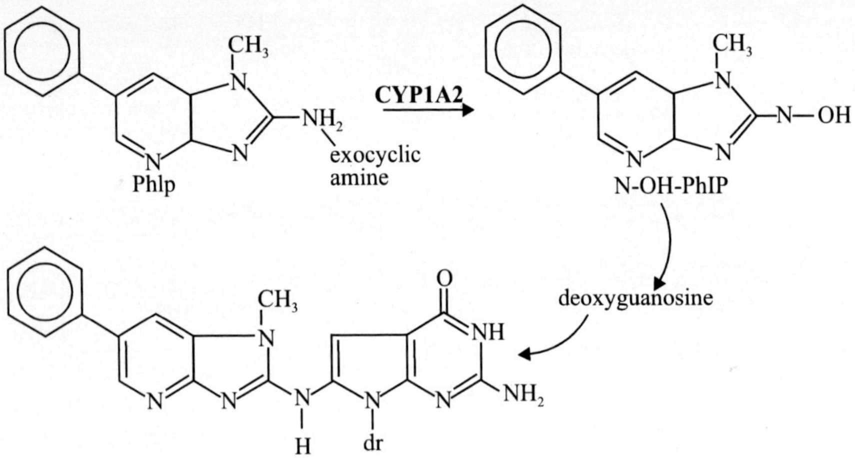

Fig. 1.17. Arylamination 8th position of deoxy guanine by a heterocyclic amine

1.5.2.4 Aralkylation

Carcinogens that transfer aralkyl groups to nitrogenous bases of DNA are pyrrolizidine alkaloids, alkenyl benzenes, nitro-aromatics epoxides, and polycyclic aromatic hydrocarbons (PAH)

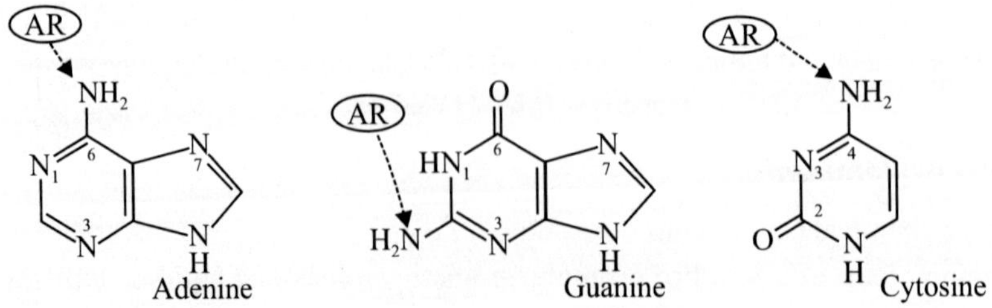

Fig. 1.18. Most frequently aralkylated (AR) region is the exocyclic amino group of the nitrogenous bases of DNA

PAH and nitro-aromatics activated (metabolized) through di-hydrodiol epoxide mechanism form adducts with DNA especially by modifying **exocyclic amino groups** of deoxy guanosine, deoxyadenosine and deoxy cytosine (shown with an arrow Fig. 1.18).

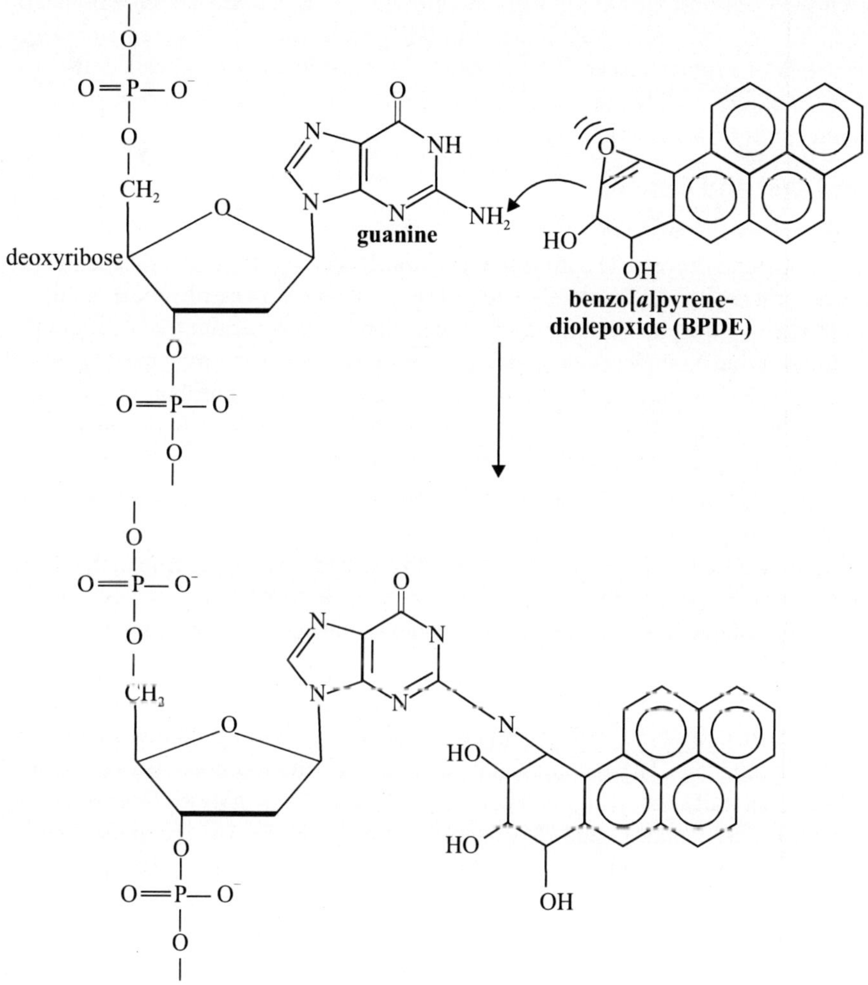

Fig. 1.19. Aralkylation of an exocyclic amino group of deoxy guanines by a metabolite (benzoic[a]pyrene-diol epoxide) of polycyclic aromatic hydrocarbon (Benzo[a]pyrene) majorly found in tobacco smoke, coal tar and smoke in the cooking area

1.5.3 Reproductive Life

Epidemiological studies showed that unmarried women are more vulnerable to breast cancer than married women. It is a very well-known fact that having children and lactating mothers reduces the risk of breast cancer for women compared to the unmarried women of marriageable age and carrier-oriented women not having children by using anti-fertility pills. The development of cancer in women is influenced by the age of the woman during the birth of the first child and the age at which the initiation and stoppage of the menstrual cycle took place. Altering the ovulation schedule by artificial means using hormonal contraceptives and fertility treatments also puts a woman in a significant risk of developing cancer. Sexual promiscuity, as observed in sex workers (multiple partners) who are more prone to HIV infection and human papilloma virus (HPV) infection, are at increased risk of the cervix or vaginal cancer. HPV is generally found in all cervical cancer tissues of sex workers worldwide. Cervical cancer incidences in nuns and women not having multiple partners are very rare.

1.5.4 Diet and Cancer

The mutagenesis caused by chemical carcinogens found in the food seemed to shed light on human cancers. The mutagenic chemicals derived from natural chemicals present in the foodstuffs or generated during cooking processor procarcinogens could also facilitate development of cancer. Foods are generally free of ultimate carcinogens but biological conversions carried out by the liver during the metabolic process or by the abundant colon resident bacteria might contribute in creating actively mutagenic and thus carcinogenic chemical species. It is observed that virtually all compounds that are mutagenic are likely to be carcinogenic as well.

In the Japanese population, most predominant cancer is found to be stomach cancer as compared to Americans, whereas colon cancer is very high in Americans. It is mainly because of the type of diet in both countries. Mediterranean diet, rich in fibers consisting of fresh fruits and vegetables, has been known to prevent gastric and colon cancer. The polyphenols, carotenoids and certain other compounds are known to be protective and prevent the development of cancer.

Heterocyclic amines (HCAs), classes of molecules that are formed in large amounts when meats of various sorts are cooked at high temperatures are known to be carcinogenic. These compounds arise through the reactions that take place between naturally occurring molecular species in cells, notably creatine, glucose phosphates, dipeptides, and free amino acids. The HCAs are undoubtedly carcinogenic. For example, the most abundant of these compounds in meats cooked at high temperature, **2-amino-1-methyl-6-phenylimidazo [4, 5-b] pyridine (PhIP)** is capable of inducing colon and breast cancer in rats and lymphoma in mice. PhIP is recognized as being the principal carcinogen in the human diet. HCAs are converted to carcinogens mainly in the liver by the cytochrome p450 system.

A study carried out by Fred Hutchison Cancer Research Center in the USA showed that habitual consumption of deep-fried foods more than once a week such as French fries, fried chicken and doughnuts is associated with an increased risk of aggressive prostate cancer.

In another study, a strong correlation was found between smoking, consumption of alcohol regularly and meat-eating regularly increased risk of cancer. The types of cancers for which meat products had the strongest correlation include breast, uteri, kidney, ovarian, pancreatic, prostate, testicular, thyroid cancers, and multiple myeloma.

Diet low in vegetables, high in nitrates and salt is known to cause stomach and esophageal cancer. Nitrates are used as food preservatives, transform into carcinogenic nitroso compounds. Similarly, a diet high in fat, low in fibers, broiled/fried foods is known to cause bowel, pancreas, and prostate and breast cancer.

Among the most potent of exogenous carcinogens is aflatoxin B1 (AFB1), which is produced by moulds belonging to *Aspergillus* genus. These moulds grow on stored foods, which have not been processed properly before storage. People exposed to AFB1 through diet are at 3-fold elevated risk of developing hepatocellular carcinoma (HCC), while those carrying a chronic hepatitis B viral infection have 7-fold increased risk of HCC. AFB1 activated by cytochrome p450 of the liver into carcinogen is known to form DNA adducts and causes G to T transition mutation.

1.5.4.1 Dietary zinc deficiency and cancer of the esophagus

Cancer of the esophagus is the eighth most common cancer in the world in the form of esophageal squamous cell carcinoma (ESCC) is the predominant subtype. Since there are no early symptoms associated with ESCC, it is frequently diagnosed at an advanced stage of the disease. Persistent inflammation in the esophageal region is one of the risk factors and the major challenge is to determine the causes of this chronic inflammation. Major risk factors for ESCC are chronic alcohol consumption, tobacco smoking and chewing, nutritional deficiencies, and exposure to environmental carcinogens such as N-nitrosomethylbenzylamine (NMBA). In many populations, including the persons with chronic alcohol consumption habit, zinc deficiency in the diet is implicated in the pathogenesis of ESCC. Individuals predominantly subsisting on a cereal diet are likely to suffer from zinc deficiency, and those who consume red meat and seafood would get a small quantity of zinc from the diet. More than 2 billion people are affected in the developing world due to dietary zinc deficiency. Zinc is a micronutrient and serves as a co-factor for many enzyme activities, regulates the functions of the immune system, maintenance of conformation of many transcription factors that control cell proliferation, apoptosis, signaling pathways. Zinc deficiency predisposes a person to disease by adversely affecting the functions mentioned above. Dietary zinc deficiency and simultaneous exposure to NMBA mimics ESCC in a high-risk population. Weanling rats kept on a zinc-deficient diet for six weeks show increased cell proliferation and changes in gene expression of squamous cell epithelium, as well as overexpression of COX2. Such a hyperplastic squamous cell epithelium of esophagus of zinc-deficient rat develops esophageal papilloma with 93% incidence of after a single exposure to low NMBA dose (2 mg/kg).

Microarray analysis of the genome of zinc-deficient mice subjected to six weeks zinc deficient diet showed distinct gene signature in the esophageal mucosa where, two pro-inflammatory genes **S100 calcium-binding protein α8 and α9** associate with esophageal epithelial hyperplasia were upregulated. Zinc plays an essential role in modulating the interaction of S100 **α8** with its receptor for advance glycation end product (RAGE) and the downstream nuclear factor NF-κB-COX2 signaling pathway, which are responsible for pro-inflammatory signals.

1.5.4.2 Increase in iron load in the body increases the cancer risk

Epidemiological studies on different populations of various ethnic groups have shown increased cancer risk in an individual with an increase in iron load in the body due to impaired iron metabolism. A study carried out by Stevens and co-workers examined the association between biochemical markers of iron stores and cancer, where more than 14,000 participants obtained from US National Health and Nutrition Examination Survey were analyzed. In this survey, evidence was pointing at the saturation of iron-binding transporter-transferrin (TF), which was found to be significantly high in men who subsequently developed cancers than in those who did not develop cancer.

Many proteins that are involved in their roles in normal iron metabolism have now been shown to contribute to malignant growth. Transferrin receptor 1 (TFR1) is overexpressed in breast cancer, leukemia, lymphoma, bladder cancer, lung cancer, glioma, and others. It has been possible to inhibit malignant growth by blocking TFR1 receptor-using antibodies developed against the receptor. Lipocalin 2 (LCN2) is responsible for alternative pathway of iron uptake, which was upregulated in breast, liver, and pancreatic cancers. LCN2 binds catechol, which is an iron-binding molecule with the properties of a siderophore, synthesized in mammalian cells as iron binding ligand (LCN2-catechol complex) facilitates circulation of iron in the blood bound. LCN2 in MCF7 are overexpressed in breast cancer cell lines, which leads to increased cell proliferation. Conversely, in mouse models for breast cancer, blocking LCN2 inhibits breast tumorigenesis.

Excess of intracellular iron is stored in the complex form with ferritin in normal cells as well as in cancer cells from where it can be easily sequestered for participation in radical-generating reactions. Iron regulatory protein 1 (IRP1) and IRP2 regulate ferritin by post-transcriptionally repression of ferritin expression and increase in TFR1 expression. In B cells when c-myc gene is expressed, which is known to induce IPR2 expression leading to repression of ferritin gene expression. It has been suggested that the increase in TFR1 could enhance the intracellular availability of iron for metabolic and proliferative purposes consequent to reduction in iron storage in the cell. Direct involvement of c-*myc*gene on TFR1 expression has been demonstrated in colon cancer. Down-regulation of ferritin in cancer cells expressing *H-ras* oncogene increases the labile iron pool and stimulates cell proliferation. On the contrary, the tumor suppressor gene, p53 inactivates IRPs by inducing ferritin production leading to growth arrest. Sensitivity of breast cancer cells to the chemotherapeutic drugs like doxorubicin and carmustin can be increased by down-regulation of ferritin, presumably due to increase in intracellular oxidative stress.

Signaling NF-κB, an important transcription factor involved in inflammation and cancer is intimately connected to ferritin. Upregulation of ferritin may support the survival of inflammatory and stromal cells in the microenvironment of cancer, which may contribute to tumor survival, whereas down-regulation of ferritin may increase the metabolic availability of iron in the cancer cells by increasing the iron uptake and decreasing iron storage and iron efflux. **Ferroportin-hepcidin** regulatory axis is one of the most important recent discoveries because these two proteins play a key role in cancer. Down-regulation of ferroportin is observed in breast cancer cell lines and human breast cancers, where decreased ferroportin levels were associated with increased levels of labile iron pool in cultured breast cancer cell lines. Therefore, in breast cancer prognosis, ferroportin and hepcidin levels are used. Ferroportin levels are known to play a significant role in the growth of primary tumors but also in metastatic spread. In addition, hepcidin is known to be synthesized by many tumors, and many cancer patients suffer from anemia due to iron deregulation. There is a straightforward conceptual link observed between cancer and proteins that regulate iron uptake or efflux because levels of these proteins directly affect intracellular iron content.

Tumors microenvironment is enriched with endothelial cells and macrophages, in which M2-polarized macrophages, that resemble tumor-associated macrophages, were known to show gene expression profile for iron efflux, an increase in ferroportin and a decrease in ferritin. In this way, macrophages may facilitate tumor growth by providing tumor cells with iron or by secretion of ferritin in the tumor microenvironment. Secreted ferritin by binding to cleaved high molecular weight kininogen, which is an endogenous inhibitor of angiogenesis may promote tumor angiogenesis.

Frataxin, a protein produced by mitochondria, is implicated in the neurodegenerative disorder (Friedrich ataxia) and the young suffering from this disease are known to develop cancers involving different tissues. The accumulation of iron in mitochondria due to frataxin dysfunction leads to oxidative stress and the production of ROS. Hypoxia-inducible factor-α (HIF1α) protein is a transcriptional regulatory protein of vascular endothelial growth factor (VEGF) is also regulated by iron levels in the cell. HIF upregulation is associated with tumor growth and progression; therefore, its activity is increased in many tumors. Cellular high iron levels can activate HIF, which may contribute to enhanced iron accumulation in tumors. Activated HIF1 has been shown to promote colorectal cancer.

Cells starved off the iron stagnate in the G1 phase of the cell cycle, which indicates the involvement of iron in DNA synthesis. Wnt signaling pathway plays a crucial role regulation of β-catenin in normal cells, which is altered due to mutation in Wnt or β-catenin in cancer cells and accumulation of β-catenin is responsible for the maintenance of stem cell characteristics in cancer cells. Cellular iron levels were found to show two effects: 1) augments Wnt signaling in colorectal cancer cells having APC mutation or β-catenin mutation, 2) down-regulation of E-cadherin in an APC independent manner. Mechanism by which how iron facilitates intestinal tumorigenesis by affecting Wnt signaling is obvious from the two explanations given above particularly in a background of APC mutation. Dietary iron and not the free iron found in systemic circulation was found to be crucial for intestinal tumorigenesis.

1.5.5 Alcohol Consumption and Cancer

Over more than 2 billion people, consume alcohol regularly as a habit or as social commitment. In 2007, International Agency for Research on Cancer (IARC) classified alcohol as a carcinogen. It is very essential that, there is a great need to publicize among the general public the cancer-causing nature of alcohol to prevent specific cancers. From the epidemiological studies it is evident that 3.6% of cancers worldwide, of which 7-19% of oral cancers are due to habitual drinking of alcohol. The mechanism of alcohol-induced cancer depends on its metabolic products it produces in the body. In the liver, the alcohol is metabolized by alcohol

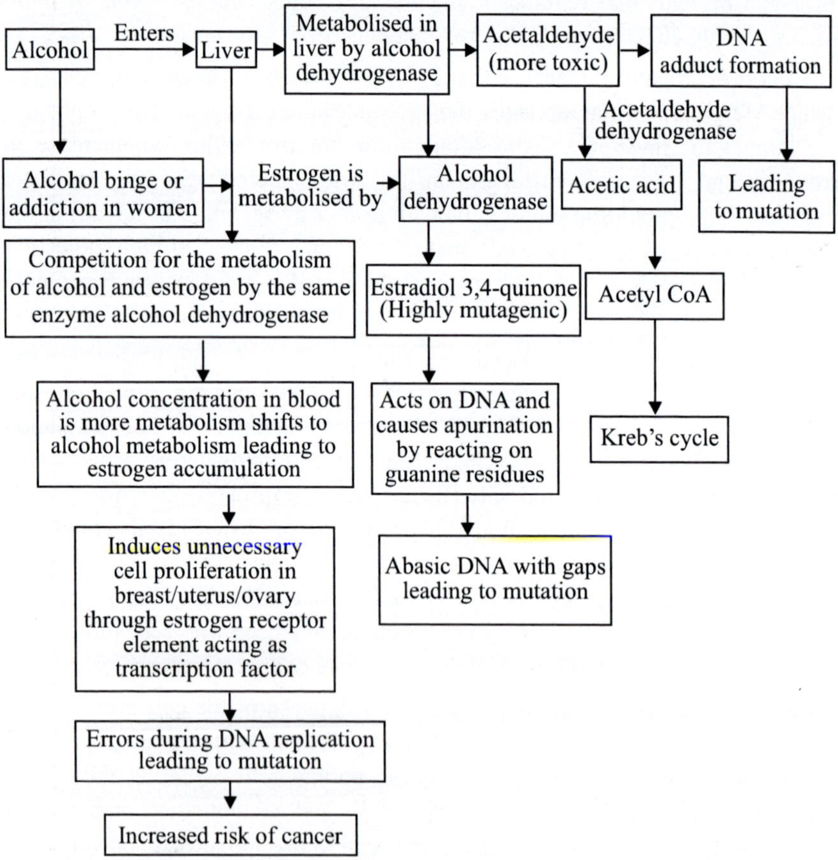

Fig. 1.20. Schematic representation of carcinogenesis due to alcohol consumption

dehydrogenase to form acetaldehyde, which is more toxic and reactive than alcohol. Acetaldehyde can directly interact with DNA and form DNA adducts, which causes mutations. In chronic alcohol consumers (addicts and binge drinkers), acetaldehyde-DNA adducts can be easily detected in their tissue samples. Bacteria in the mouth is also known to produce additional acetaldehyde such that the concentration could get enhanced to 10-100 times higher than in blood, thereby increasing the risk of mouth cancer. The enzyme acetaldehyde dehydrogenase in the liver further metabolizes the acetaldehyde to acetic acid by oxidation reaction (Fig. 1.23). In Asians, a single nucleotide polymorphism for acetaldehyde dehydrogenase gene is observed, which is responsible for alcohol intolerance due to low enzyme activity. Individuals with low aldehyde dehydrogenase activity are at increased risk of developing alcohol-related esophageal cancer. In women, alcohol consumption increases the risk of developing breast cancer because of enzyme alcohol dehydrogenase involved in estrogen metabolism and alcohol metabolism are the same. Since alcohol and estrogen share the same enzyme for metabolism, alcohol will compete with estrogen in this metabolic pathway and lead to increased estrogen concentration in the body (Fig. 1.20). Some epidemiological data suggest that there is 7% increased risk of developing breast cancer with one alcoholic drink per day.

1.5.6 Obesity and Cancer Risk

IARC has classified obesity as another major risk factor for several human cancers. Individuals with body mass index [weight (in kg) /height (in m) squared] greater than 30 (kg/m^2) are considered to be obese. Epidemiological evidence indicates that due to obesity, there is increased risk of developing cancer of the colon, breast, endometrium, kidney, pancreas, liver, and esophagus. Adipose tissue behaves like an endocrine organ capable of releasing peptide hormones, free fatty acids, and steroid hormones that can affect the functioning of other tissues. Several mechanisms of action of obesity as a cancer risk factors or as tumor promoter have been schematically depicted in Fig. 1.21.

Studies on obese mice revealed that obesity causes a chronic inflammatory response with an increase in the production of tumor-promoting cytokines such as IL-6 and TNFα by the adipose tissue that acts as a promoter of hepatocarcinoma. Indirectly, obesity due to excessive abdominal fat is responsible for acid reflux due to pressure exerted on the stomach when the person lies down, which damages the epithelium of the esophagus and constant irritation leads to inflammation, which culminates with adenocarcinoma of the esophagus. Obesity is the end result of abnormal fat metabolism, which leads to increased fat deposition in adipose cells. The fat deposits may be used for the synthesis of estrogen from androgen by the action of aromatase produced in the adipose tissue, which increases the risk of breast cancer. Adipose tissue in obese people releases large amounts of fatty acids, which chronically increases the levels of plasma insulin, which subsequently has tumorigenic effects such as increased cellular proliferation and inhibition of apoptosis mediated through insulin receptors and insulin like growth factor

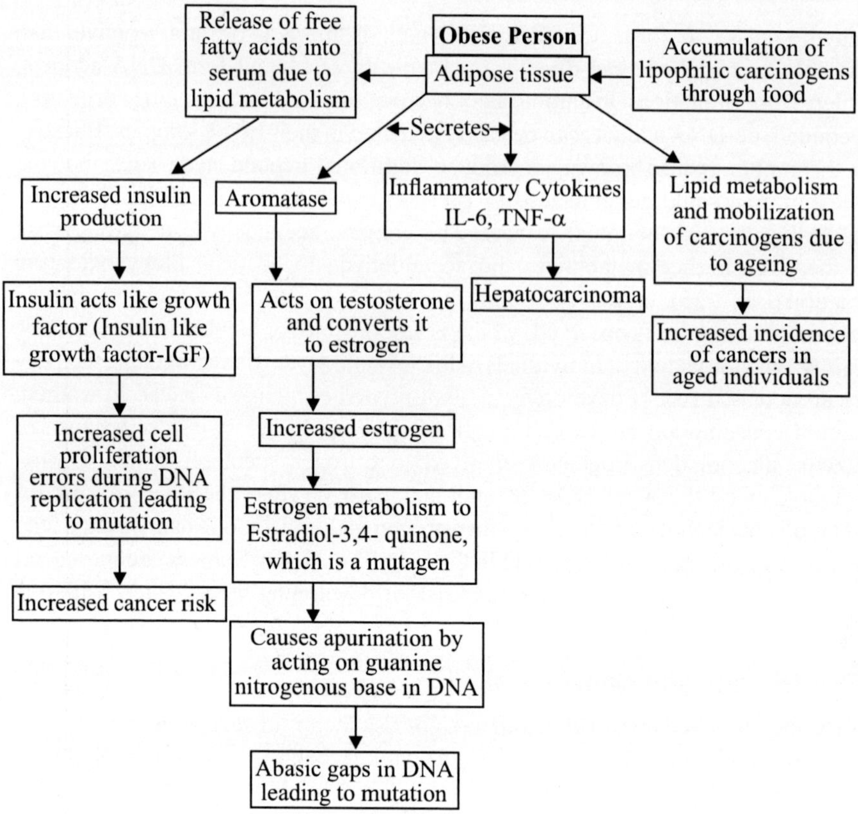

Fig. 1.21. Schematic representation of the mechanism of cancer development in an obese individual

(IGF).Adipose tissue is also a storehouse of lipophilic environmental pollutants, such as polycyclic aromatic hydrocarbons (PAH), organochlorine pesticides, etc. These pollutants enter human system through food of sea origin or animal origin (meat). Pollutants washed off into rivers and marine environment are taken up by the fish and stored in the fat, which in turn, enters the human system when fish is consumed. Similarly, meat producing animals accumulate it in their fat through their food chain, which finally finds its way into human system. Lipophilic pollutants deposited in the adipose tissue are mobilized as the person starts ageing. As these pollutants are slowly released in an aged person, where DNA is most vulnerable for mutagenic effects of these pollutants leads to tumorigenesis in aged individuals.

1.5.7 Hormones and Cancer

Other than chemicals, viruses, or radiation, there is evidence to implicate endogenous hormones as initiators of carcinogenesis. The major organs that develop hormone-related cancers are the breast, endometrium, ovary, prostate, testis, and thyroid. In women who are habitual smokers and drinkers, breast cancer is the most common cancer known to develop. As shown in the schematic representation (Fig. 1.22), estrogen (estradiol and estrone) plays a major role in the initiation and progression of breast cancer. In some women, life events like early menarche (the start of the menstrual cycle) provides an opportunity to prolonged exposure to estrogens is considered to be a risk factors for breast cancer. An extended period of production of estrogen by ovaries due to early and late menarche is considered to be one of the contributing factors for the high incidence of breast cancer. Exposure time to estrogen is affected by a pregnancy and with increased age, the site of estrogen synthesis in the body also changes: ovaries are the main source of estrogen production in the pre-menopausal women. In post-menopausal women, obesity adds to the burden because adipose tissue becomes the primary source of estrogen at this stage in life. In obese women, aromatase enzyme present inherently in adipocytes produces increased amount of estrogen by its action on androgens. Thus, obesity becomes a contributing factor for increased risk of breast cancer through increased estrogen production by adipose tissue in obese women. As shown in schematic presentation (Fig. 1.22) alcohol consumption by women puts them at greater risk of developing breast cancer because of increased levels of estrogen due to sharing of the same enzyme, i.e., alcohol dehydrogenase for the metabolism of estrogen as well as for alcohol. The mechanism of increased concentration of estrogen because of alcohol consumption by women has already been explained in the schematic presentation (Fig. 1.20). The use of oral contraceptives, the exogenous source of hormone and hormone replacement therapy increases the risk of breast cancer in women. Men also are known to develop breast cancer due to excessive production of estrogen hormone.

Two predominant models have been proposed to explain the mechanisms by which estrogen shows its effects on tissues having estrogen receptor (Fig. 1.22), and both mechanisms likely contribute to breast cancer.

One of the proposed models for estrogen-mediated promotion of cancer is: estrogen promotes cell proliferation in the breast tissue and the high rate of cell division makes the DNA vulnerable for mutation during DNA replication and at the same time less time for DNA repair, which creates an opportunity for errors to occur in DNA base pairs. The increased rate of error promotes increased accumulation of somatic mutations in the cell DNA that leads to carcinogenesis. Estrogen, indeed a mitogenic agent, acts as a growth factor breast cells that contain estrogen receptors leading to breast cell proliferation. There are two types of estrogen receptors (ERs), namely, α and β, belong to steroid hormone receptor superfamily. Estrogen mediates the effects through these receptors which bind as dimers to the estrogen response element (ERE) and regulate estrogen-responsive genes. During carcinogenesis of the breast, the estrogen receptor isoforms expression changes remarkably and estrogen receptor-α is significantly upregulated, whereas estrogen receptor-β is down-regulated in the majority of breast cancers. The reasons are unknown for these two different responses by two estrogen receptors-α.

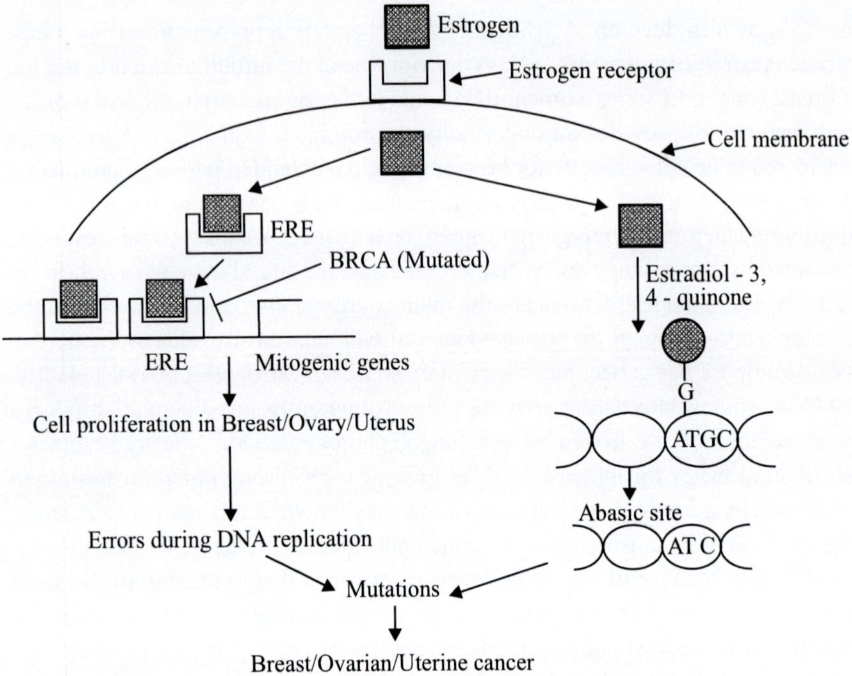

Fig. 1.22. Estrogen mediated promotion of cancer development in tissues having estrogen receptors

Detailed studies of the breast cancer suppressor genes, *BRCA1* and *BRCA2* and their involvement in increased susceptibility to breast cancer are supported by studies on estrogen signaling. *BRCA1* and *BRCA2* are considered tumor suppressor genes that regulate transcription and cell cycle as well as are involved in DNA repair. BRCA1 inhibits estrogen receptor signaling thereby inhibiting the transcriptional activation activity of estrogen receptors and suppression of proliferation of cells. It has been suggested that, inherited mutation of *BRCA* leads to loss of modulation of estrogen signaling, which contributes to the increased risk of breast cancer in women.

Another model suggests that estradiol-3, 4-quinone a metabolite of estrogen is genotoxic, which covalently binds to purine nitrogenous bases of DNA and forms adducts leads to destabilization of the bonds linking the base to the DNA backbone resulting in **abasic (apurinic)** site that ultimately leads to mutations. Estradiol quinones are known to be present in the human breast tissue of breast cancer patients who had the habit of consuming alcohol regularly indicating the involvement of alcohol in increased metabolism of estrogen due to enhanced alcohol dehydrogenase activity to metabolize alcohol (Fig. 1.22). Human breast epithelial cells exposed in vitro to estradiol-3, 4-quinone showed transformation in vitro and the metabolite was also capable of inducing loss of heterozygosity at chromosomal regions in primary breast tumors.

As to support the second model, the normal role of BRCA tumor suppressor proteins is to facilitate DNA repair and loss of BRCA tumor suppressor proteins may cause breast cells more vulnerable to the genotoxic effects of estrogen metabolites. Predispositions of women to breast cancer may involve germ-line mutations in *BRCA1* and *BRCA2* tumor suppressor genes and the genes involved in estrogen biosynthesis and metabolism.

1.5.7.1 Oral contraceptives and breast cancer

One of the leading causes of cancer deaths in women is breast cancer, accounting for 25% of all cancers. There are multiple factors involved in the etiology of breast cancer and one among them is oral contraceptives. The predominant factor responsible for higher incidence of breast cancer is estrogen levels in women from early menarche to menopause. Other factors responsible for breast cancer are nulliparity (having no children), early onset of menarche, delayed first birth, late menopause, oral contraceptives (exogenous hormone), hormone replacement therapy are a few risk factors, which are responsible for increased level of exposure to estrogen. Oral contraceptives (OCs) are hormone-containing medications, introduced in 1960 to prevent unwanted pregnancies. Over 300 million women take OCs every day worldwide and according to some studies there is increased incidence of cervical and breast cancer due to the use of oral contraceptive pills.

Breast tissue and uterine tissue are rich in estrogen and progesterone receptors, which when stimulated by respective hormones lead to proliferation, differentiation, and apoptosis of cells in that area. Exogenously administered steroid hormones in the form of OCs can cause abnormal proliferation of breast and uterine tissue due to unnecessary stimulation of these estrogen and progesterone receptors.

According to a study in 2018, there was strong correlation between regular use of OCs and predominance of breast cancer in women . With every use of OCs, the risk of breast cancer increases by 2.77 times than the non-users. In a study carried out by All India Institute of Medical Sciences (AIIMS) in 2013, it was reported that the breast cancer risk was 9.5 times higher in women who had a long history of using OCs. In women who are carriers of familial *BRCA1* mutation, which is an important tumor suppressor gene are at greater risk of developing breast cancer with the use of OCs.

In women below 40 years of age, who used OCs for more than a year, the relative risk of developing triple-negative breast cancer was 4.2 times. According to an analysis, the use of OCs increases the risk of pre-menopausal breast cancer especially with use before the first full term pregnancy. Women who had used high dose contraceptive pills, which had high dose of estrogen, are at greater risk of developing breast cancer than those who used low-dose OCs.

1.5.8 Cytotoxic Mechanisms in the Induction of Tumorigenesis

The mouth and throat cancer often classified under head-and-neck cancers is a striking example of a cytotoxic mechanism in human tumor promotion. These carcinomas are mostly seen in tobacco smokers who are also habitual alcohol consumers. There is a strong correlation between serious smoking habit together with frequent consumption of distilled alcohol, which shows 100-fold increased risk for certain types of head and neck cancers.

Tobacco smoke consists of a variety of about 60 mutagenic carcinogens, like, 3-methylcholanthrene (3-MC), benzoic(a)pyrene, dimethylbenzanthracene, etc. Ethanol after metabolism would produce acetaldehyde, which is a mutagenic agent because it can form DNA adducts. In addition, ethanol parse has toxic effects on the mouth and throat epithelial cells. Drinks containing a high percentage of ethanol kill any of these mouth and buccal epithelial cells. Therefore, stem cells found beneath the epithelium respond by dividing to regenerate and replace the lost epithelial cell layer within the mouth and throat. Under normal circumstances, these stem cells divide at a low and steady rate to replace the damaged epithelium. The damage might have occurred due to abrasion of food particles. On the contrary the stem cell mitotic rate increases substantially due to widespread denuding (stripping) of epithelium by ethanol.

As the stem cells proliferate in the mouth and throat triggered by alcoholic injury, the individual with smoking habit will induce mutations in the proliferating stem cells caused by tobacco tar mutagens, thereby making the proliferating stem cells to carry mutant alleles. The clonal expansion of these mutated cells is promoted by alcohol, which acts as co-carcinogen, thereby enabling their descendants to acquire yet another mutation that ultimately leads to clinically aggressive head-and-neck cancers. This is a good example of a toxic agent like ethanol acting as a tumor promoter.

Mitogenic agents can also function as tumor promoters, such as steroid hormones like estrogen, progesterone, and testosterone. In the female body, for example, estrogen and progesterone are involved in programming and proliferation of cells in the reproductive tissues. The monthly menstrual cycle of women between menarche and menopause results in the proliferation and then regression of the cells forming the epithelia of the ducts in the mammary gland and endometrial lining of the uterus.

Epidemiologic studies have shown that women are at higher risk of developing breast cancer if they go through more menstrual cycles'experiences in their lifetime. By one estimate, if the menarche is delayed during adolescence, lifetime breast cancer risk decreases by 20% for each year. The risk of breast cancer is only about one-half in women who stop menstruating before the age of 45 compared to those who continue to menstruate at the age of 55 or beyond. Breast cancer risk can be decreased by ovariectomy, because ovary is the prime source of estrogen in the female body and one of the main causes of breast cancer in postmenopausal unmarried women. In a study of postmenopausal women who suffered from breast cancer on an average a 15% higher level of circulating estrogen was found in them compared to unaffected women. This is a classic example of tumor promotion by estrogen, which is endogenous to the human body rather than being an agent of foreign origin, the actions of this hormone closely resemble the properties of classic tumor promoters.

Chronic inflammation led cytotoxicity also has a major role in the pathogenesis of human carcinomas. For example, gallstones lead gall bladder inflammation due to continuous irritation of glass stones on the epithelial lining of the gall bladder. Similarly, hepatocellular carcinomas (HCCs) arising out of chronic hepatitis B virus (HBV) infections and accompanying inflammation caused by the virus in the liver, which is common in East Asia. HBV induces liver cancer through its ability to cause continuous cell proliferation and this proliferation is required to replace hepatocytes that are continually being killed by HBV infectious cycles. In addition, HBV infection activates the cells of the immune system, namely; NK cells and cytotoxic T cells, which are responsible for eliminating virus-infected cells through cytotoxic mechanism, leading to chronic inflammatory state in the liver. Both mechanisms likely conspire in the pathogenesis of the hepatocellular carcinomas that so frequently afflict individuals with chronic HBV infections.

Yet other indications of infectious agents inducing inflammation like *Helicobacter pylori* led inflammation, which in turn, leads to human malignancies like lymphomas arising in gastric mucosa-associated lymphoid tissue (MALT). Seventy-five percent of MALT lymphomas are because of *Helicobacter pylori* bacterial infection and inflammation, which is curable if patients are treated with antibiotics capable of eradicating the bacterial population in the stomach (more details are given in the section "inflammation and cancer". The 25% of lymphomas that do not respond to this treatment have evolved beyond this dependence to become "promoter independent," possibly because they have sustained the chromosome 11 to 18 translocation that is frequently observed in these lymphomas.

1.5.9 Cancer from Tobacco

According to the WHO report, more than 7 million people die world over each year because of smoking tobacco and use of other tobacco products like snuff and chewing. 7000 chemicals are inhaled with every puff of cigarette or bidi by a smoker, of which about 70 of them are classified as carcinogens by IARC. These dangerous carcinogenic chemicals found in the tobacco smoke are potent mutagens too. They interact with DNA to form DNA adducts and alter the expression of certain essential genes that prevent cancer (tumor suppressor genes) and increase the risk of multiple types of cancers in a tobacco consumer. Tobacco smoking causes almost 9 out of every ten cases of lung cancers and other tobacco products can cause cancer almost in any organ in the body. According to epidemiological studies, up to 16 different types of cancers can be directly linked to tobacco consumption in one form or the other.

Indian Council of Medical Research (ICMR) reported that cancer incidence doubled in India over the past 26 years, where breast, cervical, oral and lung cancer incidences are altogether constitute 41% of the cancer burden. Epidemiological studies have clearly shown that tobacco consumption leads to lung, esophageal, larynx, mouth, throat, kidney, bladder, pancreas, stomach, and cervical cancer.

Benzo (a) pyrene is among the one of the mutagens found in tobacco is known to form DNA adduct predominantly with guanine and induce G – C → T – A mutations. Similar type of mutation can be expected from 8-oxo-guanine, which results from reactive oxygen species generated from tobacco smoke. G – C → T – A mutations are the major class of base substitution mutations observed in p53 tumor suppressor gene, whole-genome sequencing (WGS) and whole-exome sequencing (WES) of lung cancer patients and the predominance of this class of mutation correlates with smoking history. In bladder cancer patients with smoking history, most frequently found mutation was in apolipoprotein B mRNA editing enzyme catalytic polypeptide (APOBEC) as signature mutation.

1.5.10 Carcinogenic Contaminants and Dietary Deficiencies

Carcinogenic effects of food that we consume can be variable. Salmon, a fatty rich fish known to contain omega-3-polyunsaturated fatty acids, which is an essential component of a healthy balanced diet. Salmon is a carnivorous fish, known to accumulate fat-soluble pollutants acquired from its diet and the surrounding water in its fat. These accumulated pollutants can be genotoxic, are transferred to humans on the consumption of salmon. A study conducted on farmed and wild salmon from different regions of the world found that in farmed salmons of Scotland, polychlorinated biphenyls (PCBs) and other pesticides are present in greater quantities indicating that regular consumption of these farmed salmons increases the cancer risk. Eskimos diet predominantly consists of fish and seal meat. They also use seal blubber (fat) for cooking purpose. It was observed that in recent times incidences of cancer have increased in Eskimos because of a large number of carcinogenic contaminants found in their diet (seal meat, seal blubber and fish).

There could be other additive factors such as dietary deficiencies, which will contribute to increased risk of cancer. Most compelling evidence for dietary deficiency and cancer comes from a folate-deficient diet, there is an increased risk of developing colorectal cancer. During nucleotide synthesis and DNA methylation folate plays a critical role as co-enzyme and both these processes have a direct bearing on carcinogenesis. There are experimental evidences which prove that depletion of folate in the diet contributes to tumorigenesis by interfering with both nucleotide synthesis and DNA methylation. Depletion in nucleotide synthesis affects DNA synthesis leading to DNA instability that favors mutation and disruption in DNA methylation may cause hypomethylation of certain tumor favoring oncogenes leading to their activation. Low-folate diet is known to inhibit deoxy thymidylate synthesis, and the nucleotides imbalance facilitates the incorporation of uracil into DNA. In order to replace uracil incorporated in DNA, the DNA strand break occurs, which increasesthe cancer risk. In folate-deficient humans, both uracil misincorporation and DNA strand breaks are observed, and both effects are reversed on the administration of folate. Hypermethylation of tumor suppressor genes and hypomethylation of genomic DNA at specific locations are some of the epigenetic changes observed in cancer cells. For DNA methylation, methyl groups contributed by folate and folate deficient diet causes a decreased synthesis of methionine, which leads to genomic hypomethylation of DNA. In several studies, it has also been observed that folate depletion causes hypermethylation of specific 5′ gene loci. Studies carried out in rodents have shown that dietary methyl deficiency leads to changes in the hepatic DNA methylation patterns and induces hepatocarcinogenesis in the absence of carcinogen.

1.5.11 Influence of Ageing Process on Cancer

The increase in the rate of age-related cancer incidence varies between cancer types. For example, prostate cancer incidence accelerates much faster than brain cancer. Some cancers osteosarcoma, acute lymphoblastic leukemia and testicular cancer have early-life incidence peaks, at approximate 30 years of age and then sharply declines. The cervical cancer incidence also levels of at middle age. Exposure to various risk factors in early life, such as infectious diseases caused by viruses and certain species of bacteria could influence early-life cancer incidence peaks and the probability of developing malignant cancers is expected to increase with age. Apart from accumulating mutations during the normal course of life of an individual, normal ageing process also causes many changes in cells that may increase the susceptibility to cancer initiation and create tissue microenvironment suitable for the growth of malignant cells. The ageing process thus favors cancer progression and metastasis. With ageing, immune response and endocrine systems are also altered, which may also contribute as factors to cancer development. Disruption in DNA repair and/or damage response associate with ageing, cancer, or both. It has been argued that pathways and cellular processes that favor the accumulation of DNA damage and mutations, such as failure in nucleotide excision repair (NER), predisposes to cancer.

It is a well-known fact that DNA damage, mutations and genome instability increase with age. Disruption of DNA repair pathways leading to loss of cell proliferative ability or increased cell loss and transcription-coupled NER, often accelerate ageing. It is evident from studies that the accumulation of mutations with ageing is organ-specific. Some organs like the intestine, liver and lung show the highest amount of accumulation of mutations and some like testes and brain were found to show the least amount of accumulation of mutations with ageing. Role of epigenetic changes has been highly emphasized in both ageing and cancer because global hypomethylation and promoter hypermethylation are the common features observed in both the cases. For example, hypermethylation of the *ras* association domain family 1 (RASSF1) promoter is observed in cancers and is also found to increase with ageing without adiposity. Age related changes in the susceptibility to carcinogens owing to the changes in the enzymes involved in carcinogen metabolism leading to activation of carcinogens or tissue-specific manner changes in proliferative activity that occur with ageing are some of the reasons. Since mutations accumulate with age, there is every chance that aged tissues will tend to have large number of cells in an advanced stage of carcinogenesis, which is the major factor observed for increased incidence of cancer with age.

Telomeres (repetitive sequences at the end of chromosome that prevent chromatid fusion or joining) become shorter with every cell division in normal human somatic cells, thereby limit the replicative potential of the cell. Because this feature of the telomeres, they have long been hypothesized to be a causal factor in ageing. DNA damage response pathways is activated by short telomeres that cause cells to undergo irreversible growth arrest (cell senescence). It is thought that shortening of telomere evolved as strategy for tumor suppressor and disruption of this mechanism by various factors may favor cancer development. Shortening of telomere and telomere dysfunction contribute to cancer susceptibility by increasing the incidence of chromosomal aberrations caused by breakage-fusion-bridge (discussed in detail in chapter 2) cycles. In spite of its basic role as a tumor suppressor, replicative senescence may render old tissues more favorable ground for cancer development. Reports indicate that senescent cells secrete pro-inflammatory cytokines, extracellular matrix components and other factors that disturb the tissue microenvironment and promote tumorigenesis.

With ageing, remarkable changes occur with endocrine hormones level such as sex hormones like estrogen and androgen level decrease thus certain cancer risk also decreases. Growth hormones (GH) and insulin-like growth factor (IGF) levels decline with ageing; low GH and IGF1 have been associated with decreased cancer incidence.

In cancer etiology, it is recognized that inflammation has a significant role to play because it has been shown to have tumor-promoting effect (discussed in the next section of this chapter). With ageing the circulating levels of inflammatory cytokines, such as interleukin-6 (IL-6) and tumor necrosis factor α (TNFα) are found to increase, therefore, inflammation considered to be a significant contributing factor in ageing. Higher levels of IL-6 and TNFα have been associated with obesity and adipose tissue mass (discussed in the previous section 1.5.6) contributing factor for increased incidence of cancer among obese individuals because body-mass index increases with age. It is also interesting to note that higher levels of inflammatory cytokines are associated with the prevalence of colorectal adenomas in aged individuals.

Solid tumors for their survival require vascularization, for which they secrete growth factors favoring vascularization (angiogenesis – discussed in chapter 3) by especially switching on the genes of those growth factors. Vascular ageing is a normal phenomenon observed in ageing individuals, which contributes to decreased angiogenic potential of aged tissues, which suppresses the progression of solid tumors in old age.

1.5.12 Vitamin D Deficiency and Carcinogenesis

Vitamin D is produced from pre-vitamin **7-dehydrocholesterol** by skin upon exposure to sunlight.7-dehydrocholesterol derived from the skin or obtained from seafood diet or egg yolk undergoes metabolism in the liver to form 25-hydroxyvitamin D, which is a biologically inert compound. In the kidney, 25-hydroxyvitamin D is converted into biologically active 1, 25-dihydroxyvitamin

D. An individual's requirement for vitamin D up to 90-95% is met from exposure of skin to UV radiations of sunlight, where pre-vitamin D is synthesized, and the remaining requirement comes through very few foods, like oily fish (salmon, mackerel, sardines, and tuna) and in small quantity in egg yolk naturally contains vitamin D.

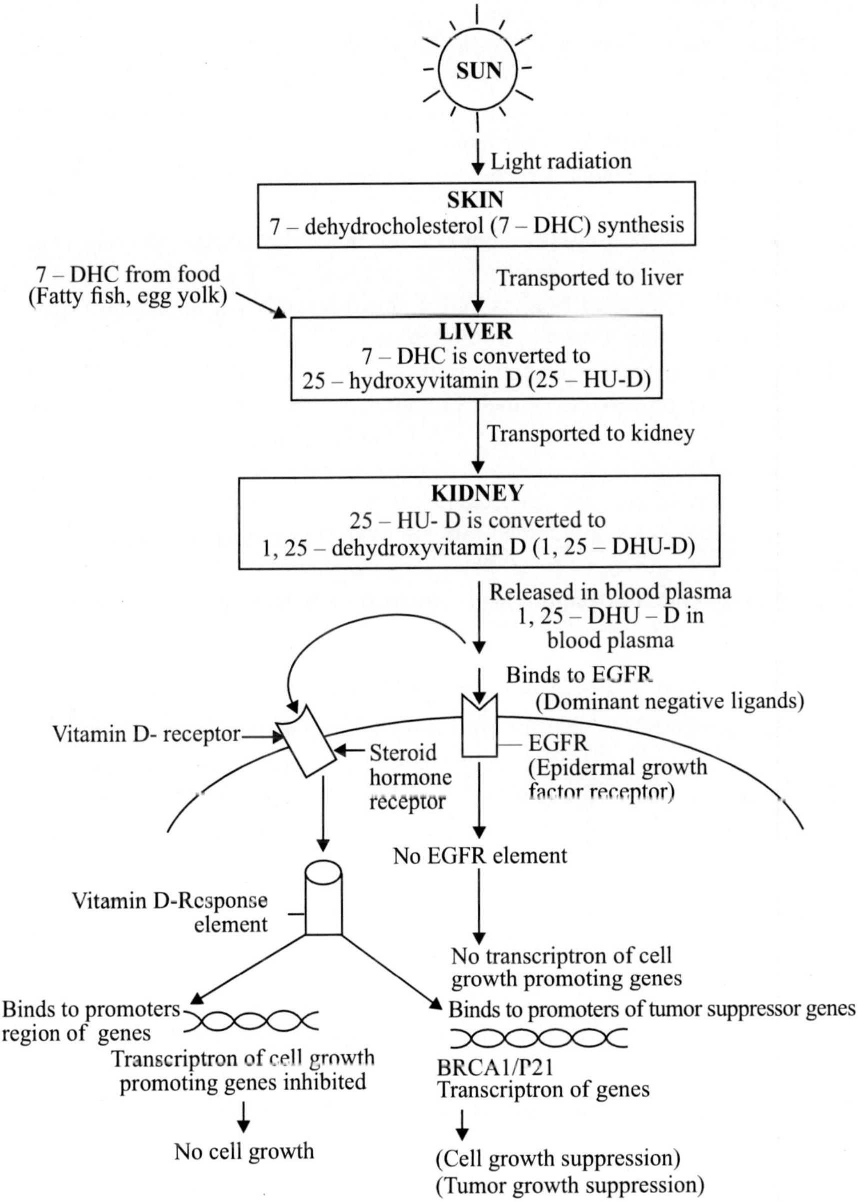

Fig. 1.23. Schematic representation of the role of vitamin D in the suppression of cancer

Epidemiological evidence indicates that people living at higher altitude are at increased risk of developing prostate, colon, and breast cancer despite the enzyme needed to produce 1, 25-dihydroxyvitamin D being present in their tissues. At higher altitude, strong UV radiations of higher frequencies coupled with vitamin D deficiency are the major factors that play a significant role in carcinogenesis. Mice deficient in vitamin D developed 80% larger tumors compared with vitamin D sufficient mice.

The molecular mechanism of vitamin D action at cellular level lies in the active form of vitamin D (1, 25-dihydroxyvitamin D), that binds to cytoplasmic vitamin D receptor, which is a member of the steroid hormone receptor superfamily (Fig. 1.23). The vitamin D bound receptor triggers signal transduction through vitamin D response element, which binds to gene promoter region, that regulates transcription of its target genes involved in inhibition of cell growth and induces differentiation and apoptosis through several molecular targets. Vitamin D can bind to EGFR (epidermal growth factor receptor) as a competitive inhibitor and prevent the binding of EGF to EGFR, and behave like a dominant-negative ligand for EGFR; this results in inhibition of cell growth. Secondly, vitamin D receptor through vitamin D response element inactivates BRCA1 and p21 tumor suppressor genes on binding to their promoter regions. p21 protein inhibits cell cycle by acting as an inhibitor of cyclin-dependent kinases (CDKs). Vitamin D is also known to promote apoptosis through mitochondrial signaling without the involvement of caspase activation. Vitamin D facilitates transport of pro-apoptotic proteins BAK and BAX from the cytosol to mitochondrial membrane, where these two proteins form the channels, that facilitates the release of cytochrome *c,* which is required for apoptosome assembly. At the same time, vitamin D down-regulates the inhibitors of apoptosis Bcl-2 and IAPs (Fig. 1.23).

1.5.13 Radiation Induced Carcinogenesis

Risk of cancer in individuals exposed to ionizing radiation is very high. Some examples of occupational and accidental exposure to ionizing radiation and cancer induction can be cited as follows:

- Uranium miners are known to suffer from lung cancer, and they show tenfold increase in incidence.
- High mortality from leukemia and other cancers were reported from the victims who survived Hiroshima and Nagasaki atom bomb.
- Chernobyl nuclear reactor disaster in April 1986 resulted in the dispersion of radioactive cloud to vast areas including neighboring European countries resulted in an increased incidence of blood cancers, and other deformities of the body.

α and β particulate radiations emitted by radioactive sources are considered to be direct-acting carcinogens because they are charged particles, which interact with DNA directly without causing ionization in their pathway when they travel through the cellular milieu. On the other hand, ionizing radiations cause ionization of materials that come in their pathway resulting in the production of highly reactive species of ions. These reactive ions interact with the substance of immediate vicinity and bring about an alteration in their nature. It is this property of ionizing radiation that makes them carcinogenic because the ions generated by them interact with DNA and bring about mutation.

Electromagnetic radiations like X-rays and γ-rays when interacting with water molecules generate highly reactive free radicals on interacting with water molecules, which interact with DNA and cause mutations. The production of free radicals on interaction with water molecules is shown below (Fig. 1.24):

$$H_2O \rightarrow e^- + H_2O^+ \rightarrow\rightarrow H^+ + OH^+$$

$$H_2O \rightarrow H_2O^- \rightarrow\rightarrow H^+ + OH^-$$

Fig. 1.24. Production of free radicals from water due to radiation effect on water molecule

The free radicals generated by water molecule due to ionizing radiation will interact with DNA and disrupt the bonds between the nitrogenous bases or may cause intramolecular cross-linking or DNA strand break. The free radicals may also bring about deamination or oxidation of bases, as shown below (Fig. 1.25).

Cytosine → Uracil

Adenine → Hypoxanthine

Guanine → Xanthine

5-methylcytosine → Thymine

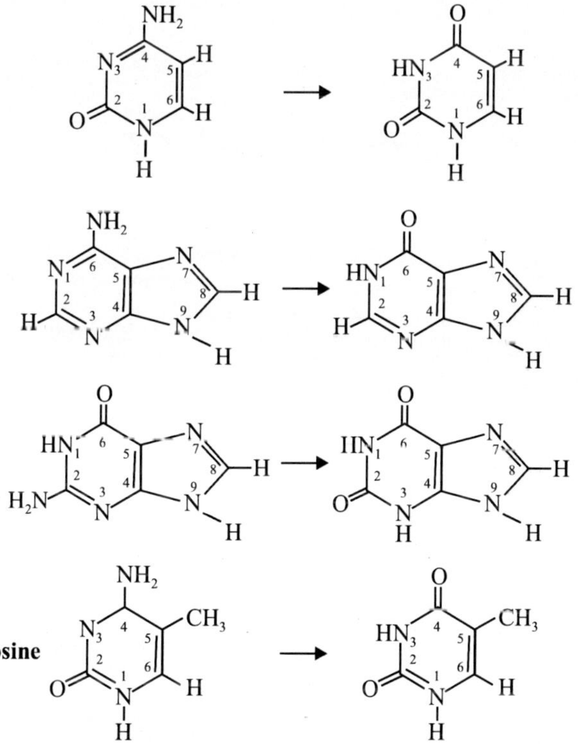

Fig. 1.25. Deamination of purines and pyrimidines due to radiation gives rise to alternative nitrogenous bases

Ultraviolet radiation (UV) is a non-ionizing type of radiation, which generates tremendous heat on interaction with matter and excites the molecules to make it chemically active. UVB (280 – 320 nm) and UVA (320 – 400 nm) present in the sunlight, are mostly responsible for melanomas, head and neck squamous cell cancers. Pyrimidine nitrogenous bases are more sensitive to UV radiation and absorb UV at 245 nm. Excited thymine bases adjacent to each other are known to undergo dimerization (Fig. 1.26). Thymine dimers (Fig. 1.27) cause distortion in DNA structure with the result the enzyme responsible for the correction of DNA molecule may not be able to read it; hence it leads to mutation.

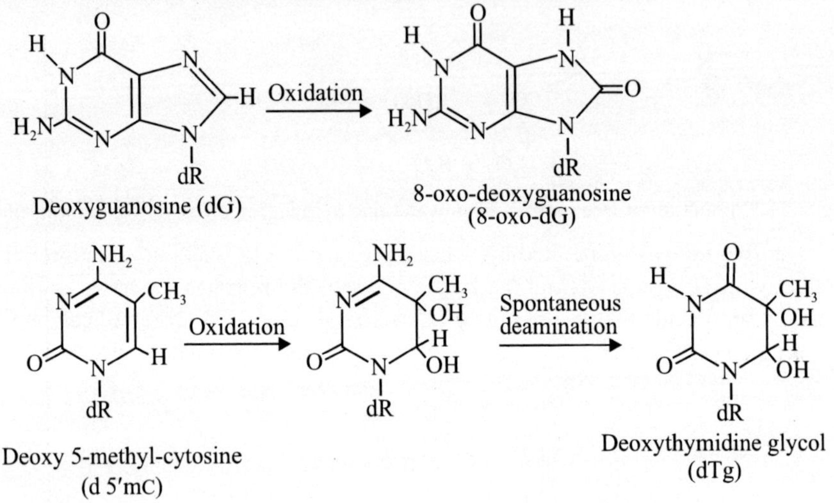

Fig. 1.26. Oxidation of nitrogenous bases due to radiation results in oxidized derivatives

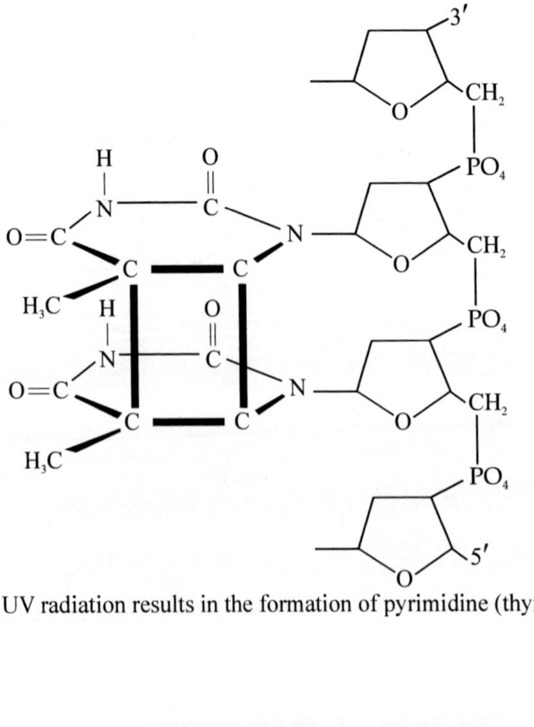

Fig. 1.27. Effect of UV radiation results in the formation of pyrimidine (thymine) dimers

UV light is readily absorbed by the nucleotides of DNA, with maximum absorption – and maximum mutagenesis - at a wavelength of 254 nm. The pyrimidines are more susceptible to excitation and damage. UV light may convert single pyrimidine into **pyrimidine hydrates** (Fig. 1.27), lesions that have altered base-pairing properties.

Epidemiological evidence indicates that white race is very prone to UV rays induced skin cancer and on analysis of DNA samples from the skin cell carcinoma of such individuals; it was evident that at many places thymine dimers were found indicating it could be one of the causes for carcinogenesis.

1.6 INFLAMMATION AND CANCER

Hepatitis B virus is a DNA virus, classified as a potent carcinogen because of its strong association with hepatocellular carcinoma (HCC) post-hepatitis B virus infection. It is a fact that HBV infection increases the risk of developing hepatocellular carcinoma by 10-25-fold greater than uninfected individuals. Immune response invoked against HBV infection causes hepatocellular necrosis, inflammation and promotes regeneration, which is very common in individuals who develop chronic infection. Oncogenic mutation due to increased cell proliferation and/or oxidative stress from inflammation caused by HBV might be the cause for hepatocellular carcinoma. Inflammation caused by HBV is a contributing factor for the development of hepatocellular carcinoma, in a manner which is almost like the mechanism observed in gastric cancer induced by *Helicobacter pylori*. In hepatocellular carcinomas, it is observed that HBV is known to integrate its genome frequently at 11p and 17p site of the chromosomes, which has tumor suppressor genes in these sites.

IARC has classified *Helicobacter pylori* as a carcinogen because the bacterium induces chronic inflammation in the stomach post-infection and initiates carcinogenesis. Gastric cancer initiated by *Helicobacter pylori* is very much dependent on the bacterial strain, host response and other environmental factors and it involves multistep process of carcinogenesis where inflammation is considered to be the initial step in the process. The steps involved in *Helicobacter pylori* induced carcinogenesis are infection → chronic superficial gastritis → atrophic gastritis (cell death) → dysplasia → gastric carcinoma.

The proposed mechanism by which *Helicobacter pylori* can cause gastric cancer is as follows:

The high-risk strain of *Helicobacter pylori* produces a protein called CagA (cytotoxin-associated antigen A), which on insertion into gastric epithelial cell membrane elicits effects on cells, such as stimulation of cell growth. Member of Src family tyrosine kinases phosphorylates CagA, which leads to signal transduction initiating increased DNA replication, which in turn, increases the risk of mutation, thereby leading to transformation of cells. CagA is known to induce the accumulation of nuclear β-catenin, an important transcriptional regulator responsible for the maintenance of stem cell characteristics, which leads to metaplasia.

VacA, another important protein of *Helicobacter pylorus* linked with gastric malignancy, which is a secreted protein that inserts itself into the gastric epithelial cell membrane and mitochondrial membrane and induces vacuolation and apoptosis. The bacterium is also involved in other mechanisms like chronic inflammation and stem cell recruitment that promote carcinogenesis, which will also involve pro-inflammatory mediators through the NF-κB pathway. Inflammation induced by *Helicobacter pylori* causes hypermethylation of DNA by stimulation of methyltransferases, which is responsible for epigenetic changes in DNA. It is a well-known fact that, during inflammation, there is excessive production of reactive oxygen species (ROS) and nitrogen oxides (NOs) resulting in increased cellular damage and cell death. ROS and NOs interact with DNA and cause DNA strand break or induce mutation. Cell death triggers cell proliferation, which in turn, involves DNA replication making DNA vulnerable for mutation.

There are also several non-infectious agents that cause chronic inflammatory conditions, which may lead to development of cancer.

- Tobacco smoke devoid of carcinogens can induce chronic inflammation and also act as a tumor promoter.
- Asbestos, cement dust and stone quarry dust are known to cause inflammation in the lungs and predisposing the individual to bronchial carcinoma. Tobacco smoking would increase the incidence of lung cancer in individuals already having inflamed condition in the lung.
- Frequent acid reflux into the esophagus causes injury to esophageal epithelium and continuous irritation to esophageal epithelium causes inflammation that increases the risk of esophageal carcinoma.
- Risk of colorectal cancer is very high in individuals having inflammatory bowel disease.

Macrophages and neutrophils of the immune system are the key cells that are involved in the chronic inflammation. Tumor necrosis factor-alpha (TNF-α) produced by macrophages is a predominant inflammatory cytokine. In addition, activated macrophages and neutrophils are known to produce reactive oxygen and nitrogen species (ROS and NOs) which causes immense cellular damage and increased risk of DNA damage. Tumor promoting inflammatory cytokines are also produced on activation of certain oncogenes like *ras* and *myc*andare known to induce inflammatory cytokines. The immune response against the tumor or transformed cells continues to play a role in tumor progression once the cancer is initiated. Inflammation facilitates malignant progression, which is contributed by both tumor cells and non-malignant cells surrounding the tumor. Tumor-associated macrophage (TAMs) and the tumor cells secret certain growth factors, cytokines, and chemokines that promote proliferation and survival of tumor. Nitric oxide (NO) synthesis triggered by TNF-α is implicated in several stages of carcinogenesis, including cell transformation and growth of transformed cells. IL-6 cytokine produced macrophages residing in the liver has been shown to play an essential role in hepatocarcinogenesis (Fig. 1.28).

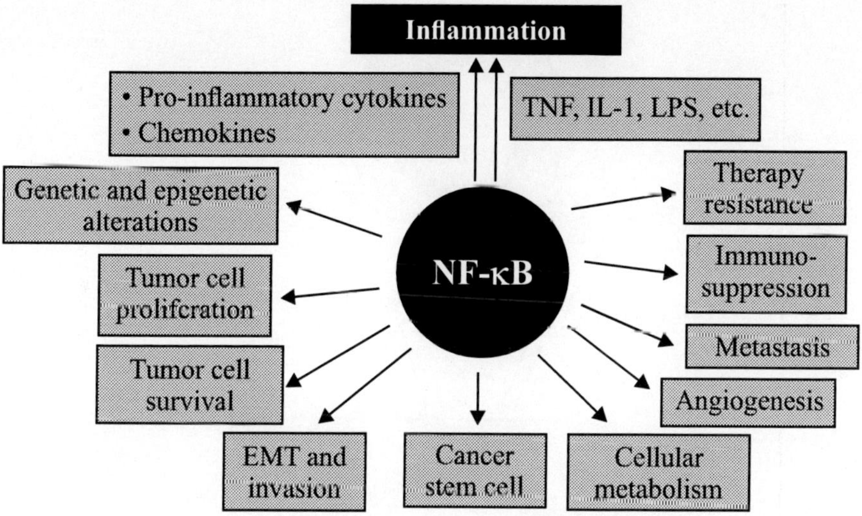

Fig. 1.28. Inflammatory response favoring carcinogenesis

NF-κB is an important nuclear transcription factor plays a significant role in the mediation of inflammatory response and does play an important role in progression of cancer. Macrophages and cancer cells induce NF-κB production to contribute to tumorigenesis by promotion of metastasis, angiogenesis, and inhibition of apoptosis in tumor cells. In certain cancers like multiple myeloma, acute lymphocytic leukemia, prostate, and breast cancers activation of certain oncogenes have a direct bearing on activation of NF-κB gene. NF-κB is an inhibitor of apoptosis by the induction of anti-apoptotic genes, which is one of the most important cellular effects exhibited on activation of NF-κB; thereby promote carcinogenesis by inhibiting an important tumor-suppressing mechanism (Fig.1.29).

Cancer-related inflammation closely resembles chronic inflammation usually observed in tissue remodeling and repair by the presence of leukocytes and inflammatory mediators.

1.7 TUMOR MARKERS (TMs)

The characteristics of tumor markers are:

1. Easily quantifiable.
2. Tumor specific.
3. Always expressed by tumors.

For the analysis of TMs generally blood plasma or serum, pleural fluid or ascitic fluid or pericardial fluid, urine and CSF are used.

TMs are broadly categorized into following types

1. Proteins.
2. Enzymes and isoenzymes.
3. Hormones.

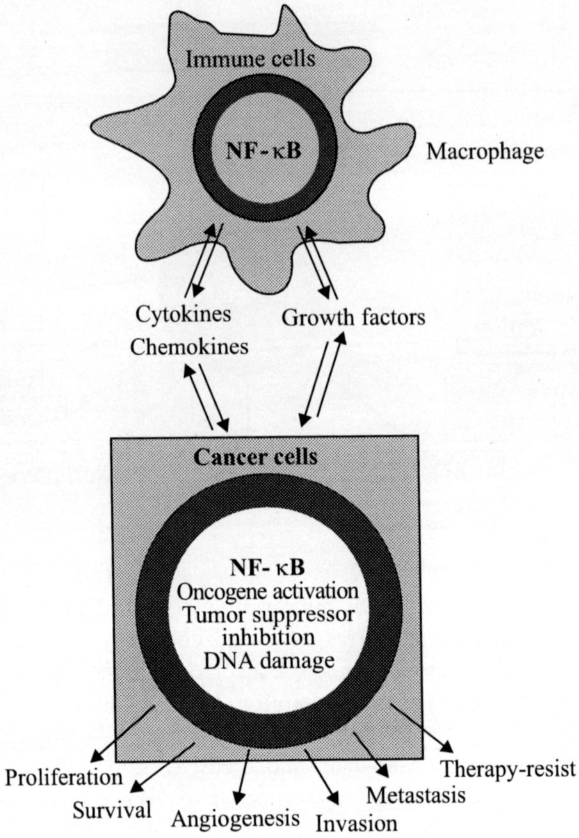

Fig. 1.29. Immune cell triggered inflammatory response

4. Immunoglobulins.
5. Antigens (oncofetal and carcinoembryonic)
6. Receptors.
7. Oncogene products.
8. Genetic markers.
9. Immune cells

1. **Proteins:** A combination of three proteins like LYVE1, REG1A and TFF1 are found in high levels in urine from which early stage of pancreatic cancer can be detected.

   P4H9-detected molecule (PDM) is expressed by spindle-shaped fibroblasts in colorectal cancer patients associated with shorter survival.

   Desmogleins were found to be prognostic biomarkers for pancreatic ductal adenocarcinomas.

   β-2 Microglobulin: It is elevated in the serum of patients suffering from lymphoproliferative disorders; nonspecific to chronic lymphocytic leukemia.

Table 1.4. Most common tumor antigens encountered and used for diagnostic purpose

Cancer	Tumor marker
Colorectal	Carcinoembryonic antigen (CEA)
Hepatocellular	Alfa fetoprotein (AFP)
Pancreatic	CA 19-9
Ovarian	CA 125
Breast	CA 15-3
Prostate	Prostate specific antigen (PSA)
Germ cell	AFP, Human chorionic Gonadotropin (HCG)
Lung (non-small-cell)	Cytokeratin fragment (CYFRA) 21-1, squamous cell carcinoma (SCC)
Lung	Neuron specific enolase (NSE), Pro-gastrin releasing peptide (Pro-GRP)
Melanoma	S100
Thyroid differentiated	Thymoglobulin

CA 15-3 (Cancer Antigen 15-3): Characteristic of metastatic breast cancers, elevated in 76% of metastatic breast cancers.

CKAP4 (cytoskeleton-associated protein 4): This protein has been identified in the blood of the patients who have lung cancer.

Gastrin: It is produced in excess by non-beta islet cell tumors of the pancreas; levels above 1000 pg/mL are diagnostic of gastrinoma; also expressed in some benign conditions.

Glucagon: It is produced in excess by tumors arising out of alpha-cells of the islet of pancreas. In glucagonoma, above 900 mg/mL in blood is observed. in severe diabetic condition also, it is detected in blood.

Calcitonin: A hormone-like substance frequently found elevated in the serum of small cell lung cancer patients; steady increase in levels indicate the progression of the disease.

PLP (Parathyroid hormone-like Protein): Squamous cell cancer and breast cancer patients show elevated levels in serum.

Alpha Fetoprotein: This protein is produced mainly by the fetal liver as a substitute for albumen in fetal condition. It is a key indicator of hepatocellular carcinoma (HCC), produced in large quantities and released in the serum.

Glypican – 3 (GPC3): It is a membrane-bound heparin sulfate proteoglycan found to be expressed by HCC found to be increased in the serum of patients in the early stage of HCC.

Serum HE4 (sHE4) protein: There is a strong correlation between serum HE4 levels with aggressive endometrial (Uterine) cancer.

Oct4A protein is expressed in VSELs will be 50-fold higher in cancer patients than in normal cells. Biomarker Oct4a protein expression in VSELs shows variations based on stage of cancer. Oct4A protein is transcription regulatory protein of embryonic condition, predominantly expressed by undifferentiated stem cells, responsible for regulation of stem cell differentiation.

2. **Enzymes: PLAP (Placental Alkaline Phosphatase or PL-AP):** Ithelpsin confirmation of malignancy in a small number of patients and the source of tumor of liver, bone, and germ cell origin can be differentiated but non-diagnostic by itself.

   LDH (Lactic Dehydrogenase): All tumors produce LDH because tumors experience the anoxic condition. Total LDH levels range from 48 to 115 IU/liter.

   Carboxypeptidase – N: Circulating peptides in the blood created by carboxypeptidase-N (CPN) help in accurately predicting the early stage of breast cancer. The peptides created by CPN originate from cancerous cells, eventually making their way into the bloodstream.

3. **Hormones:** The abnormally high amount of hormone synthesis by endocrine tumors represents unregulated cancer cell metabolism. Some examples are:
   - Insulin production by tumors of islet cells
   - Calcitonin production by medullary thyroid carcinoma
   - Catecholamines production by pheochromocytoma of adrenal.

   Sometimes, the hormone produced is not a natural product of the organ that has developed into cancer, in which case it is designated as "ectopic"hormone. For example, the production of ACTH and ADH by lung cancer cells is called ectopic.

4. **Immunoglobulins:** Multiple myeloma is characterized by production of abnormal monoclonal immunoglobulin molecules. These immunoglobulins are usually incomplete antibody molecules with isolated light chains of lambda or kappa type and rarely heavy chains. Immunoglobulins are valuable indicators for the classification and treatment of myeloma; the amount of abnormal immunoglobulin serves as an index of tumor volume. If myeloma responds to therapy positively it is indicated by a fall in abnormal immunoglobulin production, whereas a rise points to relapse.

5. **Antigens:** Tumor antigens identified by both monoclonal antibodies and polyclonal anti-sera of animal origin since they are oncofetal antigens, autologous antibodies will not be produced against them. The oncofetal antigens are predominantly expressed in embryo or fetus, but will be expressed in very low levels in the adults or not expressed at all. They may reappear and express in excess in certain tumors. For example, carcinoembryonic antigen (CEA) is expressed in colon carcinoma and found in serum in enormous quantity, which can be easily detected. Similarly, Alfa-fetoprotein is produced in copious amounts by hepatocellular carcinoma.

6. **Receptors markers:** Over expression of epidermal growth factor (EGF) receptor in many carcinomas, vascular endothelial growth factor (VEGF) receptors in almost all malignancies, platelet derived growth factor (PDGF), insulin like growth factor (IGF) receptor, protein tyrosine kinase receptor (PTK), TGFβ receptor.

7. **Oncogenic products** – ras, HER-2/neu, bcl-2, c-myc are the predominant markers in majority of tumors.

   N^1, N^{12} –diacetylespermine serves as a marker for non-small cell lung cancer.

   Catecholamines: Useful for the detection of adrenal tumor.

   Cell-free nucleic acids (cfNA): These are present in the form of cell free DNA (cfDNA) and micro-RNA (miRNA) are found in abundance in the blood serum of cancer patients indicating malignant tumor and tumor cell death. Presence of cfNA is an indicator of tumor in the body.

   MicroRNA (MiR-744) is found to be a novel diagnostic and prognostic biomarker of pancreatic cancer.

   Tumor Markers in Clinical Use

   Proinsulin C-peptide: It is levels are increased in the serum during insulinoma and islet cell tumors and it can be used for differentiating tumors derived from endocrine secreting cell type or non-endocrine cell types.

   VMA (Vanillylmandelic Acid) and HVA (Homovanillic Acid): Their levels are elevated in serum during catecholamine secreting tumor arise such as neuroblastoma or ganglioneuroma.

   Thyroglobulin: Thyroid follicular carcinoma is known to secrete it in excess and it returns to normal following the treatment or if thyroidectomy is performed. It is a useful indicator for monitoring the disease whether it is persisting and to see the recurrence of follicular carcinoma.

   Very small embryonic-like stem cells (VSELs) found in circulation in blood in large numbers in cancer patients suffering from any type of cancer, i.e., solid tumors of any tissue origin and the blood cancers.

8. **Genetic Markers**

   Philadelphia Chromosome (Ph1): Presence of chromosomal aberration due to translocation between 9 and 22 in the precursor cells of WBC, which originates in bone marrow confirms the diagnosis of chronic myelogenous leukemia.

   Translocation between 8th and 14th chromosome indicative of Burkitt's lymphoma

   Translocation between 9th and 11th chromosome indicative of T cell leukemia

   Deletion in 13th chromosome q arm is indicative of retinoblastoma

   Deletion in 5th chromosome q arm is indicative of adenomatous polyposis coli (colon cancer)

   Deletion in 17th chromosome p arm indicative of loss of tumor suppressor gene p53.

9. **Immune cells population:** Macrophages are known to suppress the tumor growth, but at the same time, certain population of macrophages in the tumor microenvironment has been found to promote tumor growth by suppressing the immune response against the tumor. From the studies carried out on breast, prostate, bladder and cervical cancer tissues, researchers have identified two types of macrophages-M1 and M2 in the tumor microenvironment. These were identified using gene markers, CCL3 gene for M1 macrophage and CD163 for M2 macrophage. M1 macrophage is immune booster against tumors, but the M2

macrophage suppresses the immune response and supports tumor progression. Therefore, in the tumor microenvironment, M2 macrophages are found in abundance in tumors that have entered malignancy, whereas low-grade tumors M1 population predominates. In high-grade gliomas, M2 population is higher than M1.

Exercise

1. What are the characteristics of cancer cells?
2. Classify the cancers based on different tissue origin.
3. List the characteristics of benign and malignant tumors.
4. By using a suitable example, explain the different stages in the development of cancer.
5. Environment and lifestyle have an important role in the development of cancer. Justify with suitable examples.
6. How does the following factors influence carcinogenesis?
   (a) Alcohol (b) Obesity (c) Hormones
7. What is the role of diet in the development of cancer? Explain with examples.
8. Does ageing have any influence on the development of cancer? Explain.
9. Explain the role of vitamin D in the prevention of cancer.
10. How chemicals behave as carcinogens and explain how they get transformed into carcinogens?
11. Write an account on the mechanism of DNA adduct forming ability of the following with suitable examples:
    (a) Alkylating agents (b) Arylaminating agents
    (c) Aralkylating agents.
12. How electromagnetic radiations induce cancer? Explain the mechanism.
13. What is the effect of UV radiation on the genetic matter? Explain with examples.
14. Explain how the following compounds are generated **or** what is the cause for generation of the following compound?
    (a) Pyrimidine dimer (b) Pyrimidine hydrates
    (c) Deaminated nitrogenous bases
15. What is the role of cytotoxicity and inflammation in the development of cancer?
16. How inflammation promotes cancer development?
17. How tumor markers help in the diagnosis of cancer?

CHAPTER

2

Process of Carcinogenesis

Recent studies carried out by Aris Katzourakis and his team at University of Oxford have shown that human DNA has roughly about one lakh pieces of viral DNA incorporated in it, which is approximately 8% of the human genome. Scientists are puzzled about this fact and they are investigating what is the purpose of viral DNA in the human genome. Most of the viral DNA in the human genome belongs to retroviruses, which includes HIV. Retrovirus on infecting a cell releases the genome into the host cell cytoplasm, which later takes over the metabolic machinery of the infected cell. Later, the viral genome replicates to form millions of copies to be incorporated into daughter viruses, which escape from the cell by causing cell lysis to infect new cells. Retroviral genome also chooses an option to incorporate its genome by first copying the RNA to form complementary single stranded DNA (cDNA) by using its own reverse transcriptase enzyme, which is activated in the host cell cytoplasm. The same reverse transcriptase synthesizes the complementary strand for cDNA to make it double stranded and then incorporate it in host genome at multiple sites.

If egg or sperm is infected by a retrovirus, its DNA gets incorporated in the haploid genome of the gametes. It can be potentially passed on to the next generation and the generation after that repeatedly, thereby becoming part and parcel of hereditary component of the individual species. Once the retroviruses become inherited stowaways, they are referred to as endogenous retroviruses. At first, endogenous retroviral genome replicates with the host cell genome and will have the ability to infect other cells when it disengages itself from the host cell genome. In due course, retroviral genome mutates and loses the ability to infect other cells but may gain the ability to transform the host cell into a cancerous cell. Retroviruses that have gained the ability of induction of tumors in mammals including humans are discussed in this chapter.

Like retroviruses becoming endogenous, some DNA viruses also have the ability to incorporate the genome in the infected host cell and become endogenous. Like mutated endogenous retroviruses that can induce tumors, endogenous DNA viruses also can transform cells to form cancerous growth. Some examples of DNA viruses responsible for cancers in humans are Epstein Barr virus (EBV), hepatitis B virus and human papilloma virus are discussed in this chapter.

2.1 TUMOR VIRUSES

They are also called oncogenic virus, which are grouped into RNA and DNA tumor viruses. Most of these viruses are host specific and selective in tumor induction with a few exceptions. Oncogenic viruses conceal themselves in infected cells genome and remain hidden or latent with no lytic and replication activity. Latent virus becomes active only when the cell is exposed to physical stress such as radiation, chemical carcinogens, hormones or even other viruses.

Relatively a large number of viruses have been implicated in animal cancers, only few of them induce cancer in humans.

The first evidence of human cancer induced by a virus was discovered in 1950 by Denis Burkitts, a surgeon working in central Africa. Many African children suffering from massive tumors of lower jaw used to visit him and he would surgically remove the tumor, which would appear again after some months. This perplexed him and he sent the tumor samples for further investigation to see whether it is malignant or benign. The tumor is named after him as Burkitt's lymphoma. On electron micrographic examination of tumor tissue by Epstein and Barr's in their laboratory, it was found that the tumor cells had large number of electron-dense cytoplasmic granules. On further investigation, it was evident that these granules are viral particles, which belonged to herpes virus family. The virus was named after the discoverers as Epstein-Barr virus (EBV). The proof of involvement of EBV in the induction of Burkitt's lymphoma was from the following evidence.

- Burkitts lymphoma cells contained proteins and transcripts (mRNA) of EBV. On adding these to normal human lymphocyte culture, the cells showed tendency of transformation but not malignancy.
- Addition of EBV to culture of human lymphocytes leads to malignant transformation.
- Injection of EBV to monkey or baboons resulted in lymphoma.

2.1.1 RNA Tumor Viruses

In 1909, Peyton Rous observed a timorous growth in the breast muscle of a hen, which was identified to be sarcoma. Rous succeeded in transplanting the tumor into the breast muscle of another healthy hen of the same breed and induced the tumor growth in the healthy hen. Later, in another experiment, Rous homogenized the tumor tissue and filtered the resulting homogenate and injected the filtrate into young birds; within several weeks the birds developed tumors. The induced tumors were subsequently found to contain an infectious agent that could be passed on through homogenate once again to another bird without getting destroyed and developed sarcomas at the sites of injection. The infectious agent was found to a transmissible virus capable of inducing tumors in birds. It was named **Rous Sarcoma Virus (RSV)**, which was later in 1970, Howard Temin proved it to be RNA tumor virus. The other RNA tumor virus to have been discovered is **Human T-cell Leukemia Virus (HTLV-1)**, which is known to cause leukemia in humans and non-human primates. At the same time **mouse mammary tumor virus (MMTV)** was discovered in certain strain of mice, which can transmit the virus through mother's milk to the offspring leading to breast cancer susceptibility in the offspring.

To show that Rous sarcoma virus (RSV) is tumor inducing virus, an experiment was conducted, where the normal chick embryo fibroblast culture was transfected with RSV in tissue culture. Within a week some cells underwent transformation and started showing the characteristics of transformed cells, such as density-independent growth, loss of contact inhibition and anchorage independent growth. From these features it was quite clear that RSV is a tumor inducing virus (Fig. 2.1).

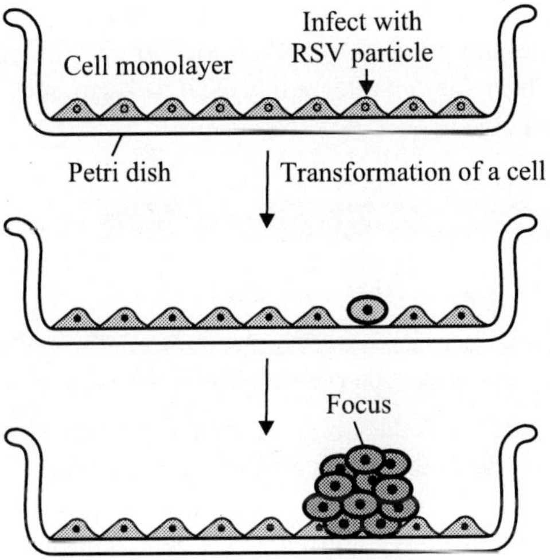

Fig. 2.1. The process of transformation of cell by RNA tumor virus

In 1974, the laboratory of J. Michael Bishop and Harold Varmus at the University of California, San Francisco, developed a DNA probe that specifically meant for recognizing *src* gene in transformation of cells, which resembled the gene found in the RSV genome. To understand *src* origin and functions, cells were infected with RSV, then *src*-specific genetic probe was used to follow the fate of the *src* gene in the infected cells presuming that RSV uninfected chicken cells would not inherently have *src*-related DNA sequences in their genomes. Following RSV infection, *src* gene sequences would readily get incorporated in the genome of the infected cell detectable by the gene probe. It was also evident from this study that the uninfected chicken cells genome also contained *src* sequences and two copies of *src*-genes exist per diploid chicken cell genome. Later it was found that almost all bird species and mammalian species have *src* sequence in their genome.

In the genome of normal organisms of vertebrate organization, the *src* gene is highly conserved and it implies that, it has important role in normal cell functioning and the cellular *src* gene is referred as c-*src* (i.e., cellular-*src*). The v-*src* gene of RSV has close resemblance to the c-*src* gene of the chicken with drastic difference between the two genes in their functions. c-*src,* found in the cellular genome, performs normal function by serving as an intracellular domain of EGF receptor, on the contrary, the very similar v-*src* gene present in the RSV genome acts as a potent **oncogene**, a gene that has the capability to transform a normal chicken cell into a tumor cell.

It is presumed that the *v-src* gene of RSV was not naturally present in the retrovirus genome of the ancestral RSV. Probably, this hypothetical viral ancestor was perfectly capable of replicating in the chicken cells without *src* gene sequence. Avian leucosis virus (ALV) is one such *src* negative retrovirus, which commonly infects chicken, being infective spreads the infection to other chickens very quickly without inducing the formation of tumors. On detailed investigation of genome of this virus, it was observed that ALV has the genomic sequence almost similar to RSV except that the genome does not contain *src* gene of RSV. It is suggested that, an ancestral virus like chicken ALV virus, after infecting a chicken cell, while escaping from the cell after cell lysis, it had acquired the gene sequence from the host cell genome (Fig. 2.2).

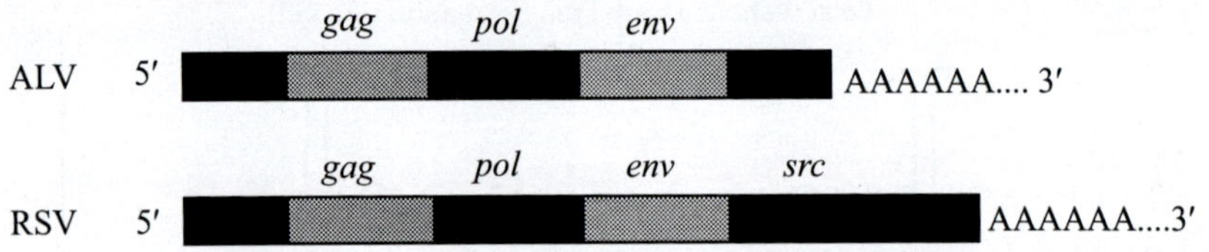

Fig. 2.2. Comparison between ALV and RSV genomes

The newly acquired cellular *src* gene sequence was readily incorporated into the viral genome, with the result a fourth gene sequence was added to the existing three genes (*gag, pol, env*), which were used by ALV-like retrovirus for its replication in infected cells. Acquiring a new gene sequence by ancestral ALV, probably, changed the virus to RSV, which is at present existing. The kidnapped *src* gene present in the genome of RSV could have been exploited by the virus to its advantage for transforming the cells infected by it. This c-*src* gene picked up by RSV is incorporated at 3′ end of the RSV genome, after some remodeling would turn into an active oncogene, therefore, c-*src* is referred to as **proto-oncogene.** It is well known that the genome of normal vertebrate cells has genes that have the potential to induce cell transformation under certain circumstances, and thus leading to cancer development. Within the RSV RNA genome, the three preexisting retroviral genes *gag, pol, env* involved in viral replication is followed by v-*src* gene downstream.

MC29 myelocytomatosis virus yet another chicken retrovirus known for inducing a bone marrow malignancy in chicken has an acquired cellular gene *c-myc* in the genome known as the v-*myc* oncogene induces rapidly growing tumors in infected chickens. Similar to v-*src*, the v-*myc* gene origin could be traced to a corresponding cellular proto-oncogene *c-myc* in the normal chicken genome. *myc* gene integration into the retroviral genome after undergoing some remodeling like *src* gene and gained oncogenic property. The gene that had essential role to play in the cells of normal chicken, after remodeling imparts potent oncogenic power to the gene for cell transformation.

Most important discovery was that the MC29 was a descendent of avian leucosis virus (ALV) like RSV. This reinforces the idea that retroviruses like ALV are quite capable of acquiring random pieces of a cells' genome. In the case of majority of hybrid viruses carrying such acquired cellular genes would not have gained tumor-inducing potential. Only when they acquire growth promoting cellular proto-oncogenes then the hybrid virus would exhibit a cancer-inducing phenotype.

Till now the two viruses that we discussed are retroviruses found in birds capable of transforming the cells. Like in birds, mammals also get infected by retroviruses that are distantly related to ALV. Like ALV, these retroviruses are also capable of acquiring cellular proto-oncogenes of mammalian cell origin, after some remodeling converts them into potent oncogenes. One of the examples is the feline leukemia virus, which probably would have acquired the *fes* oncogene in its genome from cellular *fes*, giving rise to feline sarcoma virus, and a hybrid rat-mouse leukemia virus, which probably on two different occasions acquired two distinct proto-oncogenes giving rise to transforming retroviruses, Harvey and Kirsten sarcoma viruses, which carry the H-*ras* and K-*ras* oncogenes, respectively, in their genomes.

A proto-oncogene found in the genome of mammalian or avian species can be readily detected in the genomes of all other vertebrates. For example, c-*myc* of human, mouse and chicken perform identical function in their respective hosts.

Table 2.1. Retroviral oncogenes and the host species affected

Virus	Species affected	Tumor type	Oncogene
Rous Sarcoma Virus (RSV)	Chicken	Sarcoma	src
Avian myelocytomatosis virus	Chicken	Myeloid leukemia	myc
Avian erythroblastosis	Chicken	Erythroleukemia	erbA, erbB
Harvey murine sarcoma	Mice	Sarcoma	H-ras
Kirsten murine sarcoma	Mice	Sarcoma	K-ras
Abelson's murine leukemia	Mice	Leukemia	abl

Based on cell transformation ability, retroviruses are classified into two types, namely, acutely transforming, and slow transforming. **Acutely transforming viruses** induce tumors within days or weeks, whereas slow transforming virus induce tumors over a long period of latency, i.e., months or years. Acutely transforming viruses readily possess genes for transforming a normal cell and these genes are called **oncogenes**. Oncogene carrying retrovirus becomes replication defective because to incorporate the oncogene in its genome, it will have knocked off some of its genetic sequence. In order to replicate, it requires the help from another virus. Approximately 30 different oncogenes have been identified and each has been given three letter code derived from the virus in which the oncogene was identified. Examples of acutely transforming retroviruses are given in the table.

Most acutely transforming retroviruses have only one oncogene. Except avian erythroblastosis virus ES4 contain two oncogenes (erbA and erbB). It was found that the viral oncogene sequence is almost like the oncogene readily existing in the host cell from which the virus was isolated. The host cell oncogenes are called **c-onc** or **proto-oncogene** and viral oncogenes are called **v-onc.** It is presumed that the v-onc's were created when a retrovirus picked up c-onc gene sequence entirely or in part. In most of the cases, incorporation of c-onc into viral genome resulted in deletion of important viral gene sequence, thus, rendering the virus **replication defective**. These viruses need co-infection with helper virus, which provides the structural proteins and enzymes required for replication. An exception to this is Rous Sarcoma virus (RSV) whose *src* gene does not require helper virus for replication. Most acutely transforming retroviruses are responsible for tumors in animals. To date no member of this group are know to cause tumors in humans, except human T cell leukemia virus or human T cell lymphoma virus (HTLV).

The genome of RSV is single stranded RNA, to integrate into host cell genome, it should be first converted to double stranded DNA. Evidence indicates that RSV successfully transmitted its genetic information through many successive cycles of cell growth and division, which led Temin and his team to investigate the mechanism of RSV transmission and replication. Through experimental evidence they proved that, RSV after infection of a cell, synthesizes double stranded DNA from its single stranded RNA genome with the help of its own **reverse transcriptase** enzyme. In the beginning, the RSV single stranded RNA, with the help of reverse transcriptase synthesizes a single stranded DNA and the original RNA strand is dissolved. Now the single stranded DNA copy serves as a template for the synthesis of complementary DNA strand through reverse transcriptase action. Thus, the double stranded DNA (dsDNA) derived from single stranded RNA of the RSV serves as the genome of the virus for transcription of required proteins and enzymes for the virus to complete its life cycle. The dsDNA of the virus gets incorporated in the genome of the host cell, which is called **provirus.** The cellular RNA polymerase uses the provirus as the template for transcription there by producing RNA molecules that would be encapsulated into progeny virus particles or, alternatively it could also function as messenger RNA (mRNA) to transcribe viral proteins.

As described above, each of the retroviruses that gained the tumorigenic ability might have arisen from a non-transforming retrovirus, such as avian leukosis (ALV) or murine leukemia virus (MLV), which acquired a proto-oncogene from the genome of an infected host cell as they escaped from the host cell after infection. In fact, the non-transforming original viruses could also induce cancers, but they were able to do so only after a much longer incubation period; often months or years passed before these viruses succeeded in becoming oncogenic. Such viruses are referred to as **slow transforming viruses.** In contrast to acutely transforming viruses, slow transforming viruses, such as ALV and MLV can infect the cells; the infected cells released the progeny viruses but were not able to induce apparent changes in the shape or growth behavior of cells. These viruses lacked oncogenes in their genomes, which is consistent with the fact that lack of change in cell phenotypes. Without oncogenes in them how could MLV and ALV induce malignancy? In 1981, the answer for this question was found from the detailed analysis of genomic DNAs of the leukemia's in chickens induced by ALV. The cells were found to have the copies of the ALV provirus integrated into their genomes. Surprisingly, ALV induced leukemic cell genomes contained proviral genome integrated immediately adjacent to the c-*src* (proto-oncogene) (Fig. 2.3).

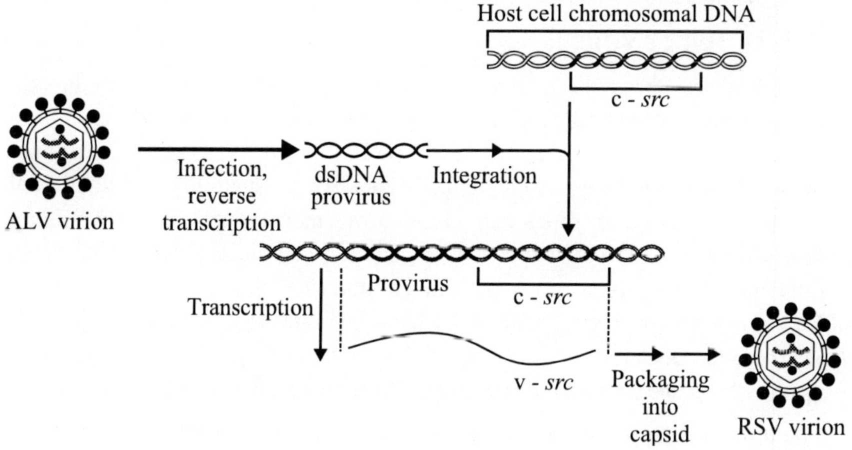

Fig. 2.3. Capture of *src* gene by avian leucosis virus

It soon became clear that, integration of provirus in close physical association with any proto-oncogene would lead to cell transformation. In the case of ALV induced leukemia, when c-*src* gene comes under the regulatory control of proviral transcriptional promoter, leading to disturbance in control mechanism that normally takes care of the expression of c-*src* gene. As a result, instead of finely tuned up and down-regulation by the control circuitry of the cell, the expression of c-*src* will be taken over by a foreign gene that results in uncontrolled expression of c-*src* at a high rate, called amplified expression. This hybrid viral-cellular gene combination that has formed in the chromosomes of chicken cells now functions much like the v-*src* oncogene carried by avian sarcoma virus. This jackpot event of changing the non-tumorigenic event of slow transforming virus to tumorigenic event occurs perhaps 1 in 10 million infections of severe viremic condition, where normal c-*myc* gene is converted to potent oncogene. This mechanism of conversion of proto-oncogene to oncogene is referred to as **insertional mutagenesis and gene amplification.** This explains the leukemogenic power of other slowly transforming retroviruses, such as MLV.

Mouse mammary tumor virus (MMTV), another retrovirus is known to show integration of its genome (provirus) adjacent to *int-1, int-2* and *int-,* all these three genes were found to be proto-oncogenes, independently responsible for cell proliferation. On integration of MMTV genome adjacent to any one of these three genes led to the appearance of mammary tumors.

Some retroviruses readily carry oncogenes, such as human T cell leukemia virus-1 (HTLV-1), which uses insertional mutagenesis to incite leukemia in humans. This virus has gene called *tax* gene, which produces certain proteins, among which one of them is responsible for the viral replication and the other is responsible for activation of interleukin-2 and GM-CSF genes. In fact, interleukin-2 is responsible for proliferation of T cells and the GM-CSF is responsible for hematopoietic cell proliferation. Since, *tax* gene is active during HTLV-1 infection and the two cytokine genes coming under its regulatory control would lead to leukemia.

2.1.2 DNA Tumor Viruses

In 1960, Richard Shope discovered **papilloma** virus, which causes benign skin warts in rabbits, on rare occasions transforms itself into squamous cell carcinomas of skin. This virus came to be named as **Shope Papilloma Virus (SPV). Polyoma virus** discovered in 1953 has been named because of its capability of induction of a variety of distinct tumor types in mice. **SV40 virus (Simian virus 40th isolate)** is closely related to polyoma virus in its size and chemical constitution, which is found in African green monkeys and chimpanzee. Shope's papilloma virus (SPV), mouse polyoma virus and SV40 have been grouped together as **papova virus,** a class of DNA tumor viruses and the term papova signifies *pa = papilloma, po = polyoma* and the *va = vacuole* forming ability of SV40 during their lytic infection.

With the discovery of **human adenoviruses**, the DNA tumor viruses group became larger, which causes upper respiratory tract infection in humans and the virus can induce tumors in infected hamsters. There is some similarity between SV40 and human adenovirus infection. SV40 lytic cycle leads to lysis of infected cells in primates. Similarly, adenovirus infection leads to lytic cycle in human upper respiratory tract cells. The natural hosts of virus are said to be permissive hosts. When these viruses are grown in cells of non-host species (non-permissive) they do not cause lysis but bring about transformation of cells leading to tumor growth.

Members of the herpes virus group (human herpes simplex virus-8- hHSV8) are the other entrant into the class of DNA tumor viruses. **Epstein Barr Virus (EBV)**, distantly related to the herpes virus family, is known to cause **Burkitt's lymphomas** in young children of equatorial Africa as well as **nasopharyngeal carcinomas** in Southeast Asia. Hepatitis B virus (HBV), human papilloma virus 16 (HPV16), Shope fibroma virus (SFV) are the other DNA viruses having tumorigenic ability.

Like RSV-transformed cells, SV40 transformed cells also show remarkably altered shape and they grow over one another because of loss of contact inhibition, which is also a characteristic of virus-transformed cells.

SV40 and polyoma are the two intensively studied DNA tumor viruses and the cell transformation by these two viruses depends on the continued presence of viral genomes in the descendents of an initially transformed cell. The proof that these two viruses are tumorigenic came from the discovery of tumor associated T antigen proteins found in the cancers induced by these two viruses. Serum antibodies found in the mice carrying an SV40-induced tumor showed strong reactivity with nuclear protein that was present in the tumors triggered by SV40 and did not react with proteins of tumors induced by polyomavirus or by other carcinogenic agents. A strong immunological response against the antigen in the SV40 induced tumor bearing mouse indicates that the viral genome present in tumor cells encoded a protein called SV40 T antigen that was responsible for induction of tumor. The presence of the virus-induced T antigen in the transformed cells directly correlates with the transformed state of these cells. Therefore, cells where the T antigen is lost would not display transformed phenotype.

The evidence for the association of SV40 viral DNA with host cell genome came in 1968, when the genome of the SV40 transformed cells was subjected to centrifugation. SV40 DNA (5 kb) from these transformed cells did not sediment separately but sedimentation occurred together with host cell genome (50 kb) indicating that viral DNA in these transformed cells does not exist separately like in non-transformed cells. Since there is integration of viral DNA into host cell DNA, it is passed on to next progeny when the cell replicates by replication of DNA, the integrated DNA also replicates with host cell genome.

After some years of this finding, this ability of papovavirus genome integration into host cell genome was also confirmed from the study on human cervical cancers induced by human papilloma virus (HPV). Almost all (99.99%) of the tumor cells genome was found to show integration of fragments of human papilloma virus (HPV) genomes into the chromosomal DNA. Interestingly, intact HPV viral genome was not integrated in cancer cell genome, instead, only the oncogenic (cancer-causing) portion of the viral genome was found in the chromosomal DNA of these cancer cells. The portion of the genome responsible for viral replication and construct progeny virus particles was almost always missing or if present, it was in fragmentary state. The genomes of DNA viruses that show successful integration into host chromosomal DNA, integration was found to be in haphazard manner that included only wild type genomic fragments (Fig. 2.4).

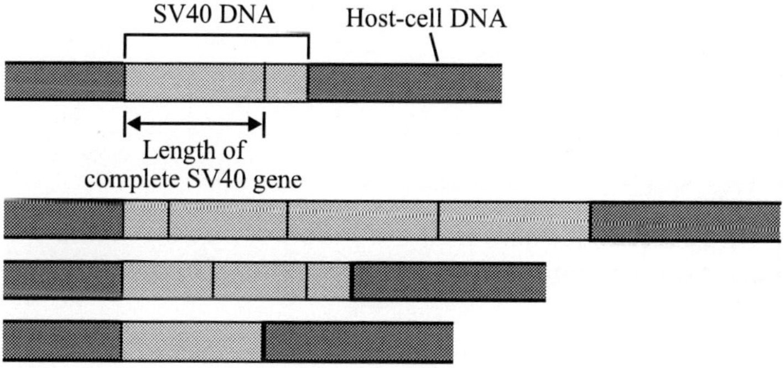

Fig. 2.4. Genome of SV40-DNA tumor virus

2.1.2.1 Mechanism of transformation by DNA tumor virus

Various steps presumed to be involved in transformation brought about by DNA tumor viruses are given below.

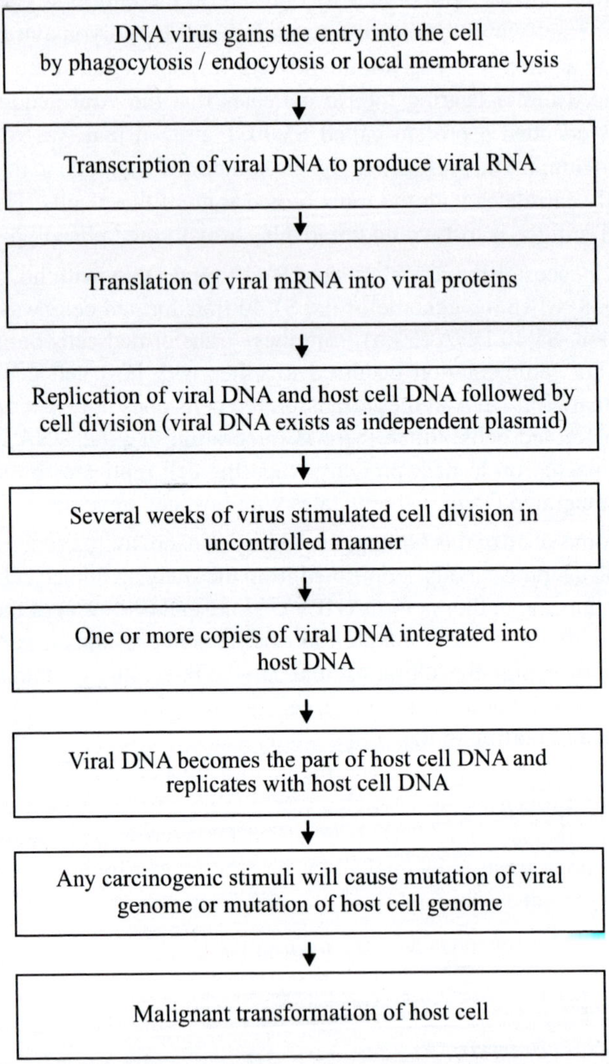

Fig. 2.5. Sequential events involving DNA tumor virus genome in developing cancer

2.1.2.2 Pathogenic mechanism of induction of hepatocellular carcinoma by hepatitis B virus (HBV) and hepatitis C virus (HCV)

Hepatitis B and C viruses are unrelated viruses that target the liver and replicate in hepatocytes. Only 5 – 10% of adult individuals contact infection and become the carriers of the virus and up to 30% is responsible for developing progressive chronic liver disease (CLD), which is characterized by hepatitis, fibrosis, and cirrhosis and finally transforms into hepatocellular carcinoma (HCC). HBV or HCV infections are responsible for about 80% of HCC world over.

HBV and HCV virus induce chronic liver damage triggering inflammation and regeneration, which favors HCC development. It suggests that the pathogenesis of HCC is immune mediated. Persistent replicative ability of HBV and HCV in hepatocytes creates an environment congenial for HCC by blunting the immune response against the virus through proteins of viral origin. Although viral-specific lymphocytes, natural killer cells (NK), NK-T cells and macrophage infiltration is generally seen in the infected liver, which is responsible for hepatocellular damage through inflammatory response but they do not facilitate virus clearance effectively. With HBV and HCV infections, there is significant reduction in IFN production, which could be one of the causes for failure in viral clearance.

HBV and HCV encoded proteins interfere with host gene expression and bring about changes in cellular phenotypes that are recognized as characteristics of carcinogenesis, which includes growth factor-independent proliferation, resistance to growth inhibition, tissue invasion and metastasis, angiogenesis, reprogramming of energy metabolism, and resistance to apoptosis due to persistent immune attack. Genetic instability in tumor cells is also promoted by chronic inflammation. HCC induced by HBV involves the expression of **hepatitis Bx (HBx)** and probably carboxyterminal truncated **Pre-S** or **S polypeptide** (Figs. 2.6 and 2.7. In the case of HCV induced HCC, the core protein and **non-structural (NS)** proteins **NS3** and **NS5A** are involved in oncogenic transformation (Figs. 2.6 and 2.7). Changes brought about in host gene expression responsible for tumorigenesis also support virus replication and protect virus-infected hepatocytes from immune attack, thus, leading to tumor promoting changes.

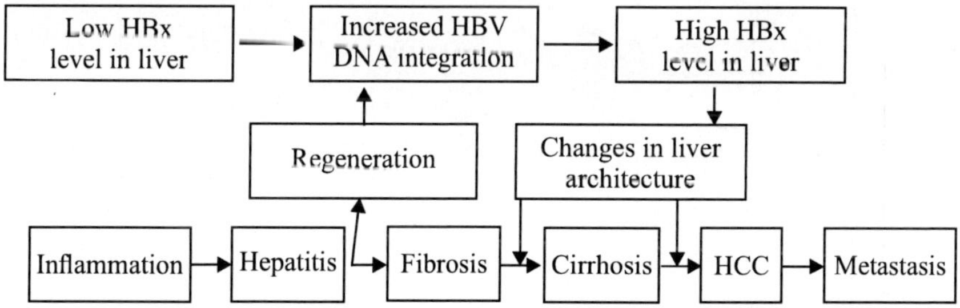

Fig. 2.6. Major steps in the pathogenesis of HBV and HCV-associated HCC

Persistent prolonged presence of HBV and HCV genome in the infected cells plays a major role in the development of HCC. HBV DNA exists in the nuclei of the infected hepatocytes as an episome in the form of a mini-chromosome. During CLD, infected hepatocytes trigger regeneration, which often results in the integration of HBx and sometimes truncated S and pre-S sequences into many sites in the host DNA and transcribe resulting in transformation of infected cells.

Each cycle of hepatocellular regeneration also favors increased intracellular levels of HBx (Fig. 2.7). On the contrary, persistent infection of HCV does not cause integration of viral genome into host genome; instead it maintains itself as an endoplasmic reticulum (ER)-associated episome. HCV virus encoded proteins promote survival and growth of virus-infected hepatocytes following each bout of hepatitis. Progressive CLD is characterized by increased proportion of virus-infected cells in the liver that acquire the characteristics of the tumor cells.

Persistent co-infection by both HBV and HCV in the same patient accelerates the pathogenesis of HCC because of simultaneous necrosis and inflammation or due to direct oncogenic activity. Both are known to induce oxidative stress and

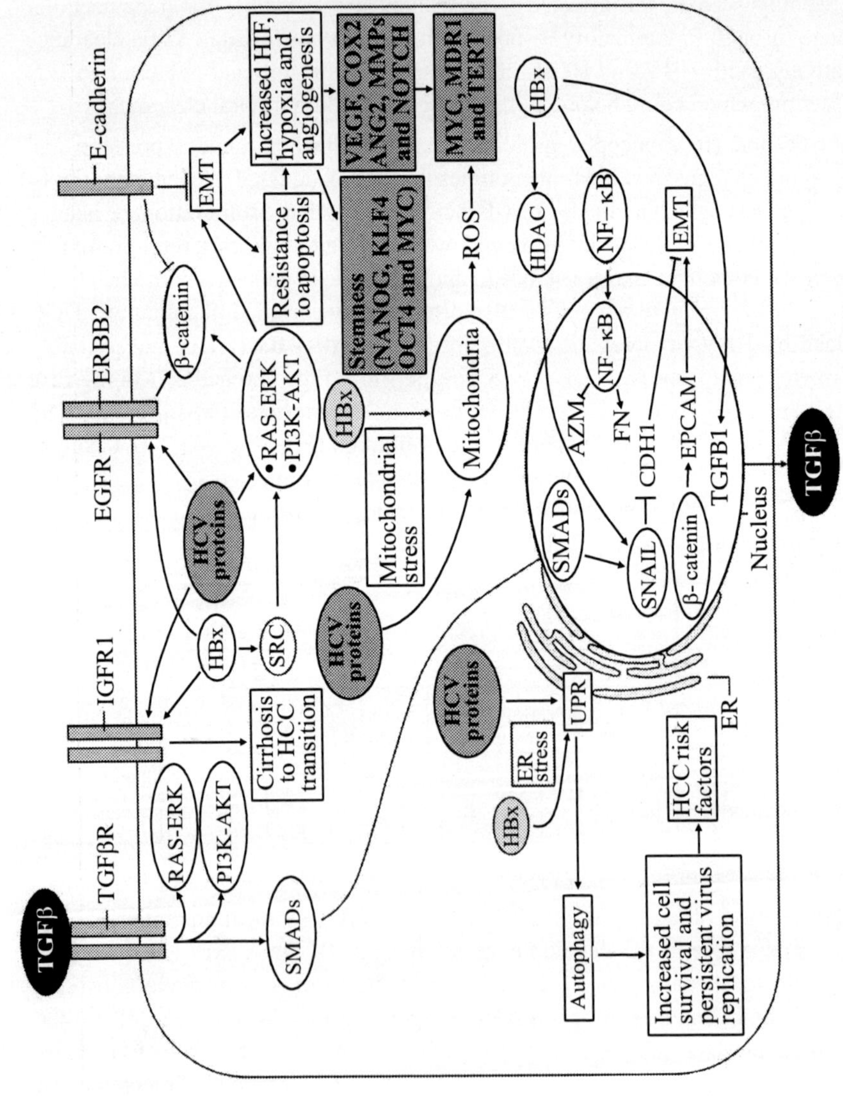

Fig. 2.7. Signaling pathway of HBV and HCV involved in CLD

production of cytotoxic cytokines. Both HBV and HCV proteins show reciprocal interference in the sense when HBV proteins are present, HCV proteins are not detectable in the liver and blood. In this case, the suppressed protein becomes the cause of an occult infection. In occult HBV infections, transactivation function of HBx is blocked by the HCV core protein, which binds to HBx. HCV core protein by binding to the HBV-polymerase and pre-genomic RNA interferes with HBV replication. HCV replication is promoted by HBV in occult infection.

HBV and HCV infected hepatocytes with low levels of virus oncoproteins exhibit cell cycle arrest and apoptosis predominate, on the contrary the cells with high levels of viral oncoproteins show strongly increased survival rate and proliferative signals, which would suppress negative growth regulation, facilitating developing resistance to apoptosis. Resistance to apoptosis directly promotes virus persistence. It is also a characteristic of tumor cells (Fig. 2.7). Presence of high level of HBx produced by HBV blocks tumor necrosis factor – α (TNF- α) and FAS-mediated apoptosis by activation NF-κB, which would facilitate survival of infected hepatocytes from immune-mediated damage. With each bout of hepatitis infection and followed by regeneration, the intracellular concentration of HBx increases with additional integration HBV genome resulting in proliferation of HBx-positive hepatocytes. In the case of HCV, core and NS5A is overexpressed resulting in the activation of AKT and NF-κB, which blocks apoptosis. During the chronic HCV infection, virus-infected hepatocytes upregulate the expression of FAS, which in turn, promotes the survival of hepatocytes by triggering apoptosis in inflammatory T cells. These events protect the virus-infected hepatocyte from immune-mediated elimination, which becomes the source of pro-oncogenic cells.

HBx and HCV proteins are known to interact with mitochondria thereby triggering oxidative stress that may end up in apoptosis (Fig. 2.7). Cytosolic calcium signaling and accumulation of calcium in mitochondria is facilitated by HBx protein of HBV, which causes increased levels of reactive oxygen species (ROS), as well as activation of the PYK_2 and SRC kinases, both facilitate HBV replication and are involved in early steps of HCC (Fig. 2.7). In mitochondria HBx binds to voltage dependent anion-selective channel protein 3 (VDAC3) resulting in membrane depolarization and the production of ROS. In HCV-infected cells, ER releases calcium, which is taken up by mitochondria, resulting in generation of ROS. In both cases, transcription factors sensitive to ROS stimulate virus replication and cell growth, which contributes to tumor development.

In chronic viral infection of the liver, cirrhotic nodules develop, accompanied by a significant decrease in vasculature leading to localized hypoxic condition. The cellular responds to hypoxia by elevated expression of hypoxia inducible factor,1α (HIF-1α), which promotes angiogenesis by upregulation of transcription of vascular endothelial growth factor (VEGF) gene, elevation of pro-inflammatory prostaglandins by stimulation cyclooxygenase 2 (COX2) and enhancement of cell migration by elevation matrix metalloproteinases (MMPs). In HBV infection, HBx binds to HIF-1α leading to HIF-1α induced transcription of VEGF gene, which promotes angiogenesis and cell achieving stem cell-like character (cell stemness). ERK and MAPK are stimulated by HBx to promote angiogenesis, which in turn, upregulates pro-angiogenic growth factor, angiopoetic 2 (ANG2) (Fig. 2.7). HIF-1α under hypoxic condition is upregulated by HCV core, E1, NS3 and NS5A proteins, resulting in increased production of VEGF, COX2, ANG2 and several MMPs (Fig. 2.7). Aggravated cell damage and inflammation is facilitated by hypoxia, which also inhibits liver regeneration, thereby providing a stimulus in the pathogenesis of HCC.

Increased signaling by insulin-like growth factor receptor 1 (IGFR1), epidermal growth factor receptor (EGFR) and PI3K-AKT are stabilized by HIF, HCV and HBx activate both PI3K and EGFR signaling (Fig. 2.7). Increased EGFR signaling by heterodimerization of ERBB2 and its upregulation by HBx is the predominant feature in HCC patients, suggesting ERBB2 activation, which is also observed in the livers of chronic HCV infected and tumor bearing patients.

HBx is known to override RAS signaling, which is associated with expression of senescence related genes. The two signaling pathways that are often disrupted in cancer AKT-ARF-p53-p21 (also known as WAF1) and RAS-MEK-ERK-INK4A (also known as p16)-RB, both are active in HCC, they are activated by HBx. They are also responsible for overcoming the senescence, which seems to be the major step in early tumorigenesis. Chronic HBV and HCV infections induce inflammation, oxidative and oncogenic stress accelerates cellular senescence, which inhibits the cell proliferation of damaged cells. This, in turn, reduces the risk of malignancy by triggering the expression of tumor suppressor genes. Unfortunately, both HBV and HCV infections overcome senescence by inhibiting the expression and functioning of tumor suppressor genes (Fig. 2.7) by upregulating DNA methyltransferases (DNMTs), which decrease the expression of genes involved in DNA repair. HBx and HCV core, NS3 and NS5A proteins inhibit several p53 functions like nucleotide excision repair (NER) and transcription-coupled repair. HCV interferes with DNA repair through the ataxia telangiectasia mutated (ATM) DNA repair pathway. HCV core protein and HBx via promoter methylation, suppress the cyclin dependent kinase (CDK) inhibitors INK4A and p21, resulting in the inactivation of RB tumor suppressor. A microRNA (miRNA), miR-221 is upregulated in HCC induced by HBV and HCV, which blocks the expression p27 (a CDK inhibitor) and promotes tumor growth and progression by activation of the PI3K-AKT-mTOR pathway.

The HBV and HCV both have the ability to alter the expression of miR122, which facilitates virus persistence, expression of oncogenes, and tumor suppressor genes in HCC. miRNA-miR122 promotes differentiation of hepatocytes and suppresses tumor growth, inhibits cyclin G1 expression as well as HBV replication by interference with enhancer regulatory pathway. HBV induced increased expression miR122 targets HBx sequences thereby promoting viral persistence. In the case of HCV infected liver, miR122 stimulates virus replication by stabilizing viral RNA, which is suppressed in HCC (Fig. 2.8).

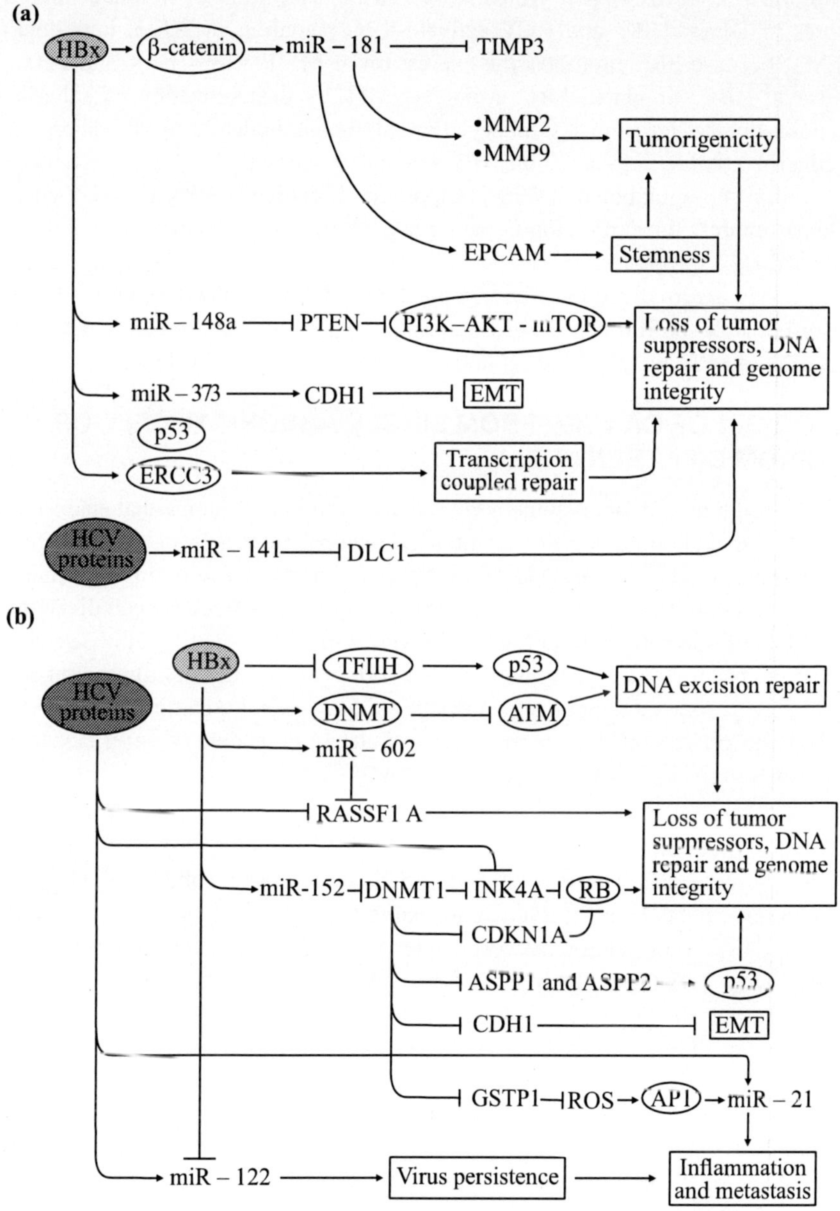

Fig. 2.8. Epigenetic alterations brought about in HBV and HCV-associated HCC

Epithelial-mesothelial transition (EMT), being the key feature of malignancy, also plays a major role in CLD because it promotes fibrogenesis, tumor progression and metastasis. In HBV and HCV associated HCC, hepatic fibrogenesis (type 2 EMT) and HCC metastasis (type 3 EMT) are also mediated by another miRNA, which is miR21, that is upregulated by NF-κB. HBx and HCV proteins activate

TGFβ and RAS-ERK—AP1, which results in the inhibition of multiple tumor suppressor genes. HBV and HCV activate SRC signaling, which is important to EMT, because SRC promotes the expression of MMPs using ERK and PI3K pathways. HBx stimulated SRC promotes EMT by destabilization of adherin junctions due to tyrosine phosphorylation of β-catenin leads to activation in E-cadherin complex. In addition, HBx-mediated upregulation of SNAIL and HCVs NS5A upregulation of TWIST2 suppresses E-cadherin. HBx and HCV core proteins suppress the expression E-cadherin by facilitating promoter methylation. HBV and HCV promote EMT by activation of RAS, WNT and VEGF signaling because they are involved in activation of SNAIL. HCV core and E2 proteins are also responsible for fibrogenesis by triggering EMT. Thus, HBV and HCV induced activation of SRC signaling contributes to the early steps in HCC (Fig. 2.8).

2.2 ORIGIN OF CANCER FROM SINGLE ABNORMAL CELL OR FROM DIFFERENT CELLS

A single cell that undergoes some heritable mutation in its genome that enables it to proliferate and outnumber its neighbors, develops into a metastasizing cancer. The origins of such cancers can be traced to an organ where a single primary tumor arises and it is presumed to be derived from mutated cell by cell division. More than billion cells will be found in a typical tumor by the time it is detected and would often include many normal cells. For example, normal fibroblasts are seen in the peripheral supporting connective tissue around a carcinoma. Is there evidence to prove that the cancer cells are indeed descendents from a clone of single abnormal cell?

One evidence can be given from the analysis of the DNA derived from leukemic white blood cells of patients with *chronic myelogenous leukemia,* which shows a characteristic chromosomal abnormality called Philadelphia chromosome. It can be used as a distinguishing character from the normal cells. It happens due to translocation between the long arms of chromosomes 9 and 22 (as shown in Fig. 2.9). On analysis of DNA from the leukemic cells of all the patients, it is found that the breakage point and rejoining of the translocated fragments is identical but differs slightly by a few hundred or thousand base pairs from one patient to another. As expected, in each of the *chronic myelogenous leukemia* a unique accident Philadelphia translocation occurring in a single cell is a common feature. We see later in chapter 3 how Philadelphia translocation leads to leukemia by producing a fusion protein, which facilitated cell transformation.

Another example to show the monoclonal origin of cancer is studying the genes located on X-chromosome and their inactivation in women. In a normal woman, random mixture, or mosaic of two classes of cells is observed. In one cell the paternal X- chromosome is inactivated and in another the maternal X-chromosome is inactivated. The inactivation of X-chromosomes is a random phenomenon in each cell, which occurs normally in the early embryonic development. Once a particular X-chromosome is inactivated, it is irreversible, so that during cell

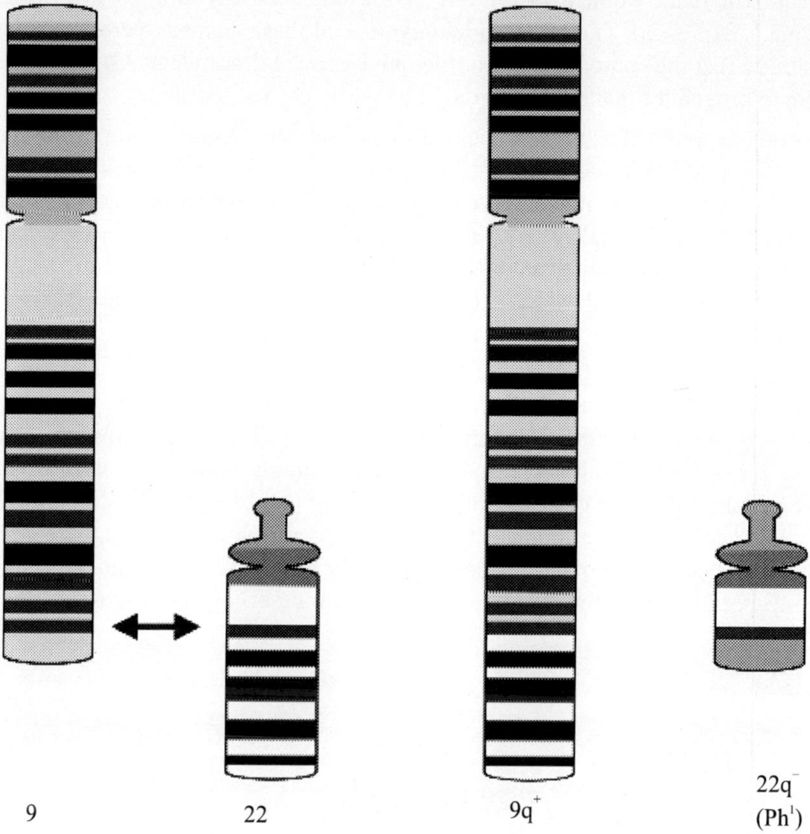

Fig. 2.9. Diagrammatic representation of Philadelphia chromosome showing translocation between long arm (q arm) of 9th and 22nd chromosome

division the same X-inactivation information is passed on to the daughter cells. Depending on the status of maternal or paternal X-chromosome inactivation, the information can be used as a heritable marker to trace the lineage of cells in the body. In the great majority of benign and malignant tumors originating in women when analyzed, all the tumor cells were found to have the same X-chromosome inactivated, suggesting that tumor is derived from a single mutated cell.

G6PD (glucose-6-phosphate dehydrogenase) gene is X-linked and it is heterozygous at this locus in more than 30% of African American woman, therefore, they carry two alleles for this enzyme in their genome. Since X-chromosome undergoes silencing by random heterochromatization, the heterozygous population of women will express in each of the cells one or the other allele of the G6PD gene. The manifestation of gene in heterozygous population, in turn, is the G6PD variant protein that these cells synthesize. With the result, in most of their tissues, half of the population of cells produces one variant enzyme and the other half of the population of cells produces another variant enzyme. **Leiomyomas** (benign tumors of the uterine wall) is common among the population of heterozygous

African American women, where one or the other variant form of the G6PD enzyme is expressed. Therefore, in leiomyomas of these women, there is a great possibility that the component cells of leiomyomas are descendents from a single common progenitor that expressed only that particular variant allele.

Another proof for the monoclonality of human tumors came from the observations of myelomas derived from B cell, which is the precursor of antibody-producing plasma cells. It is observed that, in a particular patient, all the myeloma cells produce an identical antibody molecule indicating monoclonality of the cells involved in the production of antibody. Thus, it indicates their descent from a single common cell that existed, which showed mutation amongst the heterogeneous cell population.

Majority of tumors are known to have chromosomal aberrations and tumor monoclonality can be proved from the observations of cancer cells that show different types of chromosomal aberrations that can be visualized microscopically. In the metaphase of mitosis chromosomes are highly condensed, during this stage peculiar identical chromosomal abnormality can be easily identified in all the cancer cells within a tumor mass. This indicates that all the malignant cells showing the same type of chromosomal anomaly have descended from the single ancestral cell in which the chromosomal restructuring originally occurred.

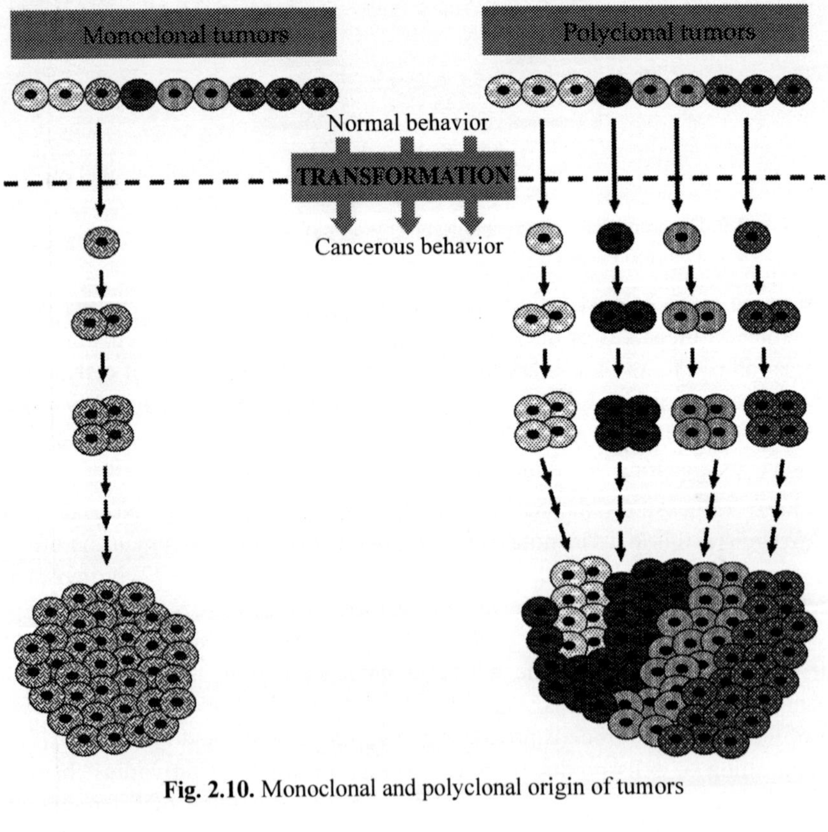

Fig. 2.10. Monoclonal and polyclonal origin of tumors

For our understanding purpose, let us imagine that ten normal cells in a tissue undergo mutation simultaneously and transform leading to malignancy and each of these cell populations underwent proliferation uncontrollably and gave rise to its descendants (Fig. 2.10). As a result, the tumor mass consisting of a mixture of these ten mutant cell populations, would be polyclonal in nature because ten different types of mutations but would contain groups of large monoclonal population of cells with similar mutations. At the same time, it is highly probable that each of these ten clonal populations varies from one another, such as type of mutations, the time required for cells to double, etc. Among this heterogeneous clonal population of cells, the cell showing slightly shorter doubling time will, sooner or later, outgrow compared to all the others, and that the descendents of this cell will be in larger number in the tumor mass, which appears to be a monoclonal tumor. Therefore, the cells in a large solid tumor mass do show monoclonality, but rarely.

Another confounding factor about tumor cell population is the genotypic and phenotypic instability. To begin with, cells within a tumor mass may be relatively a homogeneous mass, but over the course of time, different cells in this population may acquire different mutations independently and the acquisition of new mutant alleles by this population may lead to heterogeneity. The true monoclonality of this population may get masked by the resulting genetic heterogeneity only in specific subpopulations of these descendent cells within the tumor mass and the genetic markers will be present.

2.3 ORIGIN OF CANCER DUE TO ALTERED DNA SEQUENCES

If a single abnormal cell is a progenitor of a tumor, it should have the ability to pass on its genetic abnormality to its progeny in a heritable manner. There are two problems one would encounter in understanding the origin of cancer, i.e., whether the heritable aberration is due to an alteration in the cell's DNA sequence, or whether it is due to an *epigenetic* change. In epigenetic change, there will be no alteration in the DNA sequence but only the pattern of gene expression will change. Epigenetic changes or alteration of DNA involves change in the DNA structure due to hypo- or hypermethylation, acetylation or deacetylation of histone, and chemical adducts with nitrogenous bases.

There are several reasons to believe that most of the cancers are initiated by genetic changes in their DNA sequence because the genetic abnormality, exhibited by the descendent cancer cells will be identical as observed in chronic myelogenous leukemia. There are many such examples, which will be discussed in the later part of this chapter. Further, there are strong evidences to prove that genetic change can be a cause of cancer comes from studies on agents that are known to give rise to the disease. For example, consumption of tobacco in any form is known to increase the incidence of cancer and there is a good correlation between *carcinogenesis* and *mutagenesis* caused by the agents found in tobacco. There are three classes of carcinogenic agents, namely, chemical carcinogens, which will bring about local changes in the nucleotide sequence by forming adducts or complex with them; ionizing radiation like X-rays are known to cause DNA strand breaks which further leads to chromosome breaks and translocations, and biological agents like viruses are known to incorporate their genome into cell's DNA and bring about genetic change in gene expression.

In general, a cancer does not occur entirely by a single mutation or due to a single cause. As we shall see later in this chapter, cancers result from the occurrence of different mutations in one of the cells as several independent accidents at different time intervals, showing cumulative effects. These mutations are usually induced by carcinogenic chemicals, biological agents like viruses and spontaneous mutations in the genome that increases the likelihood of cell transforming into cancerous growth. High enough dosage exposure to some chemical carcinogens leads to mutation in at least one cell in the body, which will turn cancerous. For example, the chemical compound 2-naphthylamine used in the chemical industry is known to be highly carcinogenic for men who are employed in distilling it eventually develop bladder cancer.

Alkylating agents are among the most potent class of mutagens that are capable of transferring an alkyl group (methyl or ethyl) covalently to bond with the DNA bases to give rise to 1-methyl adenine, 1-methyl guanine, 3-methyl cytosine, 5-methyl cytosine, 3-methyl thymine as modified nitrogenous bases in DNA. This causes destabilization of covalent bond of nitrogenous base with deoxyribose sugar, resulting in the loss of the purine (depurination) or pyrimidine (depyrimidination) base from the DNA. This will lead to alteration in DNA structure, therefore, there is also a possibility that the alkylated bases may be misread by the DNA polymerase machinery during DNA replication.

There is sufficient evidence to indicate that the cytosine methylation in DNA controls the expression of many genes in eukaryotes. Methylation patterns are symmetrically distributed in CpG domains and are tissue specific. Methylation is brought about by methyl; transferase enzyme soon after DNA replication. Several studies have shown that active genes show **hypomethylation** and inactive genes show **hypermethylation**. Hypomethylation is associated with abnormal gene expression. Feinberg and Vogelstein (1983) observed that in human colon cancers, 4 out of 5 cases show substantial hypomethylation of certain sites of growth hormone and globin genes. They extended their studies to *ras* oncogene family in primary colon and lung cancers, and observed 6 out of 8 tumors showed hypomethylation. In this study, it was found that the degree of hypomethylation was greater in metastatic tumors than the primary nodules. Therefore, it is presumed that progressive hypomethylation in some caners is the cause of metastasis. Hypomethylation of specific sites in *c-myc* oncogene in human tumors are a common feature. Widespread hypomethylation and hypermethylation will result in alteration of DNA structure and this may lead to inhibition in expression of critical genes such as tumor suppressor gene, which plays an important role in suppression of tumor development.

Hypermethylation of **11p13** and **11p15** site is associated with Wilm's tumor (kidney tumor) and the site contains **WT1** and **WT2** tumor suppressor genes. Similarly, **3p14-23** is hypermethylated in lung carcinoma.

Many human cancers are known to have fragile sites on chromosome, which are prone to recombination with viral genome, deletion of large fragment, translocation, and chemical mutagenesis. Familial adenomatus polyposis coli (FAPC) is associated with deletion of **5q21** (-5q21). This segment of the chromosome contains a tumor suppressor gene, **adenomatus polyposis coli (APC)**. Deletion of **18q21-22** is observed in colorectal cancer, and the site is known to contain another tumor suppressor gene-**deleted in colorectal cancer (DCC)**. The most common deletion in human cancer involves **3q14-23**, which is known to contain one or more tumor suppressor genes. Deletion at **13q14-23** is implicated in the development of **retinoblastoma (retinal cancer) (Rb)**, Wilm's tumor, renal cell and lung carcinoma and breast cancer. Deletion or hypermethylation of **3p25.1** location is observed to be a common feature in **nasopharyngeal carcinoma (NPC),** which is supposed to be a tumor suppressor gene.

In addition, alterations in DNA sequence of 1p, 11p, 13p, 16q or 17p are also associated with several cancers in humans and among these, chromosome 1 was found to be affected most frequently in breast cancers.

Integration of viral genome into fragile sites of human chromosome leads to alteration in DNA sequence and it is associated with several human cancers. Human papilloma viral genome integration into **8q24** site has been associated with genital and cervix cancer. Adeno associated virus (AAV) has been implicated in several different types of cancers due to integration of its genome at **19q13** site. Hepatitis B virus (HBV) was found to be integrated frequently at specific sites on chromosome 11 and 17 in **hepatocellular carcinoma** (HCC), where **Int-2** and **hst-1** proto-oncogenes are located, which are often amplified in HCC. Epstein Barr virus (EBV), responsible for Burkitt's lymphoma and nasopharyngeal cancer, is known to integrate its DNA at two specific sites, **1p35** and **2p13**. Ras oncogene is distributed on three different chromosomes, **11p15-H-ras; 12p12-K-ras; and 1p22-N-ras.**

Chemical carcinogens belong to diverse groups, but most of them are mutagenic. On metabolism, carcinogens are converted into reactive species, which will readily react with DNA nitrogenous bases to form adducts and bring about mutation. Similarly, procarcinogens on metabolic activation get converted to ultimate carcinogen and form DNA adducts. For example, benzo[a]pyrene found in cigarette smoke is converted to ultimate carcinogen by metabolic process to benzo[a]pyrenediolepoxide (BPDE), which forms the adducts with 7 or 8th position of guanosine residues in the DNA of lung epithelial cells leading to base substitutions, which is commonly found in the mutant p53 alleles of lung cancers. Aflatoxin B1 (AFB1) derived from *Aspergillus* is highly mutagenic and causes characteristic G to T mutation (transversion) in DNA leading to point mutation, where the sequence AGG gets converted to AGT in tumor suppressor gene in hepatocellular carcinomas induced by aflatoxin B1.

Yet another example for the apparent contribution of benzo[a]pyrene towards the development of breast cancer in women who were actively smoking at the time of breast cancer showed more than 10-fold increase in G to T transversions in their tumor associated p53 tumor suppressor alleles than the nonsmokers.

2.4 MUTATIONS THAT ACCELERATES THE DEVELOPMENT OF CANCER

Clinical observations and experimental evidences indicate that large number of genetic mutations and epigenetic changes accumulate in the transformed cell which brings about tumor progression. Experimental evidences reveal that many of the genetic changes are caused by the action of mutagens, the cancer progression is fueled by non-mutagenic agents (sometimes termed **non-genotoxic**). The experimental model used in such studies depended on exposing the mouse skin to high carcinogenic tar constituents, such as benzo[a]pyrene (BP), 7,12-dimethylbenz[a]anthracene (DMBA), or 3-methyl-cholanthrene (3-MC). For example, mice subjected to daily painting of DMBA on a patch of skin would develop skin carcinomas after several months of this treatment (Fig. 2.11).

In another experimental protocol, mice skin smeared with single painting of DMBA followed by smearing of same area on a weekly basis with a second agent, termed TPA (12-O-tetradecanoylphorbol-13-acetate) a skin irritant prepared from the seeds of croton plant. Repeated painting of the DMBA-exposed area with TPA resulted in the appearance of papillomas after 4 to 8 weeks, depending on the strain of mice being used. These papillomas are in many ways analogous to the adenomas observed in early-stage colon cancer progression (Fig. 2.11). The survival and growth of these skin papillomas depended upon continuous application of TPA, since cessation of TPA application resulted in regression of papillomas. However, if TPA painting was continued for many weeks, TPA-dependent papillomas eventually emerged, which would not regress after cessation of TPA application and instead persisted for extended period. Some of these TPA-independent papillomas might, with low probability, evolve further into malignant squamous cell carcinomas of the skin after about six months.

In the absence of initial DMBA treatment, however, repeated painting with TPA failed to provoke either papillomas or carcinomas. Even more interesting observations is that, an area of skin smeared with DMBA and then left to rest for a year, and then this patch of skin was smeared with a series of TPA paintings, it would respond by forming a papilloma.

These phenomena were rationalized as follows. A single treatment by potent carcinogen (DMBA) which acts as an **initiating agent** (or **initiator**) causes a stable, long-lived damage in the genome of a cell or cluster of cells and this damage was apparently genetic mutation. Subsequent to these "mutation initiated" cells TPA is repeatedly applied which serves as **promoting agent** or **promoter** will allow these initiated cells to proliferate vigorously without having any effect on nearby non-initiated cells (Fig. 2.11). Certainly, this non-genetic effect brought

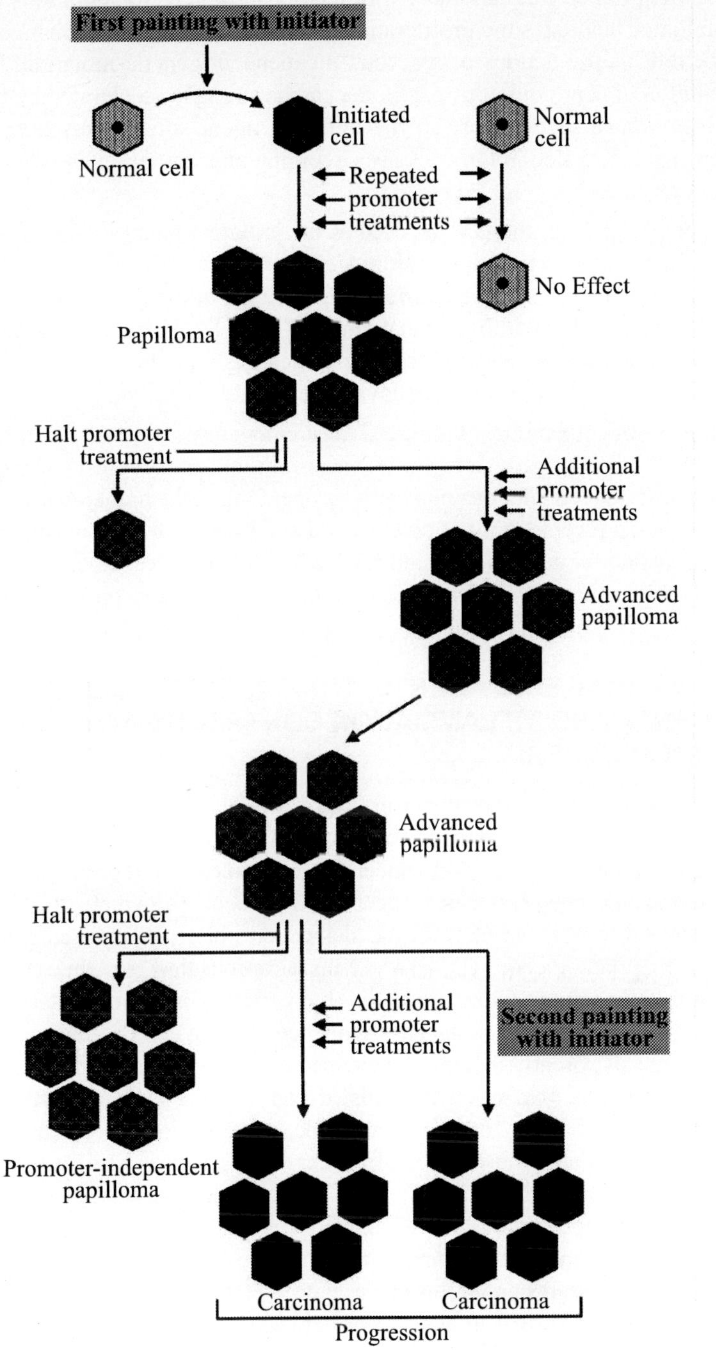

Fig. 2.11. Non-mutagenic agent favoring cell proliferation and carcinogenesis

about by the promoter collaborates with the apparent genetic alterations created by the initiator facilitates the proliferation of cells. This permanent change in cell behavior reflects the actions of a second independent genetic mutation. Indeed, this evolution of carcinomatous papilloma can be strongly accelerated by treating once again with a second dose of the initiating agent, already suspected to be mutagen. This third step in tumorigenesis (coming after initiation and promotion) is termed **progression** (Fig. 2.11).

As long suspected, the DMBA used as the initiating agent is indeed a potent mutagen in the context of skin carcinogenesis. Since it is a randomly acting mutagen, DMBA causes a wide variety of mutations in the genomes of the cells exposed to it. The skin carcinoma that emerges from DMBA initiation invariably bears point-mutation of H-ras oncogene indicating that this particular mutant allele confers some strong selective advantage on cells in the skin.

The experimental model of mouse skin carcinogenesis is useful for illustrating the principles of tumorigenesis by initiation, promotion, and progression. However, it tells nothing about analogous mechanisms operating in the human body to create cancer. In fact, a diverse array of biochemical and biological mechanisms appears to be responsible for the tumor promotion leading to human cancers. Among these are mechanisms that act in either toxic or mitogenic fashion on various human tissues.

2.5 NON-MUTAGENIC AGENTS, TOXIC AND MITOGENIC AGENTS AND INFLAMMATION CONTRIBUTE TO TUMORIGENESIS

The stages in the development of cancer from an initial mild lesion to a progressive, highly proliferative mass of cells to become a cancer can be learnt from the skin cancer model. In mice, skin cancer can be induced by repeatedly smearing highly mutagenic chemical carcinogens such as benzo[a]pyrene (a constituent of coal tar and tobacco smoke) on the shaved skin or with a related compound dimethylbenz[a]anthracene (DMBA). Single application of the carcinogen does not usually initiate tumor formation but certainly it causes mutation in the genome with altered nitrogenous base sequences, which can be detected through genomic analysis. Greatly increased incidence of cancer is observed in carcinogen smeared area of the skin when the cells of that area are exposed further to the same chemical substance or to certain other type of insults. A carcinogenic substance that initiates the process of cancer in this way is said to be a tumor initiator. Continuous irritation of the skin or wounding the skin at that initiated area or repeated exposure of initiated skin area over a period to certain mutagenic substances that are known to be tumor promoters can cause development of cancer. *Phorbol esters* (tetradecanoylphorbol acetate –TPA), the most widely studied tumor promoters is known to activate protein kinase C, which activates part of the phosphatidylinositol intracellular signaling pathway. The tumor promoters promote cancers at high frequency only after the mutagenic initiator has initiated the process of carcinogenesis.

The genetic changes caused by a tumor initiator are irreversible and invisible until they are further facilitated by a tumor promoter even after a long delay after the initiation. The tumor promoter apparently stimulates cell division from the cells that would have normally undergone terminal differentiation. Instead, it triggers the cells to continue to divide in the region that had previously been exposed to the initiator. This results in the formation of many small, benign, wart-like tumors called *papillomas.* The number and size of the papillomas induced depends greatly on the exposure to prior dose of initiator, larger the dose, larger will be the size of the papilloma. The papilloma initiated with single low dose of initiator would consist of a single clone of cells descended from a mutant cell induced by the initiator. In the resting epithelium of the skin, the genes that are directly or indirectly responsible for cell proliferation are quiescent. Some of the genes involved in cell proliferation are induced at the initiated site due to wounding and the application of the promoter. The promoter or the stimulus of wounding may enable the expression of the mutated genes, thereby influencing uncontrolled cell proliferation.

A typical papilloma would approximately contain about 10^5 cells and if their exposure to the tumor promoter is stopped, almost all the papillomas show the tendency of regression, and the skin regains normal appearance. There is a possibility that in a few of the papillomas, even after the withdrawal of promoter, further mutations occur that enable the growth to continue in an uncontrolled manner. These changes seem to originate occasionally due to spontaneous mutations in single papilloma cells which make a small fraction of the papillomas to progress to become cancers. Thus, the tumor promoter apparently favors the expansion of the population of cells that carry initial mutation to develop into cancer. As more such cells carrying mutations undergo proliferation, greater will be the chance that at least one of them will undergo another mutation pushing it forward one more step to develop into malignancy. Once the mutant cells have been created, the spread of certain types of mutant cells depends both on the frequency of mutations and factors affecting their survival and proliferation, which finally leads to cancer.

2.6 MULTIPLE MUTATIONS AND ORIGIN OF CANCER (MULTI-STEP TUMORIGENESIS)

Cancer is a disease fully dependent on genomic change. Almost all models described till date for carcinogenesis show multiple steps, successive clonal expansions, favored by the accumulation of mutations that are preferentially selected by the tumor environment. The cancer genome shows characteristic heterogeneity, which is seen across the solid tumor types. The heterogeneity is due to the action of twin evolutionary forces, i.e., generation of variation and selection. To date, almost 500 cancer genes have been identified and in a handful of cancers, specific cancer genes show consistent mutation, such as *BCR-ABL* oncogenic fusion protein in chronic myelogenous leukemia (CML) or inactivating mutations in the retinoblastoma 1 (*RB1*) tumor suppressor gene in retinoblastomas. In the development of some rare cancer type in different tissues, specific cancer genes have also been implicated. For example, the oncogenic fusion gene *MYB-NFIB* is responsible for the development of adenoid cystic carcinomas in both breast and salivary gland tissue.

Majority of common cancers are associated with mutation of many diverse cancer genes at low frequency. From the large cancer databases, the most striking evidence that has emerged is the genetic heterogeneity between cancers and even within individual cancer types. In addition to the genetic heterogeneity amongst the cancers, there is considerable diversity in the nature, number, and distribution of mutations within and across different cancers. Recent studies have revealed that the childhood cancer retinoblastoma and medulloblastoma show substantially fewer base substitutions than do common adult solid tumors such as breast cancer and hematological malignancies like acute myeloid leukemia (AML). Pattern of structural variants differs across tumor types: breast and ovarian cancers show many more tandem duplications than other tumor types. Breakage-fusion breakage bridge cycles of chromosomal rearrangements are most frequent in pancreatic cancers; prostate cancers show balanced chains of rearrangements. Similarly, depending on DNA repair defects, patterns of base substitutions differ extensively across tumors based on carcinogenic exposure.

There is good amount of evidence to indicate multi-step origin of tumorigenesis where increasing number of mutations accumulate in a cell that evolves from benign to a more malignant phenotype. Best studied example is human colon carcinomas, which is easily accessible by colonoscopy for the study at different stages of progression of cancer. On examination of the genomes of a good number of small colonic adenomas, mid-sized adenomas, large adenomas and frank carcinomas, it was observed that, there was significant progressive advancement of colonic tissues from normal appearance to a high-grade malignancy, where the epithelial cells had increasing number of mutations in various genes (Fig. 2.12).

In the early-stage colonic adenomas, loss of heterozygosity (LOH) in the long arm of chromosome 5 (i.e., 5q) is reported. Slightly larger adenomas showed mutant K-ras oncogene with LOH in 12p. High rate of LOH in the long arm of chromosome 18 (i.e., 18q) was seen in larger adenomas and about half of all carcinomas showed LOH in the short arm of chromosome 17 (i.e., 17p).

From these observations it can be said that as the colonic epithelial cells acquire increasingly large number of mutations, there is activation of a proto-oncogene into an oncogene (K-ras) and simultaneously there is inactivation of at least three distinct tumor suppressor genes, namely, APC, DCC, and p53. This was the first suggestion, now it has been found to be quite a common feature among most tumors, where inactivation of tumor suppressor genes is **larger in number** compared to **activated oncogenes.**

The APC (adenomatous polyposis coli) tumor suppressor gene, situated on the chromosome 5 in the region 5q21, is found to be often targeted for LOH, while the gene on chromosome 17 in the region 17p13 was identified as p53 tumor suppressor gene. The gene on chromosome 18q that is inactivated during colon

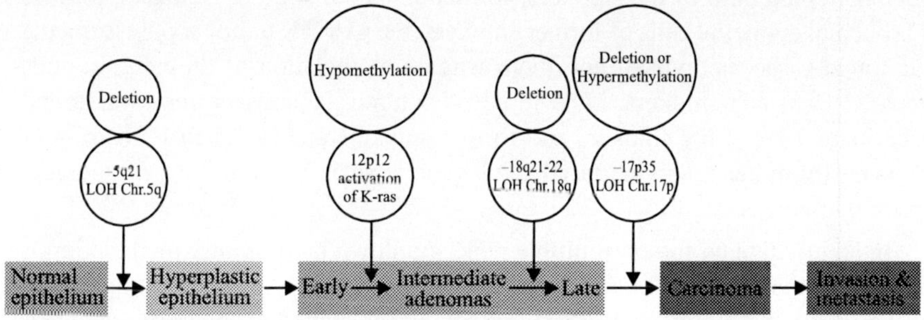

Fig. 2.12. Colon tumor progression and loss of heterozygosity in various chromosomal arms

carcinoma pathogenesis is another tumor suppressor gene called DCC (deleted in colon cancer).

The specific sequence of genetic changes taking place in the chromosome to participate in colon cancer pathogenesis can be calculated from the known evidences. Inactivation of the APC gene on chromosome 5q in approximately 90% of colon carcinomas was found to be an early step as the process of carcinogenesis begins, only about 40 – 50% were found to acquire K-ras mutation; 50 – 70% showed LOH of chromosome 17p involving p53 gene, and about 60% showed an LOH on chromosome 18q involving DCC. In addition, 12% of colonic tumors are known to have functional inactivation mutation of the type-2 TGF-β receptor.

To begin with alteration of chromosome 5 is the most predominant feature in most colon cancers followed by other alternative genetic changes that favor the development of full-fledged malignancy. Epigenetic events, such as promoter methylation for the repression of some genes and demethylation to de-repress other genes, may also contribute importantly to tumor progression. Recent evidences gathered from early adenomas indicate that hypomethylation contributes to chromosomal instability, and this state favors acceleration of the rate of tumor progression.

2.6.1 Promoter Methylation

Promoter methylation is an important epigenetic event resulting in inhibition in expression of majority of tumor suppressor genes as one of the various mechanisms of somatic mutation. More than half of the tumor suppressor genes involved in familial cancer syndromes exhibit germ-line mutations leading to silencing of TSG. In sporadic cancers, promoter methylation most often followed mechanism of gene silencing. For example, in familial retinoblastoma, the Rb tumor suppressor gene is mutated in the germ-line.

In promoter methylation, possibly two routes are followed in silencing tumor suppressor gene function. In one approach, both copies of a tumor suppressor gene might be methylated independent of one another. Alternatively, the second might be lost through a loss of heterozygosity accompanied by a duplication of the already-methylated tumor suppressor gene copy. More frequently the second mechanism seems to operate. For example, when a study is carried out on normal bronchial epithelium of the smokers, former smokers, and non-smokers, in 44% of bronchial epithelial cells of former smokers, the $p16^{INK4A}$ tumor suppressor gene was found to be methylated and there was no methylation of the gene in cells prepared from non-smokers. LOH in $p16^{INK4A}$ tumor suppressor gene was found to be 71 to 73% of the smokers and former smokers and in 1.5 to 1.7% of non-smokers. Promoter methylation BRCA1 gene is seen in 10 to 15% of sporadic breast carcinomas.

In any malignant tumor, multiple gene shutdown by promoter methylation is found to be the most common feature. For example, when a study was carried out on the methylation pattern of eight critical cancer related genes in the genomes of 107 non-small-cell lung carcinomas (NSCLCs), 37% showed one of the gene promoters methylated, 22% had two gene promoters methylated, and 2% showed five of the eight gene promoters methylated.

2.6.2 Heterogeneity of Mutations within an Individual Cancer

The sub-clonal evolution of cancer cells is facilitated by various external factors that act on the cancer genome to generate heterogeneity. The tumor microenvironment plays an important role in selecting the cells that are best adapted to the environments, which is often hostile in which they exist. Carcinogen and radiation exposure during cancer treatment and exposure to UV radiation may also play an important role in heterogeneity of cancer cell genome.

One observation that in certain types of cancer of some tissue origin there are specific genes involved in cancer development as seen in colon cancer model but it is not observed in other cancers originating from other tissues indicates that the cell of origin may be an important factor in dictating the evolutionary trajectory of cancer. Every cell in the body having arisen from a single zygote is clonal in nature. Due to difference in physiology in each organ, the same genome shows subtle genomic changes within organ systems, which are controlled by epigenome, transcriptome, and proteome of the cells in that particular organ. It follows that a somatic mutation that arises in the ground state of a cell will strongly influence how that mutation influences on the cell, because some somatic mutations are lethal and cause cell death. The concept can be explained by using the example of BCR-ABL fusion gene and its product, which is frequently seen in different types of hematological malignancies is not observed in solid tumors. The main reasons for this are the low transcriptional ability of BCR promoter in solid tumors, a lack of oncogenic interactions and the oncogenic effects of the fusion protein or failure to retain sustaining population of cancer cells.

The importance of 'ground state' of a cell is exemplified by the specific *KIT* gene mutations in gastrointestinal stromal tumors (GISTs) and its 'oncogenicity'. KIT is a tyrosine kinase receptor that gets activated by binding of stem cell factor, resulting in a signaling cascade that promotes cell proliferation, differentiation, and germ-line activation mutations of KIT results in hyperplasia of interstitial cells of Cajal (ICC) and GISTs. Genomic studies of cancer genes indicate that many of the same genes are implicated in cancer across broad range of tissue types at different frequencies.

Two independent studies have reported that the genes that were historically associated with hematological malignancies, such as runt-related transcription factor 1 (*RUNX1*) and core binding factor beta subunit (*CBFB*) are recurrently mutated in breast cancer.

2.6.3 Role of Epistasis in Evolution of Cancer Genome

A new mutation in a cancer gene will have a profound effect on the fate of the cell and it does not occur in isolation but rather enters an established genomic network. This new genomic network determines whether the cell is going to die or undergo clonal proliferation. The normal cellular function and identity are associated with the ground state of a cell, which represents normal genomic interactions, whereas interaction among oncogenic mutations involves epistasis.

Despite the extensive heterogeneity in the cancer cell genome, three major lines of evidences indicate that particular combinations of somatic mutations may co-occur more frequently than by chance, such as p53 mutation in breast cancer, *BRCA1* mutation in early onset of breast cancer, *BRCA2* mutation in late onset of breast cancer or the mutation of oncogenic K-ras and serine threonine kinase 11 (*STK11* also known as *LKB1*) in lung cancer. Second, activation mutation of K-ras oncogene can lead to a state of 'oncogene induced senescence'. This is an acute and telomere-independent senescence that can occur due to the expression of oncogenes and is protective against cancer. The second mutation in cyclin dependent kinase inhibitor 2A (*CDKN2A*) inactivation is required to ameliorate the senescence effects. Third, convergent evolution among sub-clones within the malignant tumors also implies cooperation among somatic mutations. This was confirmed from multiregion sampling study on renal cancer patients, that mutations were observed in von Hippel-Lindau tumor suppressor controlled E3 ubiquitin protein ligase (*VHL*) loss, inactivating mutation of histone modifiers can independently arise in different branches of the sub-clones. Strangely enough, independent phosphatase and tensin (*PTEN*) mutations occurred twice on one renal cancer patient in different sub-clones, despite PTEN mutations are very rarely seen renal carcinomas. This implies that, in this particular renal cancer patient some specific feature of the genomic landscape was particularly dependent on the inactivation of PTEN, which otherwise is not required for most renal carcinomas. In majority of renal cancers there is a prerequisite for early VHL inactivation. Similarly, in colon cancer, early deletion of APC gene and in retinoblastoma early deletion of RB gene is the key features.

2.6.4 Loss of Heterozygosity (LOH)

In majority of tumors, tumor suppressor genes show a tendency to undergo loss of heteozygosity (LOH) during tumor development is the only option rather than simultaneous mutation of both genes one after the other. It is highly unlikely that two successive mutational events will succeed in elimination of two copies of tumor suppressor genes. Let us presume that one of the two Rb gene copies first gets inactivated by some type of mutational event like promoter methylation or deletion of the gene at a frequency comparable 1 in 10^6 cells per generation. A cell suffering from this mutation would attain heterozygous configuration with one wild-type and one defective gene copy, which can be represented as **Rb+/-**. Suppose if a somatic recombination occurs during mitosis between the chromatid arms carrying the wild-type Rb allele and a chromatid carrying the mutant allele of the paired chromosome (Fig. 2.13).

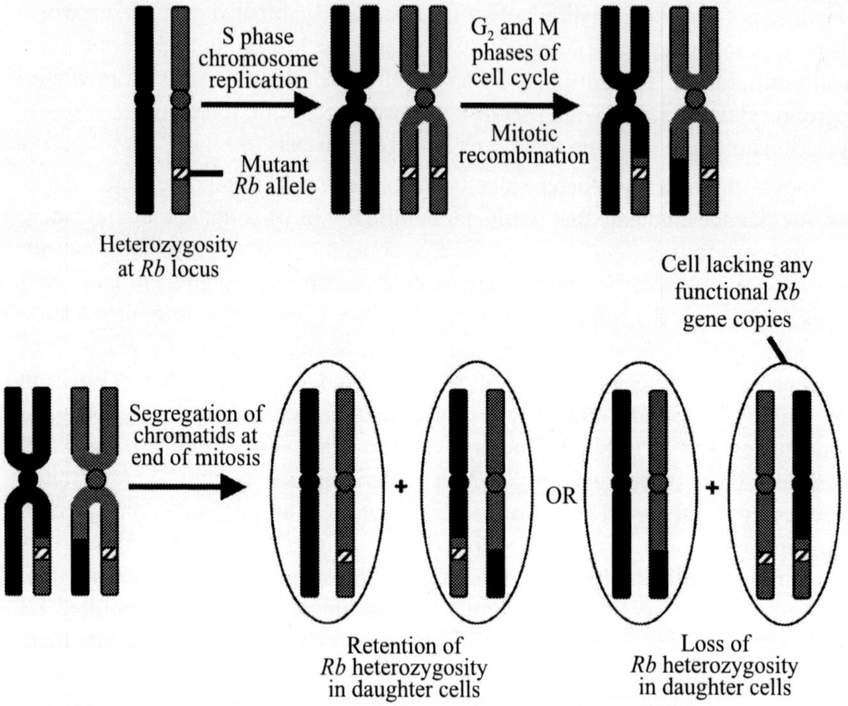

Fig. 2.13. The process of loss of heterozygosity due to mitotic recombination

Meiotic recombination events that shuffle maternal and paternal chromosomes prior to gametogenesis are a common feature but mitotic recombination during somatic cell proliferation is a strange phenomenon observed only in cancerous cells. Because of this mitotic recombination, chromatid carrying the wild-type (normal) Rb allele might get replaced with a chromatid carrying the mutant allele present in the paired homologous chromosome leading to homozygosity at the Rb locus, that would result in either Rb–/– or a Rb +/+ genotype (Fig. 2.13). This type of genetic change in a gene on a chromosome is known as **loss of heterozygosity (LOH).** Interestingly, this type of mitotic recombination leading to LOH occurs at a frequency of 10^{-5} to 10^{-4} per cell generation, it was therefore considered to be the easiest way for a cell to get rid of the remaining wild-type copy of the Rb gene to achieve homozygosity of a mutant allele.

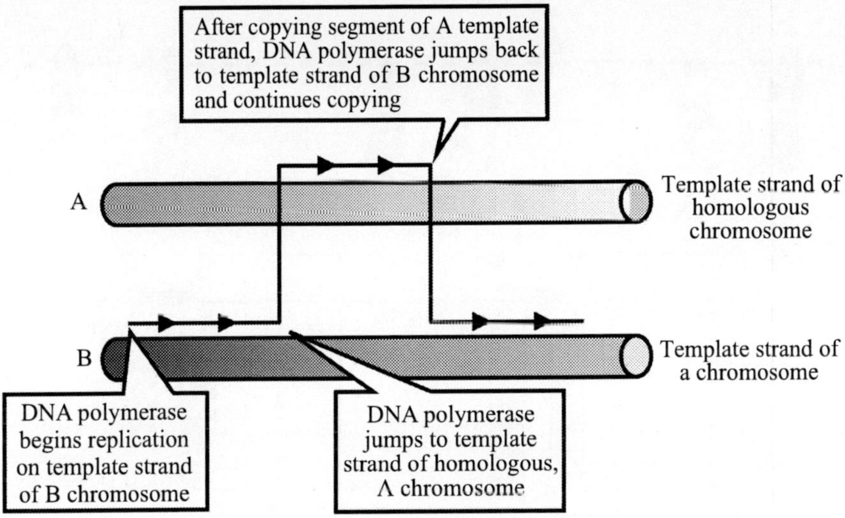

Fig. 2.14. Gene conversion leading to LOH

LOH can also be achieved by deletion of an entire chromosomal region by simply **breaking off** from the homologous chromosome. This process will lead to **hemizygosity** of this chromosomal region, where the genes on the undeleted arm of normal chromosome exist only as single copy rather than the usual two copies. Hemizygosity due to loss of a chromosomal segment is registered as LOH. Irrespective of the way in which LOH occurs, tumorigenesis is facilitated by getting rid of remaining wild-type allele of a tumor suppressor gene. In some cases of retinoblastomas, chromosome 13 showed interstitial deletion in long arm "q" at band region 14 (-13q14) (Fig. 2.15). The deletion was between 2nd and 4th band of 1st region, involving thousands of kilo bases of DNA is lost leading to loss of large number of genes in this region facilitating development of retinal tumor. In other words, to this region of the 13th chromosome, the tumor suppressor Rb gene is mapped, which was lost in one of the homologous pair resulting in hemizygosity or LOH.

In different human tumors analyzed, deletions were very frequent in chromosome 17p and chromosome 18q resulting in LOH, which provided strong evidence that both these chromosomes in the deleted region harbored tumor suppressor genes.

For silencing the tumor suppressor genes, promoter methylation is the predominant mechanisms favored as somatic mutation in majority of tumors. In familial cancer syndromes, the tumor suppressor genes are silenced by promoter methylation because of germ-line mutations leading to silencing of TSG in sporadic cancers. For example, in familial retinoblastoma, in the germ-line itself the Rb tumor suppressor gene is mutated.

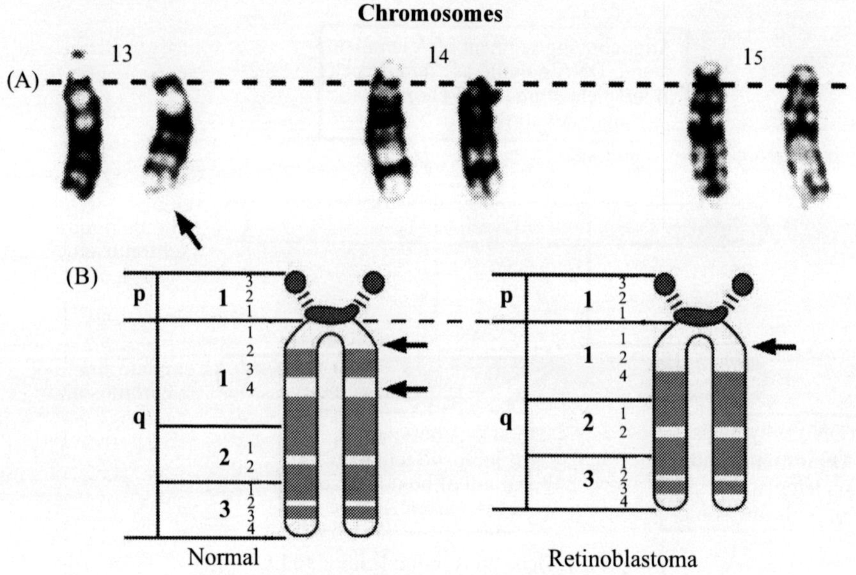

Fig. 2.15. Chromosomal localization of Rb locus

The suppression in expression of tumor suppressor gene function by promoter methylation might be achieved through two different routes and it may happen independent of one another where, ultimately methylation of both copies of a tumor suppressor gene will be achieved. The loss of tumor suppressor gene function may be gained by promoter methylation of one copy of gene and the function of the second copy might be lost through a loss of heterozygosity and further duplication of the already-methylated tumor suppressor gene copy. In majority of tumors, more frequently, the second mechanism seems to be operating.

2.6.5 Breakage-fusion-bridge (BFB)

Chromosomes have telomeres at their ends of chromatids. When the telomeres are lost due to various reasons, chromatid ends tend to fuse and such fusion may occur between the sister chromatids (Fig. 2.16). When chromosomes with fused chromatids participate in the mitosis, the mitotic spindle attached to their two centromeres will pull the chromatids in the opposite directions, which leads to creation of a dramatic anaphase dicentric bridges. Sooner or later, due to pulling force of the mitotic apparatus, **dicentric** chromatid will be randomly broken apart at some site between the two centromeres (Fig. 2.17) creating two new chromosomal ends without telomere, which will be sticky. It is highly likely that, such unprotected sticky ends will fuse with one another or with the unprotected ends of another non-homologous chromosome. This will either result in movement of the fused non-homologous chromosome to the same pole and once again a random tear will occur in the fused chromosome in the next cycle of cell division (Fig 2.17). This process will continue with every cell cycle, and it is called **breakage-fusion-bridge (BFB)** cycle. This process will lead to formation of abnormal chromosomal complexes in the cell, which is one of the features observed in malignant tumors of breast cell.

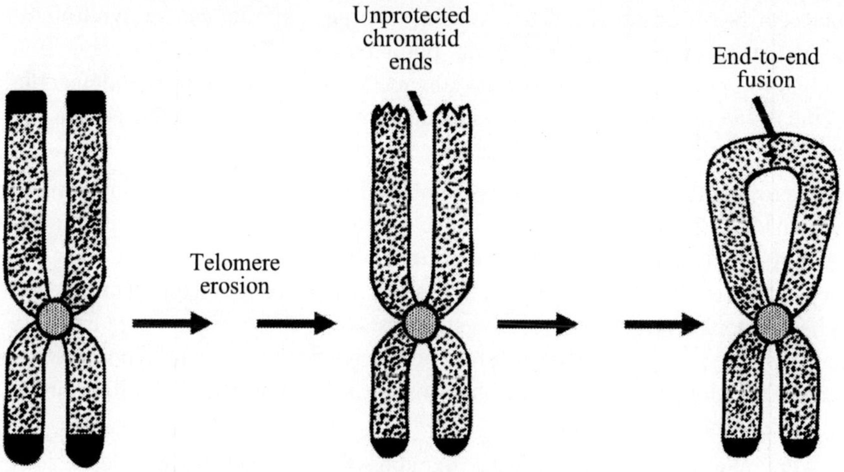

Fig. 2.16. Fusion of chromatids because of loss of telomeres

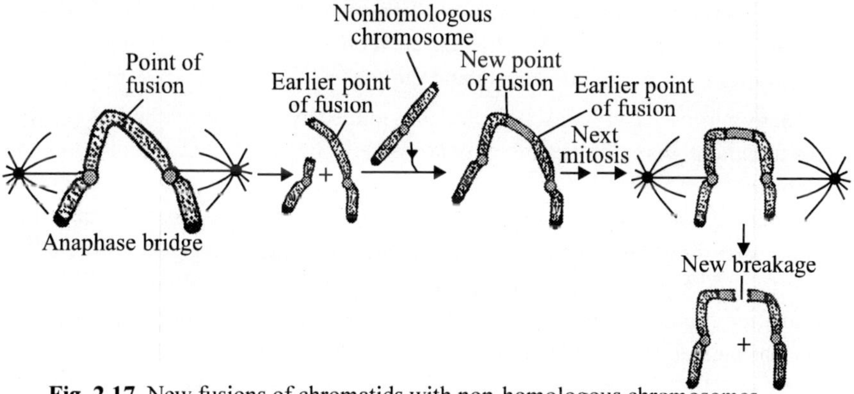

Fig. 2.17. New fusions of chromatids with non-homologous chromosomes forming new gene combinations and gene disruptions

2.6.6 Mutation Rate or 'Mutator Mutations' in Carcinogenesis

The number of **mutations** required to drive a cancer to become malignant is still not clear but it is presumed that between 2 to 20 mutations occur in common solid tumor malignancies. Some cancer types such as certain types of AML, accumulate sufficient mutations that complement each other to become malignant phenotype with a normal mutation rate. There are several lines of evidence indicating an elevated mutation rate with complementing driver mutations is observed in many cancers to achieve malignancy, which is called **'mutator mutations**. Within the cancer genes mutator mutations do occur at an increased mutation rate leading to accumulation of mutations across the cancer genome. Such mutator mutations will have tremendous impact on survival cancer and the effects of such mutations can be broadly classified into: detection of DNA damage is reduced or reduced ability to repair the DNA damage, absence of genomic surveillance mechanism, exogenous and endogenous carcinogens increase the susceptibility to DNA damage. It has been observed that several inherited familial cancer syndromes, like ataxia telangiectasia, xeroderma pigmentosum, Bloom's syndrome and hereditary non-polyposis coli (colorectal cancer) are due to germ-line defects in specific DNA repair mechanism. These mutations show elevated mutation rate and are characterized by early onset of cancers.

Microsatellite instability (MSI) involves high rate of substitutions, small insertions, and deletions, which arises due to mutations in mismatch repair genes including MSH2 and MCH1. In less than 20% of colorectal cancers and in diverse groups of tumors like gastric, endometrial, sebaceous cancers and lymphomas, MSI has been reported. A much more frequently observed pattern of genomic instability in nearly all types of common solid malignancies is chromosomal anomalies or aberrations, which involves whole chromosome segregation abnormalities during mitosis resulting in aneuploidy.

Abnormal methylation of CpG domains in promoter regions, especially multiple tumor suppressor genes is correlated with gene silencing is the most common feature in majority of cancers. This phenomenon is called CpG domain methylator phenotype (CIMP). This has been observed in many clinically distinct cancer types like colorectal cancers and gliomas.

Many aggressive clinical characteristics gained by the cancers, such as ability to resist treatment, to replenish and to metastasize, depends on the continuous genetic variation generated in the genome of the cancer cell that permits its adaptation. From the whole cancer genome sequencing studies, it is obvious that majority of tumors carry large number of somatic mutations, which correlates with elevated mutation rate. A predominance of specific base substitution mutation, such as C to T transition mutations in a CpG domain, considered a 'mutational signature' that is a clear indication of mutational process. When 21 breast cancer genomes were analyzed for these mutational signatures, major mutational processes such as base substitutions, small insertions and deletions and genomic rearrangements were observed. Mutations that occurred early and were responsible in the development of the cancer were dominated by C-to-T transitions was because of spontaneous deamination of methylated cytosines. Chromosomal fragile sites or hot spots have been documented in cytogenetic studies of several cancers, where increased rate of heterozygous and homozygous deletions at these sites were observed compared to other regions of the genome. These sites where increased rate of genomic rearrangements occurs may be because these regions have sparse origins of replication and being late replicating during the cell cycle. For example, Parkinson protein 2, E3 ubiquitin protein ligase (*PARK2*) is found to be frequently deleted and mutated in gastrointestinal tumors and deletion of APC is known to increase the incidence of colorectal cancers in humans.

The chromatin state contributes to a great extent in genomic rearrangements. During interphase stage of cell cycle, in most of the lymphomas, genes that are frequently fused with the immunoglobulin locus by translocation process are often geographically proximate. Prostate cancer being male-specific cancer, androgen induced intra- and inter-chromosomal proximity between the ETS fusion gene partners is observed. In breast cancers, 50% of somatically acquired genomic rearrangements have a characteristic gene footprint like involvement of BRCA1 gene mutation compared with 40% expected by chance.

With regards to point mutations leading to cancer development, mismatch repair deficiencies are responsible for specific distribution of signature mutations across the genome. For example, type 2 TGFβR gene is highly prone to mutation in microsatellite-unstable colorectal cancer due to frame shift mutation, whereas this gene is not mutated in microsatellite-stable colorectal cancer. Similarly, the distribution of point mutation in *p53* and K-ras in tobacco-induced lung cancer differs from lung cancer developed in non-smokers. The efficacy of DNA repair processes also plays an important role in genomic variation and mutation rate. Especially in carcinogen induced tumors, lower rates of mutation are seen in highly expressed genes compared with non-expressed genes.

2.6.7 Carcinogenic Potential of Hypermutation

A high level of genome and epigenome instability in most adult cancers is a well-known fact. The intrinsic feature of cancers, such as increased cell proliferation makes the genome vulnerable to high number of mutations without increased mutation rate. Increased genomic instability initiated during malignant transformation may mask the mutagenic processes that were responsible during early tumorigenesis. It is evident from cancer genome studies that, hypermutated cancer genomes would contain prevailing mutation signatures in genes that play an important role in cancer initiation and development.

2.7 GENOMIC INSTABILITY AND CHROMOSOMAL ANOMALIES IN CANCER CELLS

For almost a century, cancer cells have been known to often carry chromosomal anomalies. The **triradial** and **quadriradial** metaphase chromosomes (Fig. 2.18) seen in cells lacking BRCA1 and BRCA2 function are examples of these aberrations.

Two distinct classes of karyotypic anomalies can be seen in cancer cells: changes in **structure** of individual chromosomes, and changes in chromosome **number.** If changes in chromosome number occur by haploid or diploid set of entire complement of chromosomes leading to triploid (3n) or tetraploid (4n) condition, it is called **euploidy.** If changes in chromosome number occur by single or two or three chromosomes of homologous pair leading to monosomy, trisomy, tetrasomy, it is called **aneuploidy.** Certain cancers showing chromosomal instability are as follows:

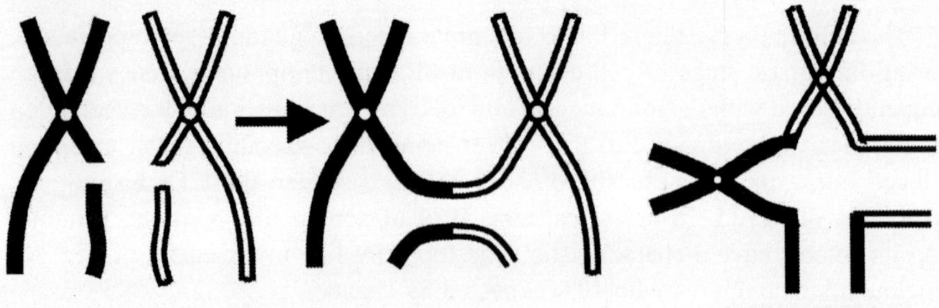

Fig. 2.18. Due to symmetric chromatin joining formation triradial and quadriradial chromosome in metaphase

Translocation between long arm of 8th to 14th long arm of chromosome is observed in Burkitt's lymphoma, translocation of 22nd long arm to 9th long arm is observed in chronic myelogenous leukemia (CML) (Fig. 2.19). In Burkitt's lymphoma, amplified expression of c-myc is observed and in CML a fusion protein of BCR-ABL is produced.

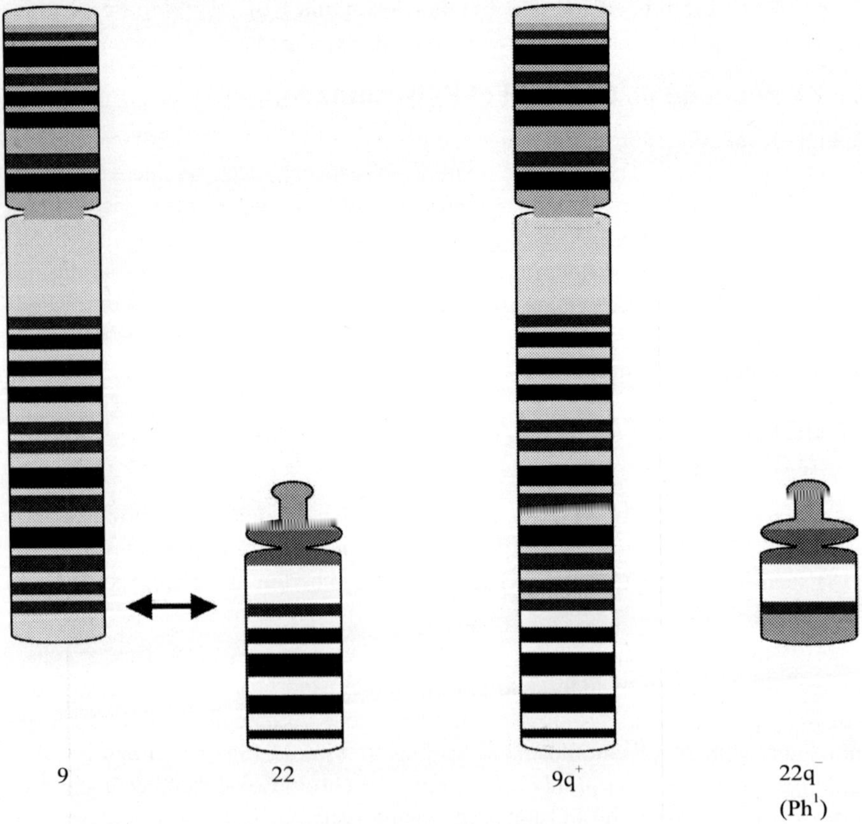

Fig. 2.19. Translocation between 9th and 22nd chromosome during chronic myelogenous leukemia

Human follicular lymphoma is associated with translocation between long arm of 14th and 18th chromosome (14q32: 18q21). T-cell chronic leukemia is because of inversion or translocation of long arm of chromosome 14.

T-cell acuter leukemia (T-ALL) is associated with recurring translocations between the following chromosomes:

t (8:14)	(q24:q32)	t (7:9)	(q35:q34)
t (11:14)	(p15:q11)	t (7:19)	(q35:p13)
t (1:14)	(p32:q11)	t (7:9)	(q34:q34.5)
t (10:14)	(q24:q11)	t (1:7)	(p34:q34)
t (11:14)	(p13:q11)	t (7:10)	(q35:q24)

Solid tumors are also known to show specific translocations:

Ewig's sarcoma (neuroectodermal tumor) t (11:22) (q24:q12)

Synovial sarcoma t (X:18) (p11:q11)

Alveolar rhabdomyosarcoma t (2:13) (q37:q14)

Myxoid liposarcoma t (12:16) (q11-14:p11)

2.7.1 Aneuploidy

- Trisomy of chromosome 12 is observed in chronic lymphocytic leukemia.
- Trisomy of chromosome 8 is observed in blast phase of chronic myelogenous leukemia (CML).
- Trisomy of chromosome 15 is observed in murine T cell leukemia induced in human T cells.
- Monosomy of chromosome 15 is observed in Syrian hamster sarcomas due to transfection by *ras* and *myc* oncogene in human fibroblast culture.

2.7.2 Importance of Genomic Crisis in Tumorigenesis

Recent direct evidences from cancer genome studies indicate that in some cancers, a significant number of mutations can occur in a considerably shorter time scale than the way in which clonal selection process operates. These mutational processes can take several forms (Fig. 2.20).

Telomere attrition (loss of telomere) is responsible for end-to-end chromosome fusion as shown in Fig. 2.16, which leads to massive genomic disruption through repeated breakage-fusion-bridge cycle (Fig. 2.17). Within a few cycles, on a shorter span of time scale than natural selection can operate, widespread chromosomal deletions and exponential new genomic combinations due to rejoining of chromosome can develop. Approximately 2 – 3% of cancers undergo catastrophic mutational process, for which a term has been coined called **'chromothripsis'.** A process that involves genome shattering and rejoining occurs in an accelerated manner localized to one or a few chromosomes resulting in a characteristic pattern of change DNA sequences up to several hundred genomic rearrangements. The damaged chromosome with altered sequences may physically get isolated in the

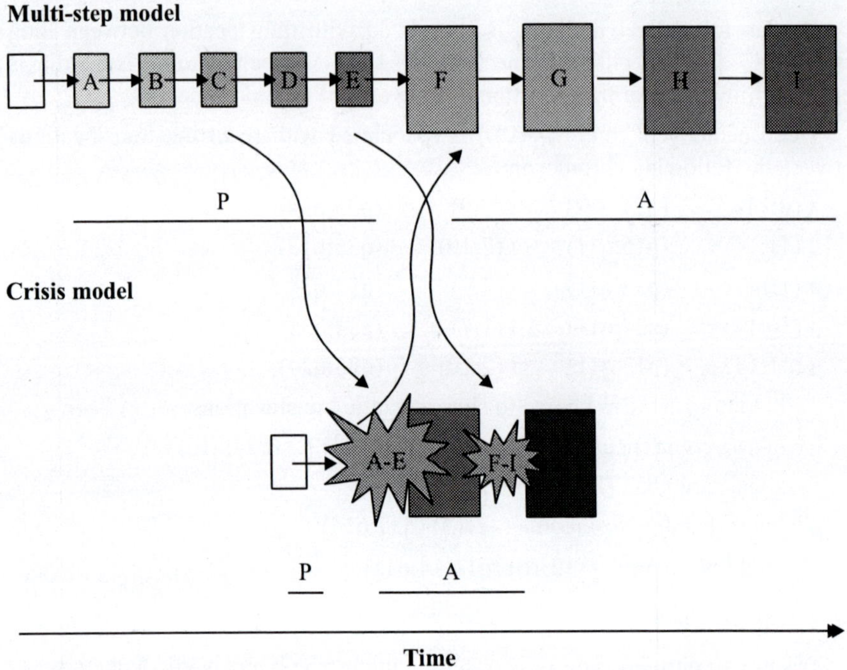

Fig. 2.20. Multistep and genomic crisis driven model of carcinogenesis. Mutations occurring from A to E are required for initiation of clonal expansion and malignant transformation and mutations occurring from F to H promote ongoing evolution and the acquisition of aggressive clinical characteristics. The pre-malignant phase (P) and the time for malignancy onset to acquisition of an aggressive phenotype (A) are reduced in the crisis **event model** compared to multistep model

form of micronuclei, which would be visible during anaphase. Chromothripsis has been known to occur at low frequency in different types of cancers, like chronic lymphocytic leukemia (CLL), neuroblastomas, myelomas, breast cancer, small cell lung cancer and non-small-cell lung cancer, renal, thyroid, and gastrointestinal malignancies. In the case of AML, medulloblastomas and bone sarcomas, high rate of chromothripsis has been reported in the presence of mutant p53 but not with normal p53.

In addition to clusters of structural variation in chromosomes, multiple point mutations are also acquired in one- o. In a large number of genomic studies of breast cancers, sizable number of point mutations in the form of clusters of cytosine mutations have been observed, the process is called ***kataegis***. These clusters of cytosine mutations can represent up to 10 to 20 base substitutions in one or two kilo bases, all occurring in both the strands of DNA (forward or reverse strand) collinear (i.e., in linkage).

All these catastrophic mutational processes in different types of cancers imply that cancer genome evolution may not always follow a gradual stepwise progression (Figs. 2.16 and 2.20). In one of the studies with chromothripsis, three tumor suppressor genes namely, E3 ubiquitin protein ligase *FBXW7, CDKN2A,* and *RecQ* helicase *WRN* were simultaneously disrupted. This suggests that the clone with such a catastrophic mutation would have taken a substantial leap along the path to malignancy soon after the catastrophic event. In multiple myelomas and neuroblastomas, chromothripsis were associated with poor survival, indicating that large scale genomic disruption may have rendered myeloma cells more malignant. In all cancers in the beginning, gradual mutation accumulation occurs to some degree, which gives a sufficient chance for the cancer cells for perpetual adaptation to the tumor environment but any time it could be disrupted by chromothripsis episode, which leads to malignancy.

2.7.3 Cancers with Minimal Mutations in Genomes

Even though there are multiple examples of hypermutations and genomic instability observed in various types of cancer, recently it has been recorded that certain pediatric cancers and some adult lymphoid cancers show relatively small number of genetic alterations. For example, in pediatric rhabdoid tumors mutation load in the order of 1 to 10 mutations per exome and only a single recurrent mutation in the gene encoding chromatin remodeling enzyme SMARCB1 was observed. Similarly, pediatric medulloblastoma, Ewigs sarcoma and adult lymphoid cancers such as acute myeloid leukemias have low mutation numbers, often with similar genetic complexity compared to normal cells. Although, increased mutation rates are the most common feature observed to deregulate cell growth and cell proliferation leading to cancer development, there are exceptions to this. The most frequently observed single-gene disruption leading to cancer are the gene encoding epigenetic modifying enzymes such as SMARCB1, DNA methyl transferase 3α (DNMT3A), TET2, enhancers of zest 2 (EZH2), and mixed lineage leukemia 2 (MLL2; also known as KMLT2D) in pediatric and lymphoid tumors suggests that single genetic change leading to global changes in gene expression can be sufficient to drive a cancer progression. Moreover, programmed genetic changes that are normally seen in certain cell lineages such as VDJ recombination, SHM and class switch recombinations that occur in lymphoid cells can inadvertently switch on cancer-associated genes. For example, recombination activation gene (RAG)-mediated deletion of ETS variant 6 (ETV6) and cyclin dependent kinase inhibitor 2A (CDKN2A)-CDKN2B observed in acute lymphoblastic leukemia (ALL), and MYC translocation in Burkitt's lymphoma leading to overexpression of MYC, which thereby promote cancer progression without the establishment of a general multiple mutation phenotype.

2.8 DARWINIAN EVOLUTION PATTERN IN TUMOR PROGRESSION INVOLVING MUTATIONS AND NATURAL SELECTION

In the process of cancer development, it is the individual cells that are evolving units and each evolving cell will be competing with its counterpart in a population of cancer cells, like the competition between the individual organisms within a species in nature during the course of natural selection. Applying the modern depiction of Darwinian evolution, random mutations that occur in cancer cell population are presumed to create genetic variability. As a result, population of cells, genetically heterogeneous, will arise and the natural forces of selection operate and then favor the outgrowth of individual cells endowed with advantageous mutant alleles having favorable traits of proliferation and survival of these cells in the microenvironment of the living tissue.

By applying Darwinian evolutionary theory natural selection to the multi-step tumor progression, it is now possible to depict tumorigenesis as a succession of clonal expansions. The scheme of understanding is like this: The random mutations that occur in tumor cell population in which a mutation that gives a cell advantageous growth and/or survival trait. This cell having this trait will proliferate and pass on the trait to their descendents having more excessive proliferative rate than their neighbors, eventually yielding a large clonal population cells with special character that dominates the tissue by marginalizing genetically less favored neighbors. Sooner or later, this cell clone of high proliferation rate and survival ability will reach a large enough size (approximately 10^6 cells), another advantageous mutation at the rate of 1 per 10^6 cell generation would take place randomly in one or another cell within this clonal population (Fig. 2.21).

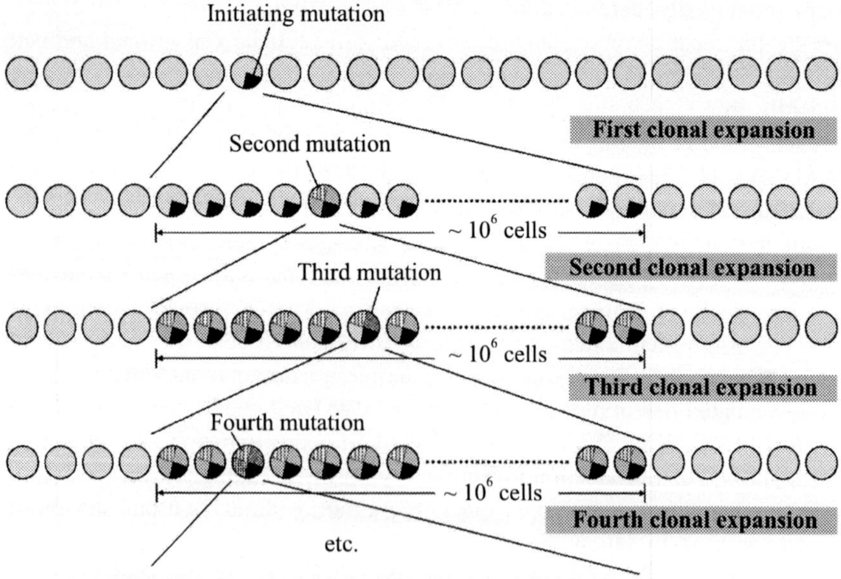

Fig. 2.21. Darwinian evolution and clonal succession of tumor progression

The resulting cells would carry double mutation, which will provide proliferative and survival ability even more effective than its 10^6 clonal predecessors. This new population of cells with new advantageous mutation will give rise to a new sub-clone that will proliferate by cell division and eventually dominate the local tissue environment by marginalizing and possibly eliminating the predecessor population from which it arose. After this doubly mutated cell clone reaches a large size, as before, a third mutation may now strike and the process of clonal expansion and succession will repeat itself.

The schematic diagram represented (Fig. 2.21) is too simplistic, where the number of distinct steps involved in tumor progression are represented by a few numbers of genetic mutations that are involved in the process. Generally, the inactivation of a tumor suppressor gene is a two-step process. First step would be mutation or methylation of one gene copy making it inactive. Thereafter, the second step would be elimination of surviving, still-intact gene cop, usually through the process of loss of heterozygosity (LOH). It is a well-known fact that elimination of tumor suppressor genes often represents most of the genomic changes occurring during tumor progression and the number of distinct genomic alterations taking place during tumor progression may be almost twice as many as the number of loci that are involved.

Since every clonal expansion is triggered by an infrequently occurring genetic or epigenetic alteration and these expansions are likely to be spaced far apart in time. During the development of sporadic colon cancers, a decade or more may separate one critical genetic alteration from the next, and in may individuals, the process may stretch over a century. For example, one of the key steps in the evolution of colon cancer from polyp to invasive cancer has been estimated to take from 4 to 11 years depending on the degree of dysplasia present in the polyp and the diet). Still, some people develop sporadic colon carcinomas in far less time, and so this schedule must be compressed in the colon of these individuals.

Not much is known about the processes that govern the rates of tumor progression in most tissues. In the case of colon cancer, certain constituents of diet may greatly increase the rate at which the genomes of their colonic epithelial cells accumulate mutations. Such increased mutation rates can, in turn, compress the time between clonal successions. Perhaps in individuals who consume certain food stuffs, 5 or fewer years intervene between successive clonal expansions rather than the usual 10 or 20. As a consequence, a disease process that usually requires a century to reach completion may reach its neoplastic end point in 30 or 40 years, well within the human lifespan.

Colon tumor progression may be accelerated through certain alterations within pre-malignant cells by the exogenous carcinogens in the foodstuff. Thus, increased mutations may be caused by defects in the complex cellular machinery that is dedicated to maintaining and repairing cellular DNA. For example, some individuals inherit mutations that compromise the functions of the enzymes and proteins of cellular DNA mismatch repair apparatus. Because of the defective DNA maintenance, colonic epithelial cells show greatly increased mutation rates leading to increased rate of formation of pre-malignant and malignant growths in the colon – the syndrome of hereditary non-polyposis colon cancer (HNPCC). More commonly, due to the defects in the DNA repair apparatus resulting from somatic mutation (or promoter methylation) occurring early in tumor progression;

the resulting crippling of the repair apparatus, and increased genome mutability guarantee that subsequent mutational steps in colon cancer progression will occur relatively rapidly. These multiple factors influencing colon carcinoma formation greatly complicate the attempts to delineate the clonal succession predicted by the Darwinian model of tumor progression.

2.9 DERANGED CONTROL OF CELL DIFFERENTIATION DURING CARCINOGENESIS

The central property of cancer cells is to defy the normal controls on cell division, in addition, the tumor cells require nutrients and oxygen for their growth, for which, they must stimulate the growth of blood vessels around them to bring the nutrients and oxygen. In many tissues organizations like skin, intestinal epithelium, and uterine epithelium even an uncontrolled increase in the frequency of cell division will not by itself produce a steadily growing tumor because, the epithelium of these tissues is normally renewed itself continuously by shedding off terminally differentiated cells from its uppermost layer by replacing it with new cells derived from the stem cells lying in the basal layer. When the normal stem cell undergoes division, it gives rise to one daughter stem cell and one cell that is programmed to undergo terminal differentiation and stops dividing. If the stem cell divides at a faster rate, equal number of terminally differentiated cells will be produced, which are lost rapidly and a balance would be maintained between genesis and destruction. Thus, if there is a need for a stem cell to be transformed to generate a steadily dividing clone of progeny, the balance maintained between stem cells and differentiated cells must be changed by tilting the balance towards having more than 50% of the daughter cells as stem cells. For this purpose, the differentiation process must be deranged so that daughter cells would retain the ability to divide indefinitely and avoid dying or being discarded at the end of the production line (Fig. 2.22).

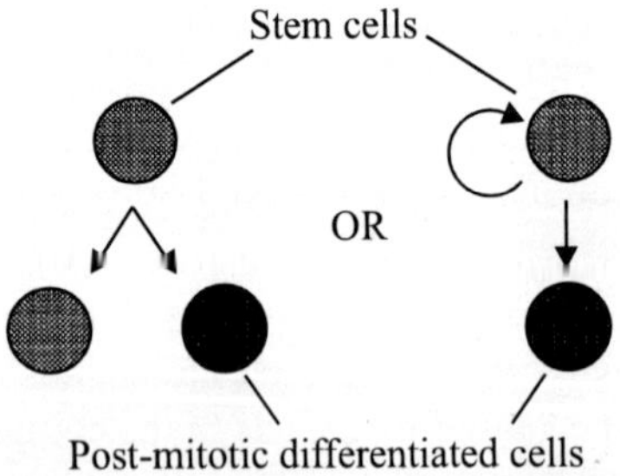

Fig. 2.22. Schematic representation to show stem cell origin of cancer

The development and retention of stem cell properties would be seen in the progression from a mild dysplasia of the uterine cervix to carcinoma in situ and malignant cancer. Similar situations apply to the development of cancer in other tissues like skin, the gut epithelium, and the hemopoietic system that relies upon the stem cells for the renewal process. For example, in several forms of leukemias, the normal differentiation process is disrupted such that a progenitor cell committed to differentiate into a particular type of blood cell continues to divide indefinitely instead of differentiating terminally in the normal way and ultimately dies after a limited number of cell division cycles. In most of the cancers, normal process of cells achieving a non-dividing state or terminally differentiated state or normal programmed cell death (apoptosis) terminally differentiated cells once their life span is over are blocked. Therefore, for the treatment of cancer, a strategy must be adopted to develop drugs that promote cell differentiation rather than targeting the dividing cells to kill them.

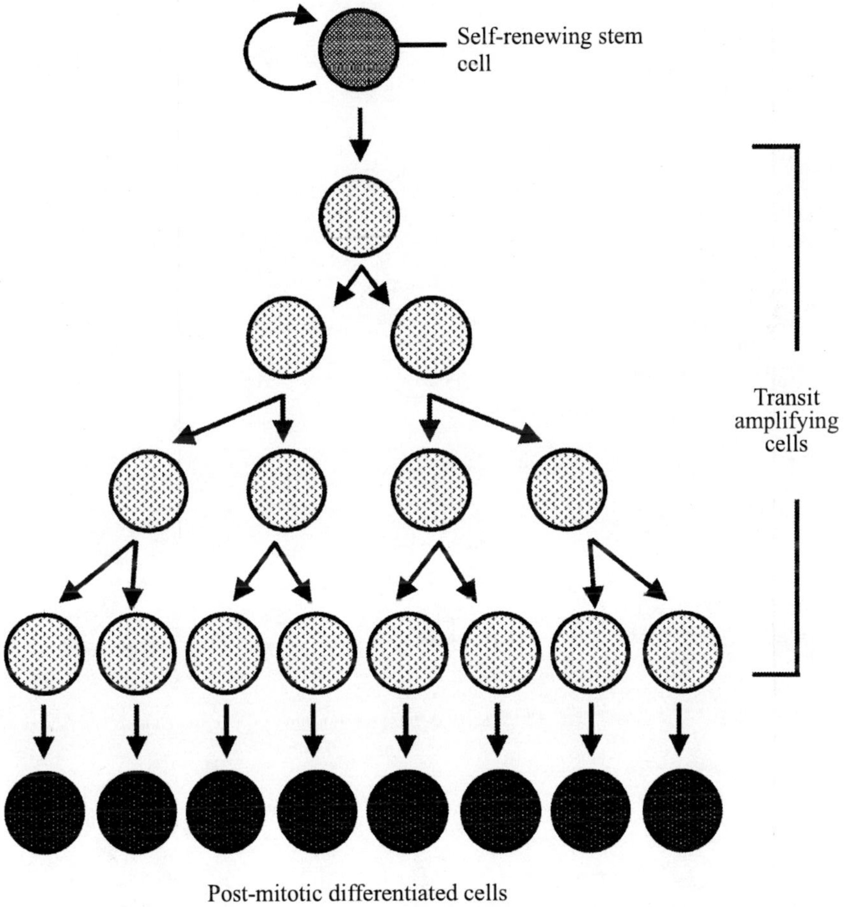

Fig. 2.23. One of the daughters of a dividing stem cells becomes a stem cell. However, others become transit-amplifying cells (progenitor cells)

Cancer cells in the majority populations behave much like transit-amplifying cells, which are also called progenitor cells, that exist in many normal tissues and they are the intermediates between stem cells and their fully differentiated descendants (Figs. 2.23 and 2.24). Experimental evidences indicate that small populations of tumorigenic cancer cells with stem cell characteristics are the prime cause of proliferation and not the much larger population of neoplastic transit-amplifying cells. The mutations that take place in the cancer stem cell population can be transmitted to the next generation of cells originating in the population through cell division while the mutations taking place in the non-tumorigenic transit-amplifying cells cannot be passed on to the next generation, because of limited proliferative ability of these cells. Therefore, the genetic evolution associated with multi-step tumorigenesis may be restricted to relatively in small population tumor stem cells.

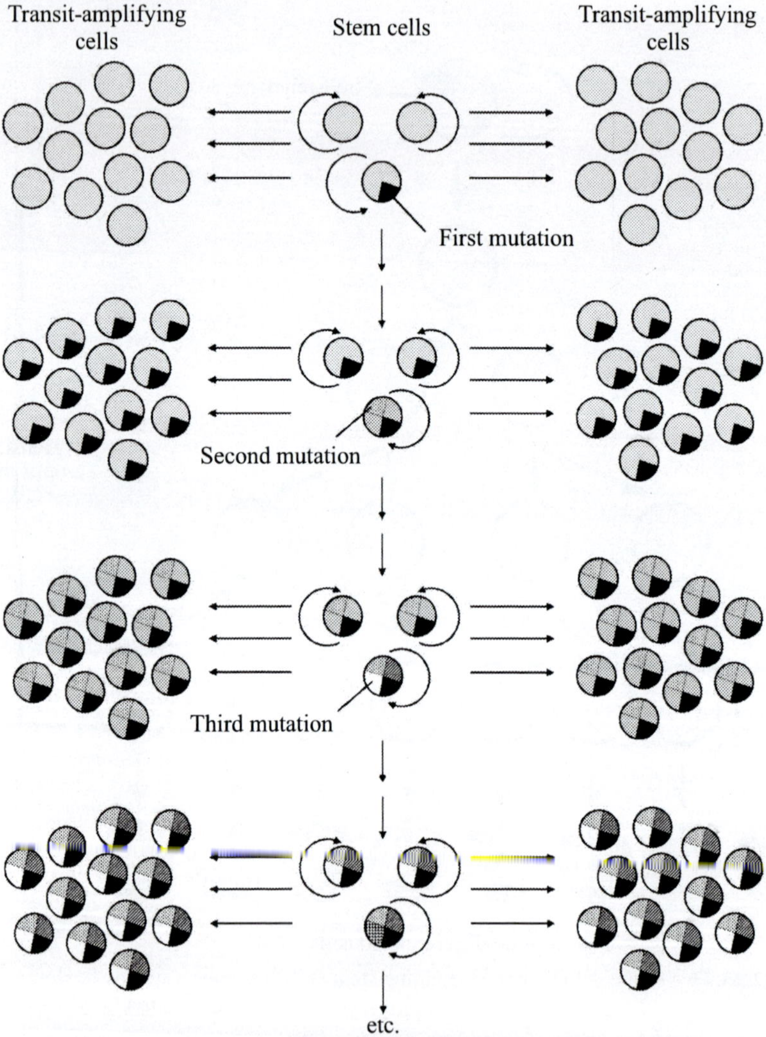

Fig. 2.24. Cancer stem cells and clonal succession

The tumor genome often becomes increasingly unstable in actual course of tumor progression, which complicates the matter and during each cell cycle, the rate at which mutations are acquired soars. The rate at which the genetic change takes place and the resulting genetic diversification soon outpaces the rate at which

Darwinian selection can occur. Consequently, actual tumor progression in many tumors looks like a highly branched scheme (Fig. 2.25) rather than linear series of clonal successions. In such a situation, a number of genetically distinct sub-clones of cells coexist within a single tumor mass.

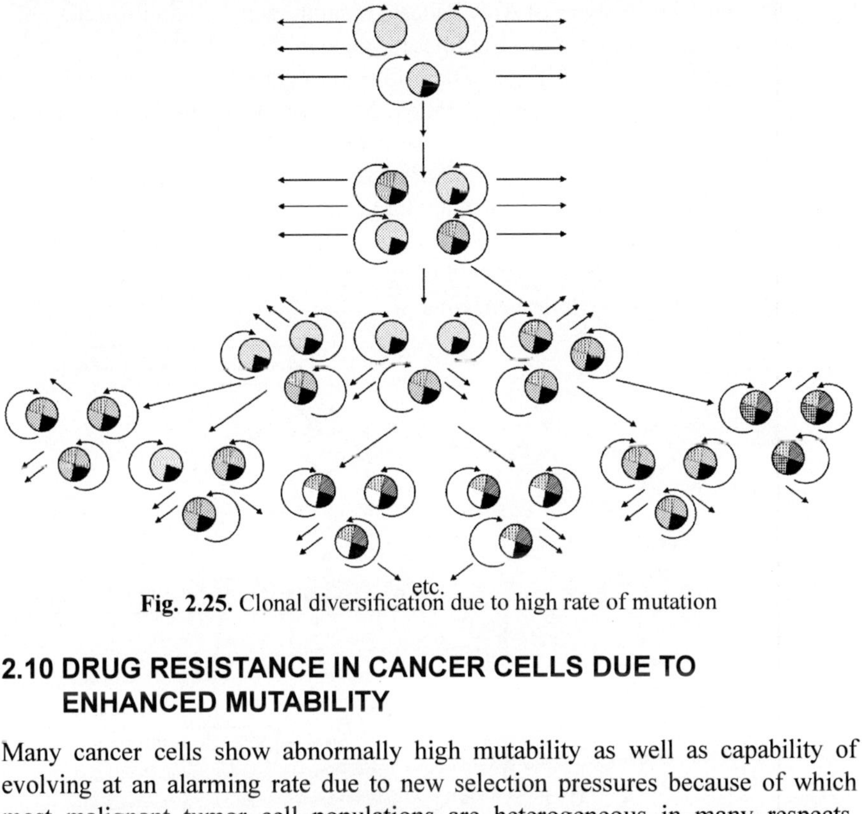

Fig. 2.25. Clonal diversification due to high rate of mutation

2.10 DRUG RESISTANCE IN CANCER CELLS DUE TO ENHANCED MUTABILITY

Many cancer cells show abnormally high mutability as well as capability of evolving at an alarming rate due to new selection pressures because of which most malignant tumor cell populations are heterogeneous in many respects. It is because of this feature cancer therapy becomes complicated and arduous. Repeated selective treatment of dividing cells with toxic drugs can kill majority of neoplastic cells in a cancer patient, but fail in killing all of them. Usually, some small population of cells survives drug treatment and become drug-resistant and such cells on further drug treatment will lead to evolution of cells with traits that promote proliferation of these cells.

It is worse that the cancer cells exposed to one drug often develop resistance not only to that drug, but also to another drug to which they were never been exposed before. This is called **multidrug resistance**, which is achieved through a change in the karyotype. Cancer cells showing drug resistance would depict the change in karyotype in the form of additional pairs of miniature chromosomes called *double minute chromosomes* or it may be depicted in the form of *homogeneously staining region* within the normal banding pattern of one of its regular chromosomes. In both these aberrations, ***multidrug resistance (mdr1)*** gene is highly amplified with a large number of copies and this gene codes for a plasma-membrane-bound transporter ATPase (P-glycoprotein) (P-gp) or the multi-drug transporter is expressed on the membrane. This glycoprotein prevents the intracellular accumulation of certain classes of chemotherapeutic lipophilic drugs by expelling them out of the cell (Fig. 2.26). The transporter is recycled and continues to increase the efflux of the drug by the second hydrolysis of ATP. Cancer chemotherapy by administration of folic-acid antagonist methotrexate amplifies the gene for the enzyme dihydrofolate reductase (DHFR) and amplification of *myc* proto-oncogene (to be discussed later) in some cancers stimulates cell proliferation. Mutation of the folate transporter results in resistance to methotrexate. Another way of developing resistance against methotrexate is by amplification of gene to increase the number of drug target molecules (Fig. 2.26). Increased alkyltransferase activity observed in some cancer cells gives rise to resistance to alkylating chemotherapeutic agents such as doxorubicin, a common chemotherapeutic drug and different tumors show highly variable levels of alkyltransferase enzyme.

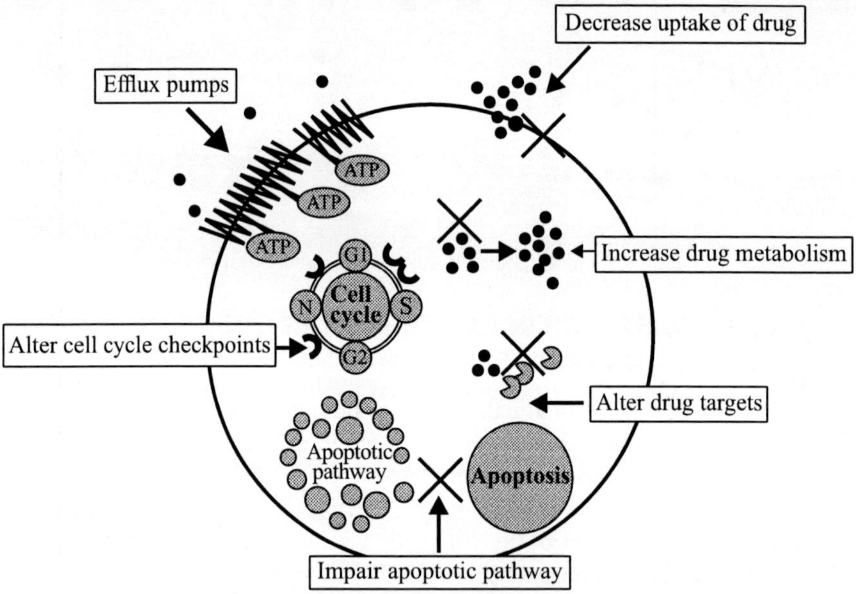

Fig. 2.26. Mechanism of multidrug resistance in a cancer cell

Many cancer cells are known to have mutations in the genes responsible for factors that assist in DNA replication, recombination or repair mechanisms leading to defects in these cellular processes, which may facilitate cancer cells to evolve further by increasing their mutability and at the same time, it may also make the cancer cells more vulnerable to attack by certain types of drugs. Taking into advantage of these vulnerable characteristics of cancer cells many tumors are killed more easily than normal cell by exposure to specific drugs that interfere with DNA metabolism. As more and more information is being gathered about the molecular mechanisms of regulation of DNA replication, recombination and repair in cancer cells, research is being carried to design new drugs to specifically target the cancer cells having effects in DNA replication, repair and recombination and spare the normal cells.

The genomic instability in cancer cells continually generates new alleles and novel genetic configurations. Evolving cancer cells can pick and choose among these genetic variations, searching for combinations that improve their ability to survive and proliferate. Variety of common human cancers like breast, small-cell-lung, and ovarian carcinomas, initially responds to commonly used chemotherapeutic cytotoxic drugs, but later, these tumors become resistant to drug treatment and therefore relapse. This drug resistance ability is acquired through genetic alterations and plasticity of cancer cell populations to adapt to newly acquired mutations.

Some of the mechanisms of drug resistance acquired by cancer cells in devising various maneuvers for eluding killing by chemotherapeutic drugs are as follows:

- By overexpression of P-glycoprotein multi-drug efflux pump the drug molecules are effluxed out of the cancer cell or cancer cell losses the ability to import drug molecules through the plasma membrane.
- Decreased drug activation due to loss of expression of cytochrome P-450
- Increased inactivation of drug.
- The dysregulation of sphingolipid metabolism is another cause for development of radiation and chemo resistance by the cancer cells. A phospholipid called ceramide-sphingosine-sphingosine 1-phosphate is a major constituent of cell membrane and its increased levels leads to cell death in normal cells. The enzyme responsible for deacetylation of ceramide called acid ceramidase (AC) is upregulated in cancer cell leading to formation of more of sphingosine 1-phosphate, which promotes cell survival or immortality. Elevated expression of AC is seen in most of the cancer patients who show resistance to radiation and chemotherapy as combinatorial therapy.

Majority of chemotherapeutic drugs act primarily by inducing DNA damage, thereby leading to apoptosis of cancer cell by triggering apoptotic pathway. However, one of the major characters acquired by cancer cells is evasion of apoptosis. Many tumors gain intrinsic ability to develop resistance to chemotherapies irrespective of whether they were previously treated with same drug. Mutations in the genes that regulate apoptosis are responsible for the development of drug resistance, which facilitates uncoupling the drug-induced damage due to activation of apoptosis. A major tumor suppressor gene p53 mutation is a common feature in almost all tumors and it is responsible for promotion of apoptosis in normal condition. Non-functional p53 in tumors contributes to drug resistance and loss of apoptosis.

Increased resistance of tumors to chemotherapeutic drugs is also brought about by upregulation of anti-apoptotic members of the Bcl-2 gene family and the down-regulation of pro-apoptotic *bax* gene. In metastatic tumors, overexpression of Bcl-2 is a common feature responsible for chemo resistance in tumors.

There is another important risk associated with treating cancer with chemotherapy for those cells that have lost functional apoptotic pathways. Genotoxic chemotherapeutic drugs cause extensive DNA damage and in the absence of apoptotic pathway, they provide an excellent opportunity for the accumulation of mutations in drug-resistant cancer cells. Consequently, this further increases the risk of carcinogenesis. Indeed, there are evidences for chemotherapy or radiation therapy related leukemia in many cases, a new cancer emerges due to the administration chemotherapy or radiation therapy.

2.11 TUMORIGENESIS CAUSED BY DEFECTS IN DNA REPAIR MECHANISM

Xeroderma pigmentosum (XP) is an unusual syndrome that involves development of high rate of squamous and basal cell carcinomas of the skin. Individuals suffering from this genetic defect are extremely sensitive to UV radiation and on minimal exposure to sunlight, infants will suffer severe burning of the skin. The skin in these individuals will have parchment-like appearance (xeroderma) and many pigmented patches or freckles (pigmentosum). In general, compared with general population, individuals suffering from XP syndrome are at an increased risk of developing skin cancer, which appears at very young age of 8 years leading to death before the adulthood. Inherited defects associated within any one of eight distinct genes of **nucleotide excision repair** (NER) can lead to xeroderma pigmentosum, because of non-repaired DNA lesions such as pyrimidine dimers.

Several other inherited syndromes are also associated with defects in NER. For example, individuals suffering from **Cockayne syndrome** (CS) appear to be defective in one of two genes that are involved in transcription-coupled NER. These patients also have increased photosensitivity like those of XP patients. **Hereditary non-polyposis colon cancer** (HNPCC) is a familial colon cancer syndrome, an inherited predisposition to 2 – 3% of all colon cancers. In addition to colon carcinomas, subclasses of HNPCC patients are increasingly susceptible to endometrial, stomach, ovarian and urinary tract carcinomas. Germ-line mutations in the genes encoding **MSH2** and **MLH1,** the two important mismatch repair (MMR) proteins are observed in majority of HNPCC cases. Because of this defect in properly detecting sequence mismatch and repair it, this contributes to high rates of mutations in genes having nested microsatellite repeats in their sequences.

2.11.1 Increased Errors during DNA Synthesis

The chances for mutations arising during DNA synthesis while copying a normal template are limited because of replicase accuracy in base selection, nearly instant proofreading by the enzyme and post-replication mismatch repair (MMR). Inactivation of any of these safeguards' mechanism would lead to hypermutation. Similarly, mutations may also get introduced during replication when small stretches of DNA that does not contain lesion is copied by error prone **translesion synthesis** (TLS) polymerase.

2.11.2 Mismatch Repair Defects

Inherited germ-line genetic defects in one of the mismatch repair (MMR) genes, namely, MSH2, MSH6, PMS2 and MLH1 predispose an individual to hereditary non-polyposis colorectal cancer (HNPCC) as well as several other types of cancers. MMR defects are most commonly due to an increase in microsatellite instability (MSI), which involves frequent deletions and insertions in arrays of very short direct repeat sequences (microsatellites). Genome-wide MSI is also common in sporadic colorectal, gastric and endometrial cancers, which often coincides with MLH1 hypermethylation or with somatic mutations in MMR genes. Increased frequency of various base substitutions is also very common in cancer samples with MSI. They form a different category of hypermutated cancers, which is distinct from somatic hypermutation that occurs in DNA polymerase gene of cancer cells.

Somatic mutations in DNA Pol ε (*POLE*) and DNA Pol δ (*POLD1*) have been linked to familial predisposition to colorectal, endometrial, and ovarian cancers. It is very well known that DNA Pol δ synthesizes lagging strand and DNA Pol ε synthesizes leading strand in a bidirectional replication fork. Samples with hypermutated *POLE*, which is even higher mutation loads than MSI positive MMR-deficient tumors have been reported, whereas sporadic mutations in *POLD1* were less frequent among ultra mutated tumors, which mostly carried mutations in the proofreading exonuclease domain of *POLE* and these samples had two separate characteristic signatures TCT→A and TCG→T.

Error-free copying of cyclobutane pyrimidine dimmers (CPDs) can be done by DNA Pol η. In multiple myeloma, the DNA Pol η [T̲ (A|T)] mutation motif was significantly enriched in A- or T- coordinated clusters. Enrichment of this motif was also found in chronic leukemia's and B cell lymphomas. Another signature mutation, [AT̲ →C] detected in hepatitis C virus (HCV)-positive hepatocellular carcinomas was due to error prone synthesis by one of the TLS polymerases because of over expression of DNA pol ζ and DNA pol ι in this type of cancer.

The gene encoding type II TGF-β receptor (TGF-β RII) was found to be mutated in majority of cancers due to deletion of one or two A's from homopolymeric stretch of ten A's normally present. The deletion of A's leads to changes in the normal reading frame of coding sequences of the TGF-βII gene called frame shift mutation, as a result nonfunctional TGF-βRII protein is produced (Fig. 2.27)

One can imagine that once tumor cell precursor fails to express functional TGF-βRII, these cells can escape the growth-inhibitory effects of TGFβ, which is an important anti-mitogenic factor. Tumor cells endowed with this highly advantageous trait acquired very early will facilitate tumor progression by epithelial cells. In the great majority of tumors, the MMR defects and the resulting mutant alleles were discovered in sporadic cancers. MMR genes, like tumor suppressor genes, can be made non-functional either by somatic mutation or by promoter methylation resulting in transcriptional silencing. In fact, the second mechanism is responsible for the major share of defective MMR in about 15% of

Table 2.2. Human familial cancer syndrome due to inherited defects in DNA repair

Name of Syndrome	Cancer phenotype	Enzyme or process affected
AT (Ataxia telangiectasia)	Leukemia, lymphoma Ataxia telangiectasia mutated (ATM)	Response to double strand DNA breaks
Familial breast, ovarian cancer	BRCA1, BRCA2 gene mutation	Homology directed repair of dsDNA breaks
Werner	Several cancers	Exonuclease, DNA helicase
Bloom	Solid tumors	DNA helicase
Fanconi anemia	Acute myelogenous leukemia (AML), head and neck squamous cell carcinoma (HNSCC)	Repair of DNA cross links and double strand breaks
Nijmegen breaks	Mostly lymphomas	Processing of double stranded DNA breaks, nonhomologous end joining (NHEJ)
Li-Fraumeni	Multiple cancers	DNA damage alarm protein
Li-Fraumeni	Colon, breast	Kinase signaling DNA damage

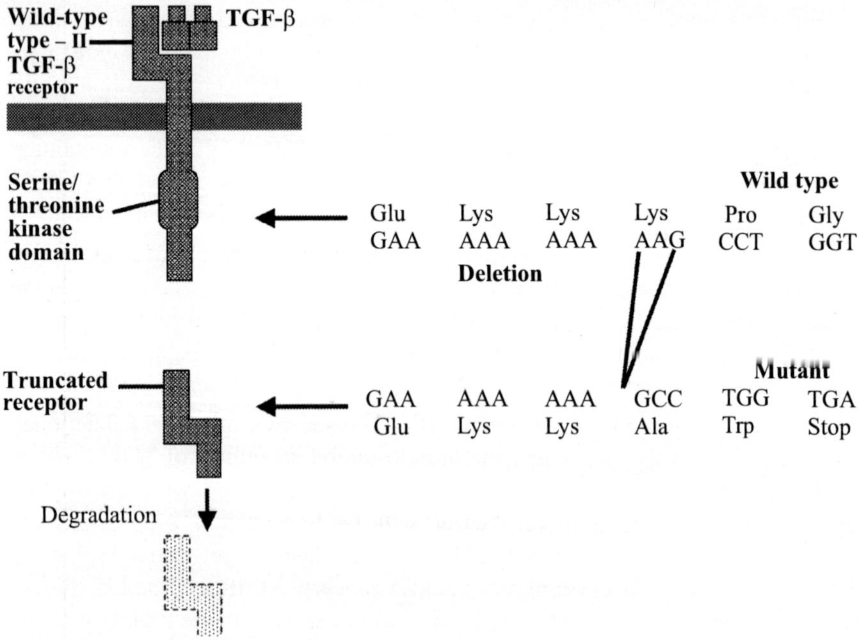

Fig. 2.27. Defects in DNA repair mechanism resulting in truncated receptor

sporadic gastric, colorectal, and endometrial tumors and in almost all of these, the observed microsatellite instability is because of methylation resulting in silencing of the MLH1 gene. Interestingly, in the endometrial tissue adjacent to tumors with normal histology was found to have defective MMR, methylation of MLH1 gene is often observed, suggesting that, methylation is one of the earliest events of tumor progression in this tissue.

Repeated observation of methylated mismatch repair genes in pre-malignant cells during tumor progression provides direct evidence that a somatically acquired (i.e., non-inherited) defect in a DNA repair function conferring advantage to evolving tumor cells during DNA replication. In many of the tumor cell genomes showing microsatellite instability, there are hundreds and likely thousands of genes that are concomitantly mutated. BAX gene, which encodes an important pro-apoptotic protein, can be silenced through mutations provoked by a stretch of eight G's in its normal reading frame and an MMR defect. Even the genes that encode MMR proteins are themselves inactivated by MMR defects.

By far the two most notorious tumor suppressor genes associated with cancer are BRCA1 and BRCA2. Germ-line mutation in the alleles of either of these genes confers an inborn increased susceptibility to breast and ovarian carcinomas. Mutant germ-line alleles of BRCA1 or BRCA2 are responsible for 70 – 80% of all familial ovarian cancers. These two genes are considered to be "caretakers", produce DNA repair proteins meant for maintenance of genomic integrity.

Exercise

1. With illustration explain the role of RNA tumor virus in cancer formation.
2. How does DNA tumor virus induce cancer formation? Explain with diagrammatic presentation.
3. Explain the pathogenic mechanism adopted by HBV or HCV in induction of hepatocellular carcinoma.
4. How do epigenetic alterations facilitate hepatocarcinogenesis induced by HBV or HCV?
5. What is meant by monoclonal origin of cancer? Give a schematic or diagrammatic presentation.
6. What is meant by polyclonal origin of cancer? Give a schematic or diagrammatic presentation.
7. Alteration in DNA sequence and mutation leads to origin of cancer.

   OR

   Multiple mutations leads to tumorigenesis. Justify the statement with suitable cancer development model.
8. Non-mutagenic agents facilitate cancer development.

   OR

   Continuous mitotic stimulus leads to carcinogenesis. Justify the statement with explanation.

OR

Continuous inflammatory response leads to tumorigenesis. Explain why and how it happens.

9. Write short notes on:
   (a) Heterogeneity of mutations within a cancer
   (b) Role of epistasis in cancer genome evolution
   (c) Loss of heterozygosity in cancer genome promotes cancer development
   (d) Breakage-fusion breakage bridge formation in chromosomes contributes to carcinogenesis
10. Discuss the role of chromosomal anomalies and genetic instability in cancer development.
11. Explain the role of mutator mutations in cancer development.
12. What is the role of genomic crisis in carcinogenesis?

    OR

    What is meant by chromothripsis? How does it contribute to cancer development?
13. Defects in DNA repair mechanism lead to susceptibility to cancer development. Justify this statement with suitable example.
14. During cancer development, Darwinian evolution and natural selection of cancer cell occurs. With schematic representation, explain how it happens?
15. Elaborate on altered cell differentiation genes promotion of carcinogenesis.
16. What is mechanism adopted by cancer cell to develop drug resistance? Explain with diagrammatic presentation.

CHAPTER

3

Molecular Aspects of Cancer

3.1 EPIGENETIC CHANGES AND CARCINOGENESIS

Epigenetics refers to heritable genetic information that is encoded by the genome for modification of the genome and chromatin components. Structure and conformation of chromatin is modified due to epigenetic alterations, which affects the gene expression due to altered regulation of transcription. Nucleotide sequence of the DNA does not change due to epigenetic alterations, but only change in gene expression takes place, therefore, they are not treated as mutations. For the normal cell differentiation process, stable epigenetic changes are important. For example, gene for differentiation in stem cells is silenced by epigenetic means to retain stem cell characteristics. Cell undertakes two types of epigenetic modifications, namely, **histone modification and DNA methylation**, which are acquired or inherited and both affect gene expression due to modification of nucleotide sequences in gene promoters where the transcription factors bind to appropriate sequences.

3.1.1 Histone Modification

A histone protein when subjected to post-translational modifications such as acetylation, methylation, phosphorylation, and ubiquination, which alters chromatin structure, thereby affects gene expression. Acetylation of histone-by-histone acetyltransferases (HATs; add acetyl groups) and deacetylation by histone deacetylases (HDACs; remove acetyl groups) are responsible for modification of histone. Relaxation of the chromatin or euchromatization is brought about by acetylation of histone, making the chromatin accessible for gene action (transcription), whereas deacetylation leads to compacting of chromatin (heterochromatization) and gene silencing.

3.1.2 DNA Methylation

Transcriptional regulation of genes is affected by yet another epigenetic process called DNA methylation where methyl group is substituted in the 5th position of cytosine resulting in the formation of 5-methyl cytosine. Only 3-4% of all cytosine residues in DNA are methylated at CpG domains. 50% promoter region of human genes consists of CpG clusters, called CpG islands.

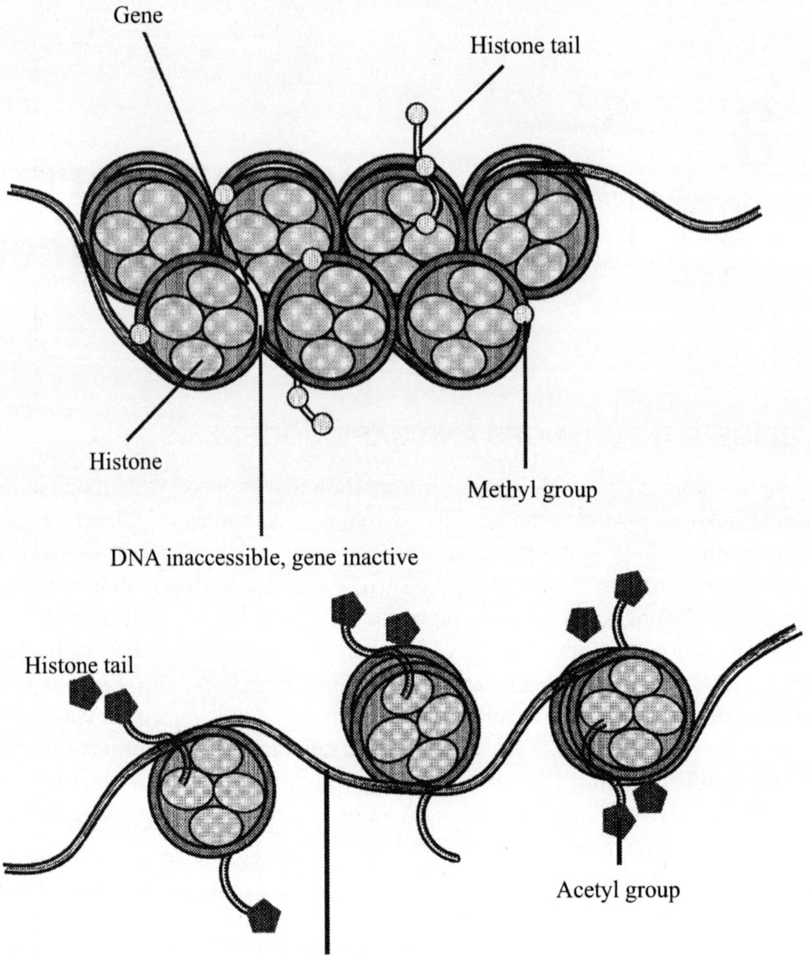

Fig. 3.1. Histone acetylation and methylation process as a means of epigenetic modification of chromatin

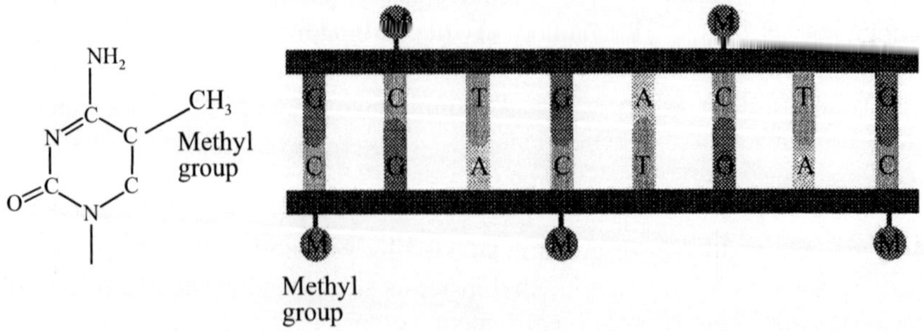

Fig. 3.2. 5 Methyl cytosine and methylation of cytosine in DNA

The enzyme that facilitates covalent addition of a methyl group to the 5th position of cytosine is called DNA methyl transferase (DNMT), which is brought about by the methyl carrier, S-adenosyl methionine. There are three DNMTs playing different roles at different times of cell cycle.

3.2 ROLE OF EPIGENETICS IN CARCINOGENESIS

In cancer, misregulation of epigenetic process plays an important role. Large groups of genes may get inactivated due to abnormal epigenetic programs. Misregulated epigenetic events can cause genome-wide alterations and genomic instability in the cell, leading to inactivation of genes, which cooperate during carcinogenesis. On one hand, due to mutations, enzymes responsible for epigenetic regulation may be disabled and on the other hand, epigenetic silencing could lead to loss of heterozygosity (LOH) of tumor suppressor genes as a means of inactivation in a recessive manner.

3.2.1 Histone Modification and Cancer

In several cancer types, HAT and HDAC activity has been observed to be predominantly altered. Interestingly, in epithelial cancers, a gene EP300 considered to be a tumor suppressor gene that codes for HAT has been found to be mutated. In several other cancers, opposite is observed where, HDAC activity was found to be increased leading to inactivation EP300.

Acute promyelocytic leukemia (PML) is characterized by production of a fusion protein called PML-RAR due to chromosomal translocation and this novel fusion protein recruits HDAC to the promoter region of RA target genes, thereby repressing the expression of these genes, which causes the blockade of differentiation gene hence, leukemia.

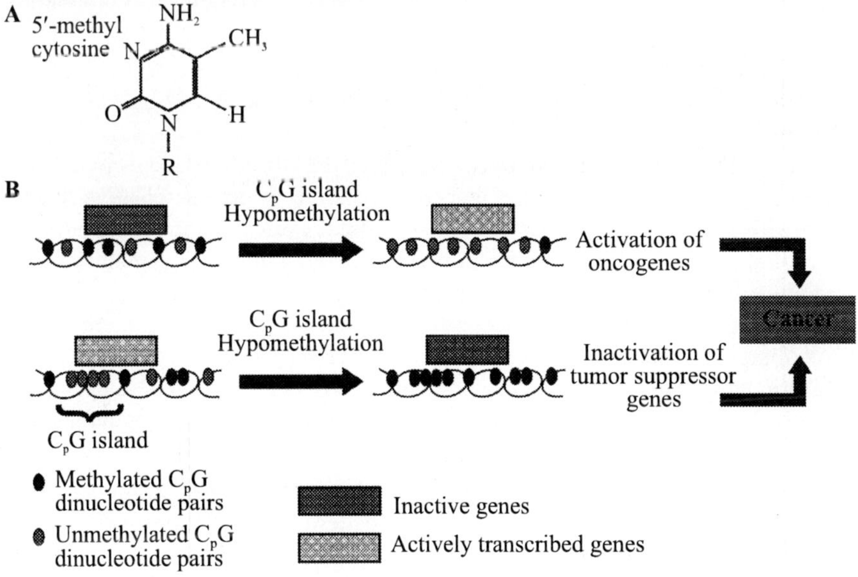

Fig. 3.3. DNA methylation pattern in development of cancer

3.2.2 DNA Methylation and Cancer

DNA methylation of certain genes specific to cancer has been recognized and many studies on different types of cancers have shown hypermethylation of CpG islands of gene promoters, which are not methylated. During carcinogenesis, gene silencing by methylation is one of the important mechanisms followed whereby critical genes normally involved in tumor suppression are silenced. In many human tumors, inactivation of gene expression is predominant due to promoter region hypermethylation and very often this is the mechanism followed for inactivation of tumor suppressor genes. For example, estrogen receptor protein is expressed on the membrane of normal ovarian epithelial cells, which is frequently lost in ovarian cancer. Many breast cancers that are estrogen receptor positive show promoter hypermethylation of the estrogen receptor-α gene. In ovarian tumors also hypermethylation may be responsible for this phenotype. As another example, in many familial breast cancers, BRCA1, a tumor suppressor gene, is often mutated in recessive manner. Thus, suppression of BRCA1 leads to inherited breast cancer, where hypermethylation is often associated with suppression of BRCA1 in non-inherited breast cancers, which is another way of silencing of a gene. Additional examples of genes affected by hypermethylation in several cancers include, the retinoblastoma (Rb) gene; inhibitor of the cell cycle p16INK4A; pro-apoptotic death-associated protein kinase (DAPK); adenomatous polyposis coli (APC); and the estrogen receptor gene. Evidence also indicates that abnormal methylation being the key feature in pre-malignant cells leading to altered signal pathways that facilitate subsequent mutational events which provide the cell with a selective advantage and promotes tumorigenesis.

Methylated DNA sites on interaction with additional epigenetic events such as histone-modifying enzymes, cytosine binding proteins, and DNMTs, in a collaborative manner play a major role in defining the structure of chromatin. PML-RAR fusion protein forms stable complexes with DNMTs at RAR promoter resulting in hypermethylation contributing to carcinogenesis. DNMTs, may also serve as platform for the assembly of chromatin-modifying factors in addition to mediating methylation.

Non-genotoxic carcinogens like phenobarbital are considered to be epigenetic carcinogens because they induce hypermethylation in tumor-sensitive mice treated with it. The data suggests that phenobarbital causes disruption of normal methylation pattern leading to tumor susceptibility and it may act via methylation. In addition, the cellular level of S-adenosyl methionine, an important source of methyl group donor, is affected by nutritional deficiencies of methionine and choline. This suggests that dietary deficiencies can cause perturbation of methylation. In normal stem cells and progenitor cells, epigenetic gene silencing is staunchly followed and it may be silenced during chronic injury and inflammation thereby contributing to carcinogenesis.

In several cancers, mutation of DNA methyl transferases has been observed, which leads directly to changed methylation pattern. Deamination of 5-methyl cytosine to thymine or hydroxylation of 5-methyl cytosine is found to be another way of altered methylation in transformation and to promote mutation.

In the cancer cell genome overall 20-60% hypomethylation in the coding region of gene and of repetitive DNA sequences is observed compared to a normal cell and at the same time certain specific genes that inhibit tumor formation are hypermethylated. This is the major reason for activation of genes in cancer cells that are not normally expressed in a normal cell. Overall misregulation of many epigenetic processes culminates in cancer development.

3.3 PROTO-ONCOGENES AND ONCOGENES

Proto-oncogenes are normal cellular genes that perform certain functions in normal cells and when they mutate will transform themselves into oncogenes and bring about transformation of normal cell into cancer. The transformation of proto-oncogene into oncogene may be brought about by virus or chemical carcinogens. There are evidences to indicate viral transformation of cell by altering proto-oncogene sequence due to insertion of viral genome very close to proto-oncogene or replacement of part of proto-oncogene sequence with viral genome sequence.

Till date, about 60 proto-oncogenes have been discovered, which perform certain functions in normal cells. Each of these proto-oncogenes can mutate into an oncogene, which plays a major role in the development of cancers. In several different types of cancers most of the proto-oncogenes with a variety of mutations have been repeatedly encountered.

Most of the proto-oncogenes are involved in cell communication and signaling pathways in a normal cell, which includes molecules involved in cell signaling-secreted proteins, transmembrane receptors, GTP-binding proteins, protein kinases, gene regulatory proteins, etc. All these molecules normally interact with one another and facilitate proliferation of cells when more cells are needed. But certain mutations alter their functions such that they deliver the signals even when cell proliferation is not required. The receptor for epidermal growth factor (EGF) is encoded by the proto-oncogene c-*erbB* (c for cellular); when EGF binds to the extracellular domain of the receptor, a stimulatory signal inside the cell is generated by the intracellular domain. A mutation in c-*erbB* where the extracellular EGF-binding domain is deleted will turn into an oncogene in such a way that the intracellular stimulatory signal is produced constantly, even if no EGF is present. Similarly, a point mutation at 12th, 13th and 61st codons in a *ras* gene produces a Ras protein that fails to hydrolyze GTP bound to it, thereby, keeping the protein abnormally in active state all the time in cancerous cells. This results in intracellular signal transduction giving signal for unnecessary cell proliferation even when it is not required.

The types of genetic mutations that can transform a proto-oncogene into an oncogene are point mutations; local DNA rearrangements due to deletion; insertional mutagenesis due to integration of oncovirus genome; gene amplification due to translocation of gene near an active promoter which need to be active all the time and chromosomal aberrations (numerical and structural alterations due to fusion of chromatids, loss of heterozygosity, breakage-fusion breakage, etc.). The change can occur in the protein-coding region of proto-oncogene adjacent to its control regions to yield a modified excessive product, because the gene is simply overexpressed. Alternatively, due to certain faults in the process of chromosome replication, the gene may be overexpressed due to its amplification to a high copy number. Some genes respond very specifically to chemical carcinogens and they would show characteristic signature mutation at the same site of the gene all the time with respect to carcinogen. For example, skin tumors induced in mice by dimethyl Benz[a]anthracene (DMBA) show A-to-T transversion mutation 90% of the time exactly at the same site in *ras* gene; this mutation caused by DMBA presumably, alters the nitrogenous base sequence at this site that efficiently induces the skin cells to form a tumor.

A middle-aged man who had been smoking for four decades developed bladder carcinoma, showed point mutation in H-*ras* oncogene. Cigarette smoke contains large number of carcinogens, which enter the lungs in large amounts, from the lungs the carcinogens are carried by the blood and distributed to different parts of the body. The kidneys being major organs for filtration of blood, help in removal of the toxicants and unwanted substances and facilitate excretion of the unwanted chemical species through urine. While these chemical carcinogens of cigarette origin pass through the bladder as urine gets collected in the bladder and retained for quite some time until it is discharged. During this residence time of the urine in the bladder, some of the carcinogen molecules present in the urine come in contact with the cells lining the bladder and enter the cells thereby attacking their DNA. Most of the carcinogens of cigarette origin are known to form adducts with DNA, which might have been responsible for point mutation in the H-*ras* proto-oncogene, which was evident from the change in amino acid sequence of the protein produced by the H-*ras* proto-oncogene. The point mutation induced by chemical carcinogen causes the substitution of **glycine** with **valine** residue in the protein encoded by H-*ras* proto-oncogene. It is a common feature that, a large number of human tumors were found to carry point mutations in one of the three *ras* family genes, namely, H-*ras*, K-*ras* and N-*ras* present in the mammalian genome. Significantly, in each of the tumors that developed in humans, the point mutation in the reading frame of *ras* family genes was seen in one of the three specific codons 12, 61 or less frequently 13, which resulted in the production of Ras oncoproteins.

The *myc* oncogene found in avian myelocytomatosis virus, is strongly deregulated by the viral transcription promoter resulting in amplified expression leading to transformation of cells. Potent transforming powers of *myc* oncogene got further enhanced due to subtle changes in the reading frame of the *myc* oncogene, which led to change in the structure of its encoded Myc oncoprotein. Members of the *myc* gene family are frequently overexpressed or amplified in majority of tumors and the Myc protein provides signal in the nucleus for cell proliferation. Amplified expression of Myc protein causes the cell to enter cell-division cycles, whereas regulated expression of *myc* as it occurs in normal cells, the cell will put a stop to cell division.

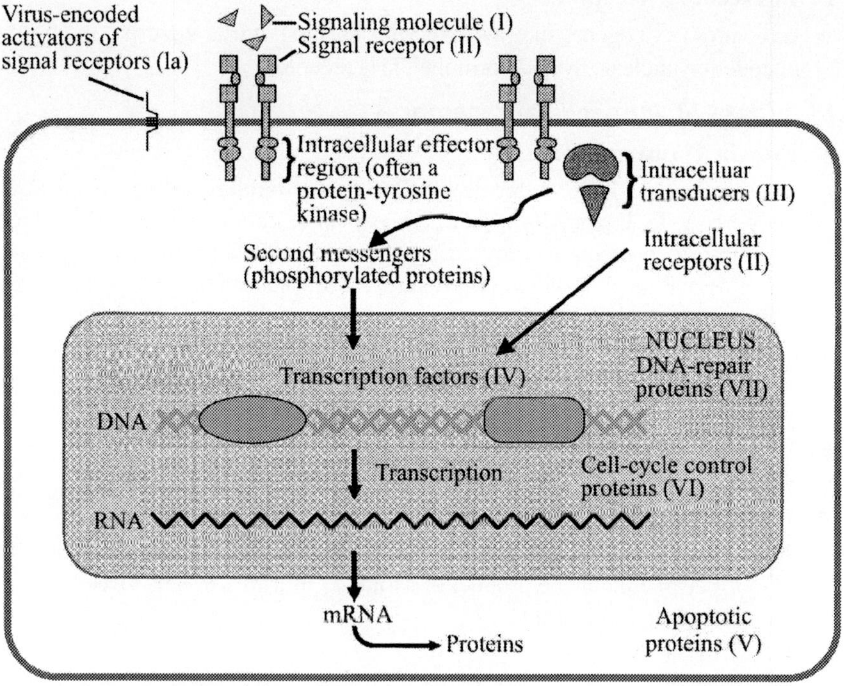

Fig. 3.4. Diagrammatic presentation of functions of the proto-oncogenes (cellular oncogenes)

3.3.1 Functions of the Proto-oncogenes in Normal Cells

The products of the proto-oncogenes mainly act as growth factors or growth factor receptors and some act as intracellular signal transducers, nuclear transcription factors and cell cycle control proteins.

Proto-oncogenic products are classified into 7 different categories (Fig. 3.4), which are as follows:

3.3.1.1 Class I. Growth factor

sis oncogene (like simian sarcoma virus) is known for secretion of platelet derived growth factor (PDGF). It is the only oncogene known so far that encodes for growth factor.

3.3.1.2 Class II. Cell receptors

A. Cell surface receptor with protein tyrosine kinase (PTK) activity

fms proto-oncogene, like McDonough feline sarcoma virus gene encodes plasma membrane colony stimulating factor-1 (CSF-1) receptor. e*rbB* proto-oncogene, similar to avian erythroblastosis virus gene is known to encode for epidermal growth factor (EGF) receptor of plasma membrane.

B. Intracellular receptor

erbA proto-oncogene, like avian erythroblastosis virus gene is known to encode for nuclear thyroid hormone (TH) receptor.

3.3.1.3 Class III. Intracellular receptor

A. Protein Tyrosine Kinase

These receptors have extracellular domain for binding to the ligand and on binding to ligand, they facilitate phosphorylation of tyrosine in the cytoplasmic protein, thereby bringing about signal transduction in the cytoplasm. Phosphorylation of tyrosine residue is brought about by tyrosine kinase enzymatic activity in the intracellular domain of the receptor. These receptors act as growth factor receptors and continuously provide growth stimulatory signals in tumor cells. Some of the proto-oncogenes involved in such activity are *src* (oncogene of avian Rous sarcoma virus); *yes* (Yamaguchi avian sarcoma virus) and *abl* (Abelson's murine leukemia virus).

B. Protein Serine-Threonine Kinase

These protein kinases are specific for serine-threonine residues in proteins of cytoplasm. Oncogene product of Moloney murine sarcoma virus, *mos* is known to function like this.

C. Ras protein

These are G-proteins with GTPase activity found as intracellular proteins in the cytoplasm, sometimes attached to intracellular domain of some growth factor receptor. Proto-oncogenes like H-*ras*, K-*ras* and N-*ras* express these proteins.

3.3.1.4 Class IV. Nuclear transcription factors

These are proteins that mainly regulate transcription by acting as transcription factors. *fos (*feline osteosarcoma*)* proto-oncogene product functions as AP1 transcription factor. Similarly, *myc* (avian myelocytomatosis virus), produces proteins that regulate transcription.

3.3.1.5 Class V. Apoptosis promoters

Tumor suppressor gene like p53 regulates the apoptosis protein genes and promotes apoptosis of abnormal cells. Proteins like Bax, Bad, caspase, IkB and Apaf (apoptosis activation factor) gene are regulated by p53.

3.3.1.6 Class VI. Cell cycle regulatory protein

These proteins are generally called tumor suppressor proteins because they do not allow the cells to divide unnecessarily by having regulatory control over cell cycle proteins. p53 is responsible for control of apoptosis and pRb protein of retinoblastoma gene is responsible for cell cycle regulation.

3.3.1.7 Class VII. DNA repair proteins

Proteins and enzymes involved in nucleotide excision repair, mismatch repair and base excision repair play a major role in DNA repair. Absence of these proteins leads to failure in DNA repair and many of them are responsible for various types of cancers in their absence.

3.3.2 Oncogenes

An oncogene is a mutated version of proto-oncogene, which shows dominant expression and it causes neoplastic transformation of cultured cells on transfection. A transgenic mouse produced by injecting into a mouse egg nucleus DNA fragment of an oncogene linked to a suitable promoter DNA sequence. This recombinant DNA molecule after getting integrated into a mouse chromosome may succeed in expressing in many tissues or it may express in only select few tissues because of the tissue specificity of the associated promoter. The transgenic mice with multiple copies of *myc* or *ras* oncogene in its genome will show amplified expression of the gene in some tissues leading to an increased growth, which after some time undergo mutation and give rise to cancers. On the contrary, most of the cells in the transgenic mouse that express the *myc* or *ras* oncogene alone, however, do not give rise to cancers, which indicates that the single oncogene is not enough to cause neoplastic transformation.

There is a strong correlation between the oncogenes associated with retrovirus and the oncogenes present in the human tumors that are non-virally induced (Table 3.1). In these cases, it was discovered that in human tumor cell genomes the retrovirus-associated oncogenes were present in multiple copies. The DNA of the HL-60 human promyelocytic leukemia cell line was found to have multiple copies of *myc* oncogene, originally discovered in avian myelocytomatosis virus (AMV). The amplified expression of *myc* gene (about 10-20 per diploid genome) results in the increased production of Myc oncoprotein, which somehow favors the proliferation of the cancer cells. The *erbB* gene belongs to avian erythroblastosis

Table 3.1. Examples of oncogenes associated with retroviruses that have been discovered in altered form in human cancers

Name of virus	Species	Oncogene	Homologous oncogene found in human tumors
Rous sarcoma	Chicken	*src*	Colon carcinoma
Abelson's leukemia	Mouse	*abl*	Chronic myelogenous leukemia
Avian erythroblastosis	Mouse	*erbB*	Gastric, lungs, breast
McDonough feline sarcoma	Cat	*fms*	Acute myelogenous leukemia
Murine sarcoma	Mouse	*raf*	Bladder carcinoma
Simian sarcoma	Monkey	*sis*	Many types of tumors of non-ectodermal cells
Harvey sarcoma	Mouse/rat	*H ras*	Bladder carcinoma
Kirsten sarcoma	Mouse/rat	*K-ras*	Many types of tumors
Avian erythroblastosis	Chicken	*erbA*	Liver, kidney, pituitary
Avian myeloblastosis	Chicken	*ets*	Leukemia
Avian myelocytoma	Chicken	*myc*	Many types of tumors

virus (AEV) (malignancy of red blood cell precursors is called **erythroblastosis**), was found to be present in the DNAs of human stomach, breast, and brain tumor cells in multiple copies showing amplified expression and it is a typical feature in majority of human carcinomas.

In many breast cancers, amplified expression (more than five copies per cancer cell) of the *erbB* gene and its related counterparts variously known as *erbB2, neu*, or *HER2* was reported, which correlates with poor survival of patients. Mutant form of *src* oncogene in the genomes of 12% of advanced human colon carcinomas is a common feature.

v-*myc* oncogene of avian myelocytomatosis virus (AMV) and its homolog *c-myc* in normal cells is transformed largely due to deregulation of its expression by creating this gene into an oncogene. In some human tumors, *myc* gene is found to be amplified many times higher than the two copies that exist in the normal human genome and its expression is controlled by its own natural transcriptional promoter. In 30% of aggressive childhood neuroblastomas, N-*myc* a close relative of *c-myc*, is been found to be amplified with corresponding increase in the level of Myc and N-Myc proteins, having potent growth-promoting powers leading to uncontrolled cell proliferation.

The overexpression of c-myc gene in Burkitt's lymphoma was validated from the observation of metaphase chromosome spreads of these tumors. These tumors frequently showed translocations between chromosome 2, 14 and 22 with chromosome 8. It was found that chromosome 8 has *c-myc* gene at the site very close to the break point lies and this sequence is translocated to downstream of the promoter sequence of antibody protein genes. For example, gene for kappa light chain of antibody is present on chromosome 2, the gene for lambda light chain is present on chromosome 22, and the gene for heavy chain is present on chromosome 14. Translocation of c-*myc* very close to any of these three antibody genes results in continuous expression of c-*myc* gene (Fig. 3.5). This causes, overproduction of Myc protein leading to cell proliferation and tumor formation.

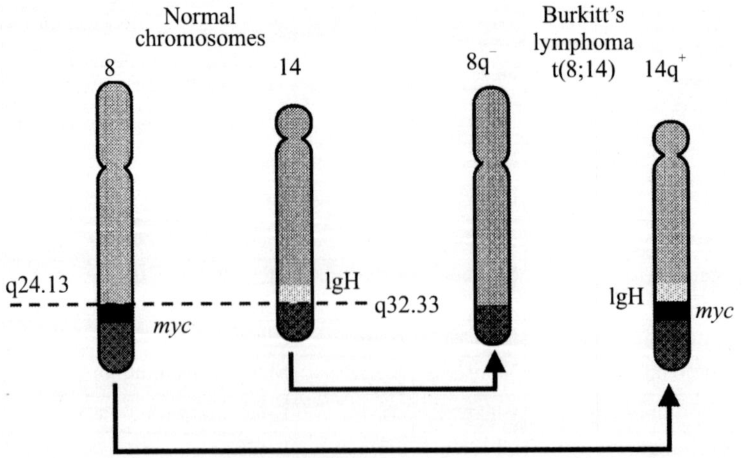

Fig. 3.5. Translocation between chromosome 8 and 14 in Burkitt's lymphoma

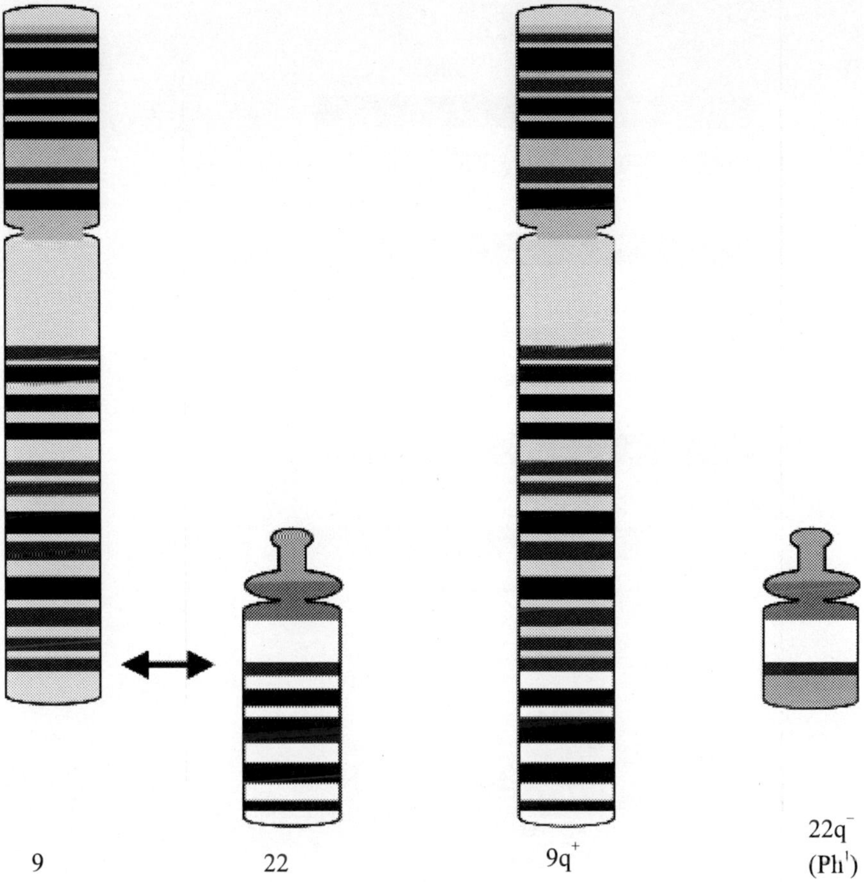

Fig. 3.6. Translocation between 9th and 22nd chromosome in chronic myelogenous leukemia

The chromosomal translocation observed in **chronic myelogenous leukemia** (CML), a bone marrow-derived malignancy results in quite different genetic expression from that found in Burkitt's lymphoma. In this case translocation causes fusion of two distinct reading frames of the genes. On one side of the break point is *abl* proto-oncogene is present on chromosome 9 and on the other side bcr gene is present on chromosome 22. Two simultaneous breaks occur in chromosome 9 and 22 and the segment from chromosome 9 is translocated to the broken region of chromosome 22 (Fig. 3.6). The resulting *bcr-abl* fusion protein (Fig. 3.7) enhances the expression of well-controlled Abl protein, causing it to emit strong growth-promoting signals in a deregulated fashion.

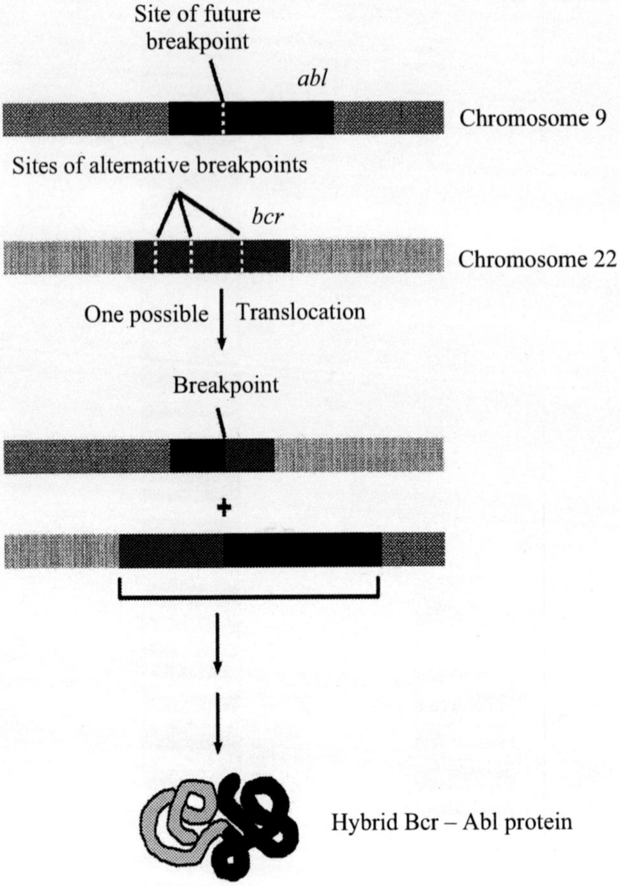

Fig. 3.7. Translocation between 9th and 22nd chromosome leads to collaboration between *bcr* and *abl* genes leading to the formation of fusion protein or oncoprotein

3.3.2.1 Origin of oncogenes from proto-oncogenes

Recent research suggests that cellular oncogene (c-onc) is derived from normal proto-oncogenes by at least five different mechanisms.

(i) Point mutation

(ii) Local DNA rearrangements

(iii) Gene amplification

(iv) Insertional mutagenesis

(v) Chromosomal aberrations (numerical and structural alterations)

(i) Point mutation: Point mutation is a simplest mechanism by which conversion proto-oncogene into an oncogene would occur single base pair change resulting in the production of altered protein, which differs by one amino acid from the protein coded by proto-oncogene. This is frequently observed with respect to *ras* proto-oncogene.

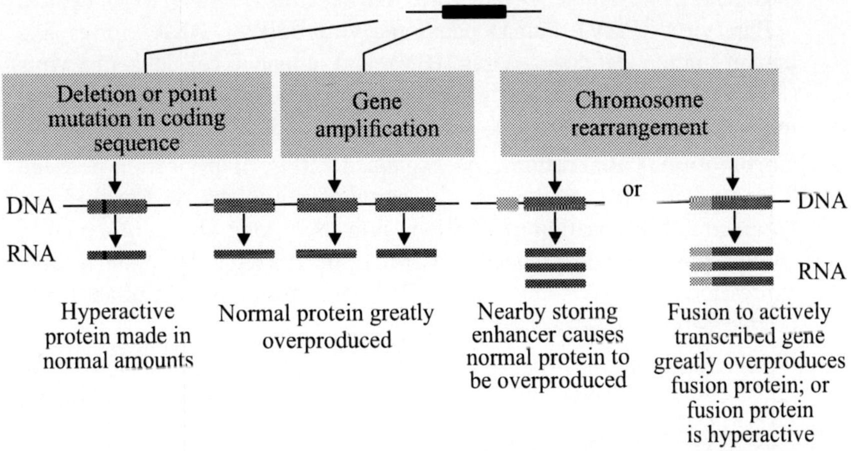

Fig. 3.8. Diagrammatic representation of transformation of proto-oncogene into an oncogene by different mechanisms. Recombination between retroviral DNA and a proto-oncogene is the fourth mechanism (not shown). The effect is like that of chromosome rearrangement, where the proto-oncogene is brought under the control of a viral promoter or fused with a viral gene that is actively transcribed

G → T transversion in the 12th codon (gly → val) of cH-ras proto-oncogene is observed in human bladder cancer. G → A transition in the 12th codon (gly → glu) of cH-ras proto-oncogene is observed in methyl nitrosourea induced rat mammary carcinoma.

(ii) **Local DNA rearrangements:** This mechanism involves deletion or base sequence exchange between proto-oncogenes and surrounding genes due to homologous recombinations. The *trk* oncogene is generated by DNA rearrangements that disrupt 5′end of trk-proto oncogene. The rearrangement results in the production of a fusion protein, i.e., a hybrid protein where NH_2-terminal end of the Trk protein is replaced by an amino acid encoded by a neighboring gene. For example, EGF receptor behaving like an erbB protein.

(iii) **Gene amplification:** Enhanced expression of a gene leads to overproduction of the normal protein encoded by the proto-oncogene. This results in disruption of various regulatory functions in the cell leading to transformation of cell. For example, c-*myc* in Burkitt's lymphoma, N-*myc* in human neuroblastoma and L-*myc* in human lung carcinoma are overexpressed. c-erbB2 is over expressed in human mammary carcinoma. L-*myc* in lung carcinoma (1p32); *erbB1* (7q12-13) in glioblastoma (50%), squamous cell carcinoma (10-20%); K-*ras* (6p12) in lung, ovarian, bladder carcinomas; N-*ras* (1p13) in head and neck cancers; *cyclin E* (19q12) gastric cancers.

(iv) **Insertional mutagenesis:** Insertion of viral DNA into a host chromosome proximity to proto-oncogene takes place, resulting in disruption in the expression of host proto-oncogene and thereby converting it into an oncogene. For example, DNA viruses like hepatitis B virus (HBV), Epstein – Barr virus (EBV), human papilloma virus (HPV); RNA viruses like human immunodeficiency virus (HIV), and human T cell leukemia virus (HTLV). Most common oncogenes that seem to be activated by insertional mutagenesis are *myc, erbB*, K-*ras, int-1, -2*, and *-3.*

(v) Chromosomal aberrations: As explained earlier, translocation between 8th long arm to the 14th long arm of chromosome is observed in Burkitt's lymphoma, translocation of 22nd long arm to 9th long arm is observed in chronic myelogenous leukemia (CML). In Burkitt's lymphoma, over expression of c-*myc* is observed and in CML a fusion protein of abl-bcr is produced.

In human lymphoid cancer, follicular B cell lymphoma, associated with translocation between long arm of 14th and 18th chromosome (14q32 : 18q21) involves deregulation of *bcl*-2 proto-oncogene; and chronic B cell lymphomas involves deregulation of *bcl*-3 proto-oncogene. T-cell chronic leukemia is associated with inversion or translocation of long arm of chromosome 14.

T-cell acuter leukemias (T-ALL) is associated with recurring translocations between following chromosomes:

t (8:14)	(q24:q32)	t (7:9)	(q35:q34)
t (11:14)	(p15:q11)	t (7:19)	(q35:p13)
t (1:14)	(p32:q11)	t (7:9)	(q34:q34.5)
t (10:14)	(q24:q11)	t (1:7)	(p34:q34)
t (11:14)	(p13:q11)	t (7:10)	(q35:q24)

Solid tumors are also known to show specific transnlocations:

Ewig's sarcoma (neuroectodermal tumor) t (11:22) (q24:q12)

Synovial sarcoma t (X:18) (p11:q11)

Alveolar rhabdomyosarcoma t (2:13) (q37:q14)

Myxoid liposarcoma t (12:16) (q11-14:p11)

(a) Aneuploidy

- Trisomy of chromosome 12 is observed in chronic lymphocytic leukemia
- Trisomy of chromosome 8 is observed in blast phase of chronic myelogenous leukemia (CML).
- Trisomy of chromosome 15 is observed in murine T cell leukemia induced in human T cells.
- Monosomy of chromosome 15 is observed in Syrian hamster sarcomas due to transfection by ras and myc oncogene in human fibroblast culture.

3.3.3 Oncoprotein as a Result of Altered Growth Factor Receptor

In 1984, it was discovered that oncoprotein encoded by the *erbB* oncogene resembles the sequence of the EGF receptor (Fig. 3.9). *erbB* oncogene is originally discovered in the genome of avian erythroblastosis virus (AEV), a retrovirus capable of transforming red blood cell precursors rapidly to leukemia (**erythroleukemia).**

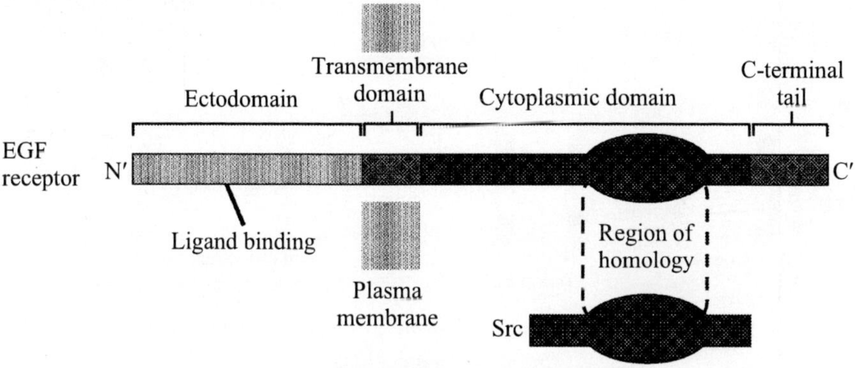

Fig. 3.9. Typical architecture of EGF receptor

On detailed examination of *erbB* oncogene encoded oncoprotein of avian erythroblastosis virus revealed deleted amino acid sequence in the N-terminal ectodomain of the EGF receptor (Fig. 3.10). Due to deletion in the N-terminal sequences of the ErbB oncoprotein it cannot recognize and bind to EGF, but still it stimulates cell proliferation by auto activation. The cytoplasmic domain of the EGF receptor is homologous to Src oncoprotein of Rous sarcoma virus and it is tyrosine kinase domain, which facilitates signal transduction through phosphorylation. The truncated ectodomain EGF receptor protein sends growth stimulating signals to cell in a constitutive manner by self-activation (self-firing) of tyrosine kinase domain without binding to EGF. It is called ligand–independent firing.

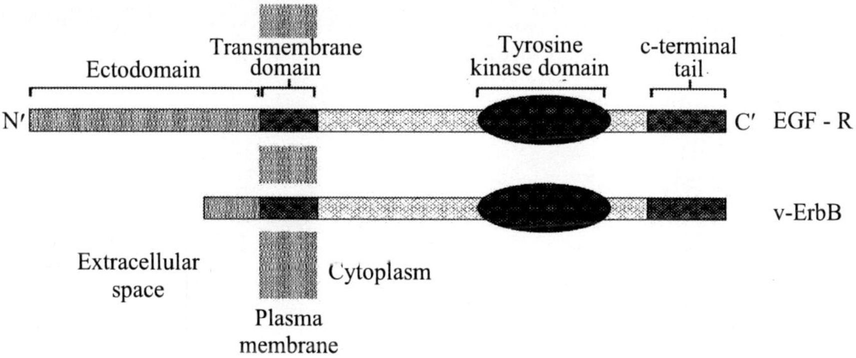

Fig. 3.10. EGF receptor and *v-erbB* gene product (EGF-like receptor)

A point mutation in the genes encoding growth factor receptors resulting in change in amino acid residue in the transmembrane domain, or in the ectodomain and cytoplasmic domain of some receptors, which can provoke ligand-independent self-firing of the receptor (Fig. 3.11).

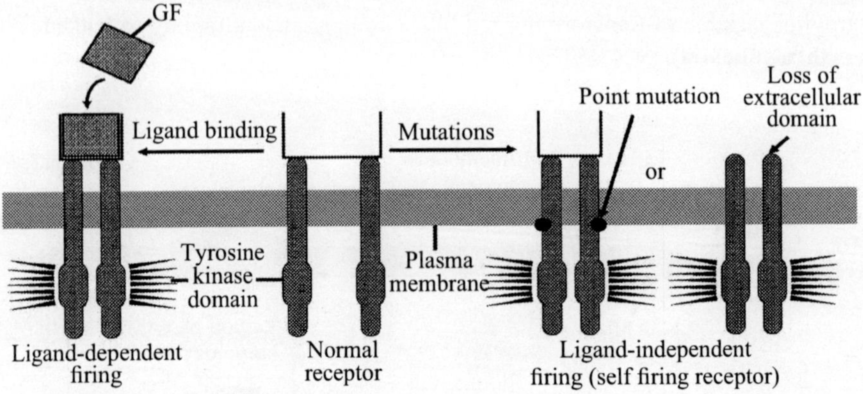

Fig. 3.11. Growth factor receptors showing two types of ligand independent firing due to mutations

3.3.4 An Oncogene Derived from a Growth Factor Gene: The *sis* Oncogene

In 1983, it was discovered that the B chain of platelet derived growth factor (PDGF) resembles the simian sarcoma virus oncogene v-*sis* encoded oncoprotein. PDGF serves as growth factor for mesenchymal cells, such as fibroblasts, adipocytes, smooth muscle cells and endothelial cells. The underlying important mechanism between PDGF and the *sis*-encoded oncoprotein in transformation of cells was understood from the detailed study of simian sarcoma virus infected cells. Infected cells having *sis* oncogene release copious amounts of *sis* protein into the surrounding medium, which resembles PDGF. PDGF-like factor attaches to PDGF-R (receptor) displayed by the same cell that has just synthesized and released it. This results in strong self-activation (auto-activation) of the cell's PDGF receptors, in turn, stimulating the cells with continuous growth-stimulating signals by the ligand-activated PDGF-R (Fig. 3.12).

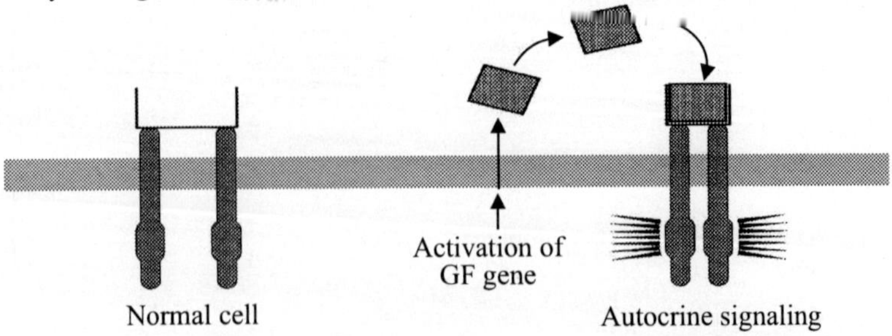

Fig. 3.12. *Sis* oncoprotein transformed tumor cell expressing autocrine growth factor and firing the receptor

In fact, there are varieties of human tumors that are known to produce and release substantial amounts of self-stimulating growth factors to which the tumor cells respond (Table.3.2).

Table 3.2. Most commonly involved receptors in tumors

Name of receptor	Main ligand	Types of alteration	Types of tumors
EGF-R/ErbB1	EGF, TGF-α	Overexpression	Breast, head and neck, non-small cell lung cancer, ovarian cancer
EGF-R/ErbB1	EGF	Truncation of ectodomain	Glioblastoma, lung and breast carcinoma
ErbB2/HER2/ Neu	NRG, EGF	Overexpression	Breast adenocarcinoma
FGF-R3	FGF	Overexpression, amino acid substitution	Multiple myeloma, bladder and cervical carcinomas

Some human lung cancers are known to produce as many as three distinct growth factors like transforming growth factor-α (TGF-α), stem cell factor (SCF) and insulin-like growth factor (IGF), at the same time, simultaneously express the receptors for these three ligands, resulting in establishment of three autocrine signaling loops simultaneously, which stimulates tumor growth.

3.3.5 Ras Protein Functions Almost Like a G Protein

Ras protein binds to GTP and gets activated to bring about downstream signaling. GTPase acts on GTP bound to Ras protein and converts it into GDP, which results in inactivation of Ras protein. Inactive Ras protein once again gets charged with GTP by displacing GDP with the help of **GEF (guanine nucleotide exchange factor)** and the cycle of Ras protein activation and inactivation continues resulting in signal transduction within the cytoplasm of the cell (Fig. 3.13). Ras oncoprotein encoded by Harvey sarcoma virus showed point mutation in *ras* oncogene, which

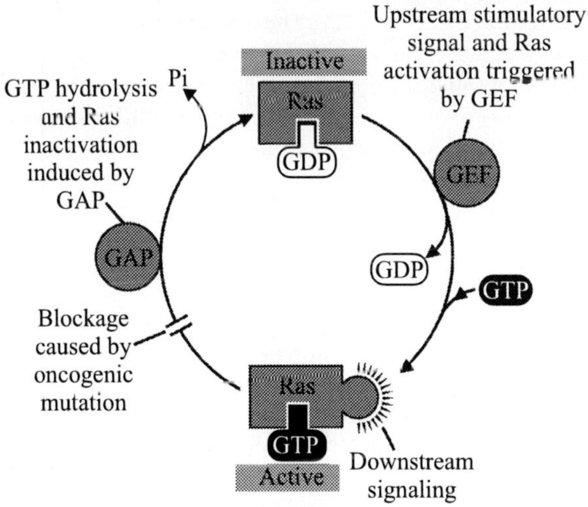

Fig. 3.13. Amplified Ras signaling leading to oncogenesis

could bind to GTP like normal Ras protein, but this oncoprotein virtually have lost all GTPase activity because of loss of **GAP (GTPase activating protein)** function (Fig. 3.13). In such a condition, it will be an actively emitting signal and activated Ras oncoprotein cannot turn itself off. The negative feedback loop that is so essential to the operations of the normal Ras protein is damaged due to point mutation resulting in amino acid substitution.

Prolonged signals emitted by Ras oncoprotein for indefinite period floods the cell with these signals resulting in oncogenesis. Only those rare cells gain proliferative advantage over their wild-type counterparts because of the acquired mutations affecting one of the three amino acid residues of Ras (residues 12, 61 or rarely, 13), thereby become the ancestors of the cells in a tumor mass.

3.3.6 Some Integrins are Necessary for Tumorigenesis

β1 integrin overexpression seems to be responsible for development of tumors. Especially in mammary tumors, it has been observed that β1 integrin overexpresses in ductulus of the mammary gland which has undergone transformation.

3.4 CELL PROLIFERATION FACILITATED BY Wnt-β-CATENIN PATHWAY

Wnt proto-oncogene is one of the first to have been discovered. Integration of viral genome in cellular Wnt gene (insertional mutagenesis) resulting in alteration in genetic sequence of cellular Wnt gene leading to constitutive expression of Wnt pathway or the mutation that results in constitutive expression of Wnt signaling pathway have been commonly observed in several types of cancers. For example, in colorectal cancer, constitutive activation of Wnt pathway is responsible 90% of the time together with inactivation of APC gene function by deletion (-5q21) or activation of β-catenin.

There is a strong link between stem cells, Wnt pathway and cancer of the small intestine or colon because intestinal tissue is highly regenerative tissue which on daily basis has to renew its epithelium. The stem cells and epithelial progenitor cells, which are also called transit amplifying cells residing in the crypts of villi give rise to more differentiated cells that migrate up along the villi (Fig. 3.14). Fully differentiated cells upon reaching the top of the villi undergo apoptosis and this process of rejuvenation of intestinal epithelial cells takes place on day-to-day basis. In the normal cells Wnt signaling maintains the stem cells and the progenitor cells status in the crypts.

β-catenin is an important protein found attached to the intracellular domain of cell adhesion receptor E-cadherin molecule (Fig. 3.15a). In the cytoplasm β-catenin also exists in soluble form and its turnover rate is less than 20 minutes. β-catenin acts as an important component of the transcription factor in the nucleus. In a normal cell, soon after the synthesis of β-catenin it combines with two other cellular proteins–Apc (the adenomatous polyposis coli protein) and axin to form multiprotein complex. These two proteins facilitate β-catenin to be brought closer to GSK-3β executioner. GSK-3β facilitates phosphorylation of β-catenin and ensures that it is ubiquitylated after phosphorylation and destroyed.

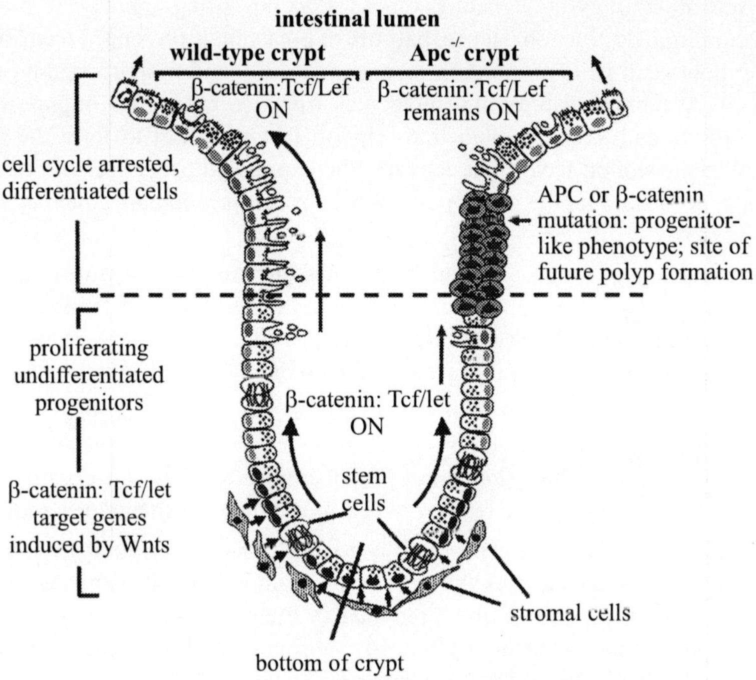

Fig. 3.14. Contribution of stem cells in the crypt area of the intestine for the replacement of dead cells at the top of the villi by the migration of transit amplifying cells toward the top of the villi and final differentiation into epithelial cells

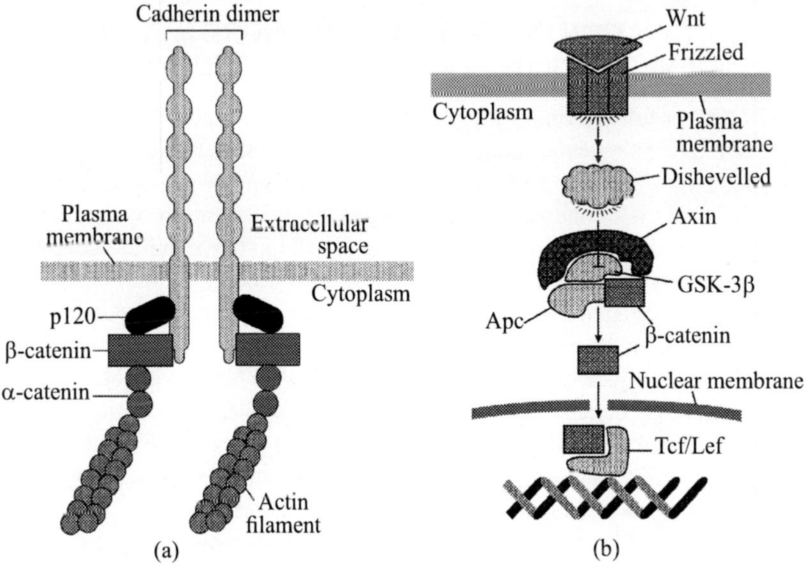

Fig. 3.15. (a) The role of β-catenin in the cell adhesion molecule. (b) Intracellular role of β-catenin

Activation of Wnt signaling blocks GSK-3β firing thereby it prevents β-catenin from destruction. Hence, half life of β-catenin is prolonged from 20 min to 1-2 hours and its concentration increases steadily and proportionately within the cell. Accumulated β-catenin molecules from the cytoplasm migrate to the nucleoplasm and associate with transcription factor Tcf/Lef to form the multi-subunit transcription factor that activates the expression of number of important target genes including the genes responsible for cell proliferation, such as **cyclin D1** and **myc.**

Excessive expression of β-catenin in intestinal stem cells ensures that these cells maintained in an undifferentiated state, rather than differentiate into a specialized cell lining the wall of the intestinal villi. Such high levels expression of β-catenin is very important for the formation of colon carcinoma.

It is very well known that in many cancers showing metastasis, E-cadherin is shed off or gene of E-cadherin is mutated. In such a condition, due to non-availability of intracellular domain of E-cadherin for binding of β-catenin, it will accumulate in the cytoplasm leading to cell proliferation as mentioned above. .

In many human breast cancers, four- to tenfold increased expression of Wnt is observed, which facilitates the operation of autocrine and paracrine growth-stimulatory pathways. It is also seen that in many cancers, β-catenin gene is mutated such that β-catenin cannot be phosphorylated, consequence of that would lead to accumulation of high levels of β-catenin in the nucleus to facilitate transcription of cell proliferation genes. In almost all colon carcinomas, β-catenin degradation is defective because of defect in APC protein which otherwise would have facilitated its degradation.

3.5 COLLABORATION BETWEEN TWO OR MORE MUTANT ONCOGENES FACILITATES TRANSFORMATION

The resistance of fully normal rodent cells to mutant *ras*-induced transformation led to certain interesting experiments with known oncogenes. Polyomavirus (DNA tumor virus), for example, bears two oncogenes, ***middle T*** and ***large T*** genes, which collaborate with one another and facilitate transformation of rodent cells. The large T oncoprotein facilitates adaptation of cells to tissue culture conditions and their immortalization, while the middle T oncoprotein elicits many of the characteristics associated with *ras* oncogene, where cells become round, loss of contact inhibition, and acquire anchorage independent growth, characteristics of all cancer cells. The genetics of transformation by DNA tumor viruses suggested that mutant cellular genes might also collaborate in cell transformation. In fact, a line of human promyelocytic leukemia cells was discovered to carry both an activated N-*ras* and an activated *myc* oncogene. This suggested the possibility that these two cellular oncogenes were cooperating to create the malignant phenotype of the leukemic cells. In an experiment, when a *myc* oncogene together with an H-*ras* oncogene was introduced into rat embryo fibroblasts (REFs) the cells readily underwent transformation showing morphologically different appearance, as well as tumorigenic abilities. On the other hand, neither of these oncogenes on its own was able to bring about transformation in REFs or in differentiated cells.

myc and *ras* cellular oncogenes clearly affected cell phenotype in quite different ways, since they were able to complement one another in eliciting cell transformation. Each seemed to be specialized to evoke a subset of the cellular phenotypes associated with the transformed state. For example, *ras* can induce the cells to undergo spherical shape, cause loss of contact inhibition and acquisition of anchorage independent growth, whereas *myc* induces the cells to become immortalized and reduce the cellular requirement of growth hormones. Similar results were found in experiments, where E1A oncogene of human adenovirus 5 was used as collaborating partner of a *ras* oncogene. Once again, the two oncogenes were found to be collaborating and complementary in effect. The *ras* oncogene is capable of collaborating with the SV40 large T oncogene, polyoma large T oncogene, but not with middle T oncogene, bcl-2, erbB, etc. Similarly, *myc* collaborates with middle T oncogene, bcl-2, and erbB but not with erbA, E1A, SV40 large T oncogene. The reason being cytoplasmic oncoproteins are encoded by *ras*-like oncogenes, whereas proteins responsible for nuclear action are encoded by *myc*-like oncogenes. It is well known that Ras-like oncoproteins constitute cytoplasmic mitogenic signal cascade and Myc-like oncoproteins perturb in various ways cell cycle control machinery. From this observation it can be said that oncogenes show pleiotropic (chain of interdependent events) effect in cell to bring about transformation of a cell.

The collaboration between oncogene was further understood by mating transgenic mice carrying a *myc* oncogene, the other one carrying a *ras* oncogene so that the progeny obtained would carry both oncogenes together. *myc-ras* hybrid offspring developed cancers at a much higher rate than either parental strain, but at the same time all the cells in the hybrid progeny did not show cancerous growth, rather there was scattered isolated tumors among normal cells. This proves that, even with the expression of two collaborating oncogenes, there is a need for cells to undergo further mutations to become cancerous.

When two or more specific oncogenes synergistically act to bring about transformation of cells to cancerous growth is known as ***oncogene collaboration***, which can be further demonstrated by in vitro as well as in vivo experiments. Rat embryo fibroblasts culture on transfection with a *ras* or with a *myc* oncogene alone will not bring about transformation of cells, on the contrary, cells continue to behave normal. If the rat embryo fibroblasts are transfected with both oncogenes together, the cells undergo transformation immediately. Cancers originating from different cell types of different tissue origins different combinations of oncogenes will collaborate with one another for transformation. In lymphocyte-derived cancer such as B-cell lymphoma, prefers collaboration between *myc* and the *bcl*-2 gene is observed. Overexpression of *myc* alone in cells drives the cell to undergo continuous cell division cycles, but it will not succeed in cancer development because apoptosis will be triggered to get rid of progeny of such abnormally forced cell divisions. On the contrary, if *bcl*-2 is overexpressed at the same time in those cells, it results in survival of progeny cells and they will further proliferate because *bcl*-2 acts as an oncogene and protein product Bcl-2 is an inhibitor of apoptosis.

The cancer is a phenomenon, which puts in place fail-safe mechanism of the complex network of regulatory controls on cell proliferation and survival. Multiple control mechanisms that operate in parallel are put in place, so that a single faulty component does not lead to disastrous end to cancer cell. In this control system, proto-oncogene's role is only half and the tumor suppressor genes counterbalance them. Deletions and point mutations or hypermethylation of tumor suppressor genes has a significant role in human cancer as do mutations of proto-oncogenes into oncogenes.

Table 3.3. Oncogenic collaborations and their mechanism of action

Oncogene pair	Cell type	Mechanism of action
ras + E1A	Mouse embryo fibroblast	**ras:** induces proliferation and senescence **E1A:** prevents senescence
TGF-α + myc	Mouse mammary epithelial cells	**TGF-α:** induces proliferation and blocks apoptosis **myc:** induces proliferation and apoptosis
ras + myc	Rat fibroblasts	**ras:** induces anchorage independent growth **myc:** induces immortalization

Contd...

3.6 ANGIOGENESIS IS THE KEY FOR CANCER PROGRESSION

As early as 1950s, pathologists noted that cancer cells grew by stimulation the blood vessels to grow around them and the process is called angiogenesis. Tumor cells do not grow if they are located more than about 0.2 mm away from blood vessels and those tumor cells that are even farther away will dye because of lack of nutrition and oxygen. This threshold of 0.2 mm in the living tissue represents the distance at which oxygen can effectively diffuse through the living tissues. Cells located within 0.2 mm radius from the blood vessel can rely on guaranteed supply of oxygen and those situated farther away suffer from moderate to severe hypoxia. In hypoxic condition, tissue cells become necrotic and may suffer apoptotic death triggered by p53 gene. Inactivation of p53 in cancer cells is the most common feature, which enables them to survive even though they are under extreme stress in the small perimeter surrounding each capillary.

Hypoxia is the only price paid by the cells lacking proximity to the circulatory system. Effective interaction of vasculature with cells is important to get the constant supply of nutrients and to throwaway the metabolic waste products, including carbon dioxide. More specifically, capillaries appear to form wherever they are needed by the assistance of non-vasculature parenchymal cells in a normal tissue. Tumor cells cannot rely upon genetic information to aid them in configuring their blood supply and must design their own layout of blood vessels for their survival, because hypoxia will trigger the death of tumor cells.

Angiogenesis is triggered by one of the important growth factors known as **vascular endothelial growth factor (VEGF)**. The VEGF gene expression is controlled by the oxygen tension in the cell environment, which in turn, regulates the expression of **Von-Hippel Lindau (VHL) gene. HIF1 (hypoxia inducible factor)** protein is the product of VHL gene, which regulates the expression of VEGF gene (Fig. 3.16). The production of VEGF is associated with tumor cells, macrophages, and myofibroblasts and it depends on the stage of progression of tumor and tumor type. VEGF and another important angiogenic factor called **basic fibroblast growth factor (bFGF)** binds to its cognate receptor on the endothelial cells and triggers their proliferation. Proliferating endothelial cells arrange themselves to construct blood capillaries. Moreover, several other cell types like pericytes and stromal cells in addition to endothelial cells contribute to the construction of capillaries and larger vessels.

In addition to VEGF and bFGF, other growth factors such as **transforming growth factor β and χ (TGFβ and χ), acidic fibroblast growth factor (aFGF), angiogenin, tumor necrosis factor β (TNFβ), platelet derived growth factor (PDGF), granulocyte colony stimulating factor (GCSF), placental growth factor (PGF), Interleukin-8 (IL-8), hepatocyte growth factor (HGF), proliferin, angiopoietin** and **leptin** also facilitate growth of blood vessels.

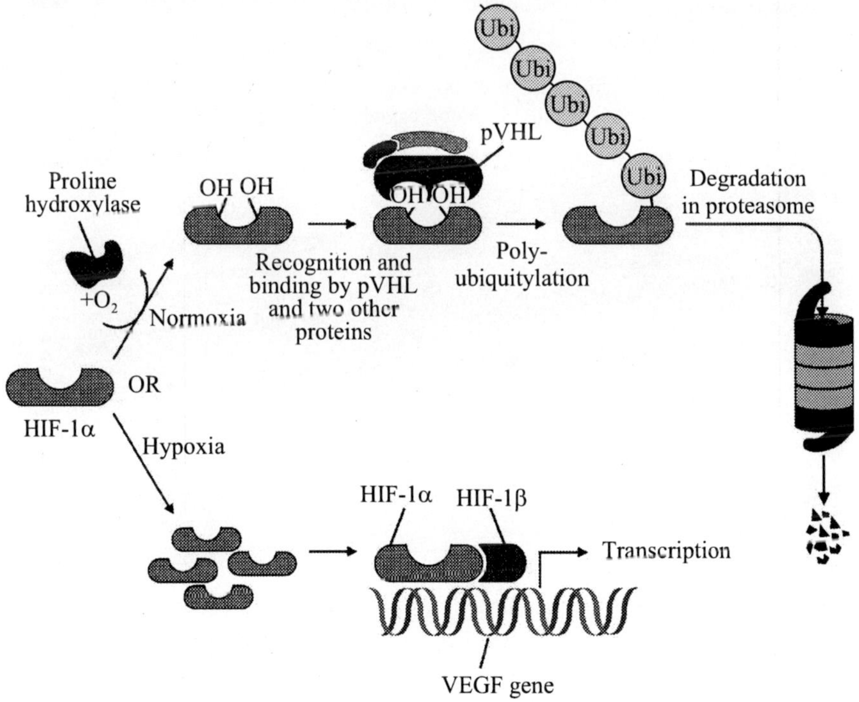

Fig. 3.16. HIF-1 and its regulation by pVHL

The systematic covering of capillaries by pericytes seen in normal tissue is altered to chaotic arrangement in the capillaries associated with tumor tissue. Capillaries in tumor tissues have three times greater diameter than their counterparts in normal tissue. In addition, the overall architecture of the blood vessels surrounding the tumor masses and within is quite haphazard (Figs. 3.17 and 3.18). Often the blood vessels stop abruptly or circle back to end up in a loop. The haphazard architecture of the blood vessels in tumors is because of loss of contact or adhesion between the endothelial cells of blood vessels associated with tumors, which otherwise in normal tissue would have resulted in seamless lining of the lumen of capillaries. Due to several microns-wide gaps between the endothelial cells, capillaries in tumors become highly leaky and gain ten times more permeability than normal capillaries. The leaking capillaries cause the deposition of fibrin in the tumor parenchyma.

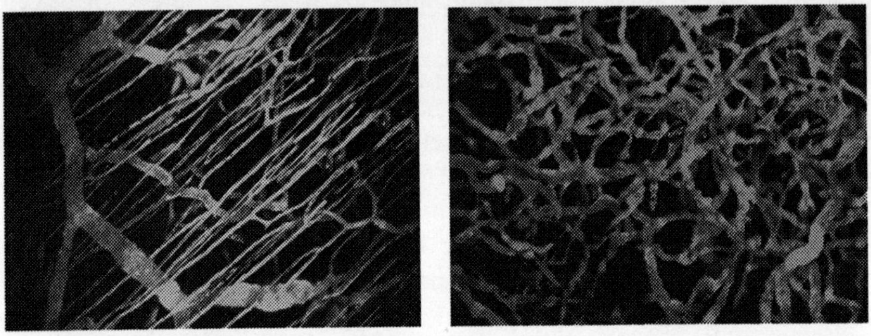

Normal tissue　　　　Tumor

Fig. 3.17. Normal architecture of blood vessels in normal tissue and abnormal architecture of blood vessels in tumors

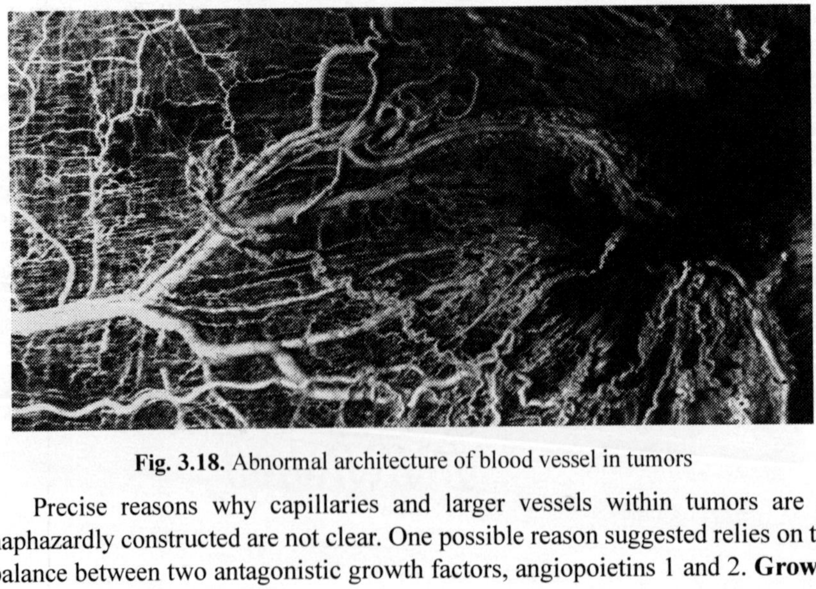

Fig. 3.18. Abnormal architecture of blood vessel in tumors

Precise reasons why capillaries and larger vessels within tumors are so haphazardly constructed are not clear. One possible reason suggested relies on the balance between two antagonistic growth factors, angiopoietins 1 and 2. **Growth**

of blood capillaries is initiated by VEGF, which is responsible for attracting and stimulating endothelial cells and a mix of angiopoietins 1 and 2 induces endothelial cells to recruit the pericytes and smooth muscle cells to arrange properly for the construction of blood vessel with appropriate proportion of these cell types. An imbalance of these two antagonistic angiopoietins, together with the greatly elevated levels of VEGF within tumors is suspected to be responsible for construction of defective capillaries of larger dimension within neoplasm.

Lumen of the blood vessel is lined by endothelial cells, which in turn, are surrounded by pericytes and vascular smooth muscle cells (Fig. 3.19).

Accumulation of substantial amounts of fluid in the parenchymal spaces within a tumor occurs due to leakiness of tumor-associated blood capillaries. In normal tissues, the lymphatic vessels facilitate draining of fluids, which eventually gets emptied into the venous circulation. The ongoing expansion of the cells in solid tumors exerts pressure on the lymphatic vessels leading to collapse of the lymphatic system.

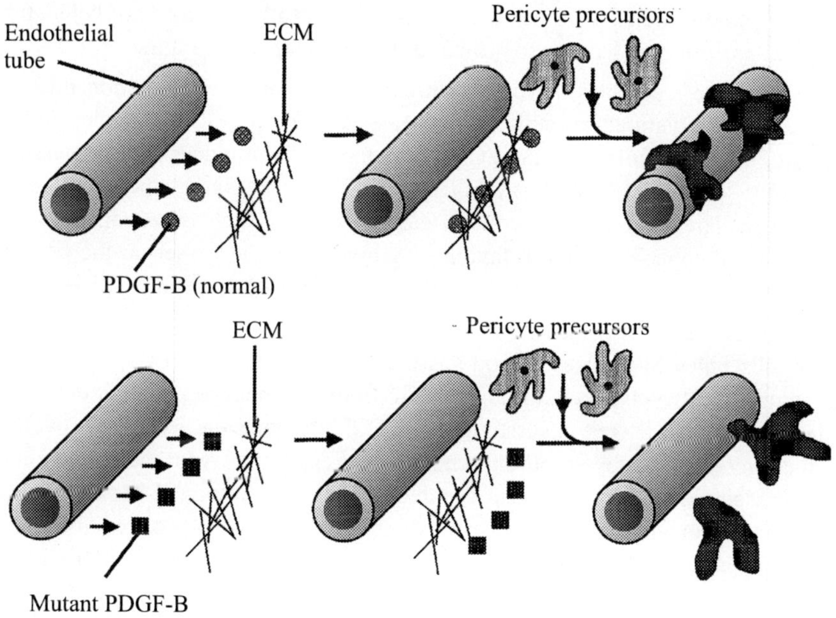

Fig. 3.19. Pericytes, smooth muscle cells, and endothelial cells of the micro-vessels getting assembled for the construction of blood vessel

3.6.1 Tripping the Angiogenic Swltch

Whenever groups of cells, including cancer cells suffer from hypoxia, automatic release of **angiogenic factors I** takes place, thereby provoking the growth of capillaries in their midst. This relieves the cell from clutches of hypoxia and results in an appropriate density of capillaries in the tissue harboring these cells.

In fact, as tumors progress, the ability to attract or grow blood vessels around tumor becomes very important for the tumor's survival, which many tumor cell populations initially do not possess and must acquire. Those tumor cells that are within 0.2 mm distance of the blood vessel grow quickly and become metastatic, whereas those that are farther away from blood vessels grow slowly and show apoptosis and necrosis to a great extent. At some stage of progression when apoptosis favoring gene is switched off due to mutation in tumor cells, it provides an environment for the growth of blood vessels by favoring the expression of genes VEGF and angiopoietin.

In an experiment conducted on transgenic mice transfected with large T and middle T oncogene of SV40 to induce pancreatic islet cell tumors, it was observed that it took more than 7 weeks for the hyperplastic (neoplastic) nodules of islet cells to induce the blood vessel formation. Initially, the transformed islet cells showed high rate of proliferation and death, where the tumor size remained the same for a long period because of balance between cell death and cell proliferation. Suddenly after 10th week there was increase in the size of tumors islet cell and growth of blood vessels around the tumors of islet cells indicating switching on of "angiogenic switch". This resulted in decreased death rate in tumor cells and increased proliferation leading to growth of tumor in size and volume.

Tumor area resembles a wounded area showing high inflammation due to infiltration of inflammatory cells like macrophage, mast cells and neutrophils. In addition, extracellular matrix (ECM) of tumor cells produces matrix metallo proteiase-9 (MMP-9), which mobilizes VEGF by cleaving the inhibitory component. The inflammatory cells release MMP-9, which is responsible for tripping of angiogenic switch in favour of growth of blood vessels at the site of tumor, which otherwise experiences extreme attrition (cell death) due to hypoxia.

In VEGF gene knock out mice, when the same experiment was repeated, the tumor cells failed to grow the blood vessels in the absence of VEGF, indicating that angiogenic switch occurs through VEGF leading to batteries of other changes in the tumor site. It is well understood that VEGF promotes the growth of already existing blood vessels by sprouting (shooting) of capillaries from the preexisting blood vessels, in addition it is also capable of initiating formation of new blood vessels in tumor areas, which have no direct contact with blood vessels. This happens by attracting endothelial precursor cells (EPC) to the site of tumor where new blood vessel is to be established. EPCs originate in bone marrow and travel throughout the body through blood. As and when VEGF secretion occurs in an area, EPC are attracted towards the area where VEGF concentration is high. EPCs undergo self- assembly in the area where VEGF secretion is found and align themselves to form the blood capillaries. Once the EPCs align, rest of the cells responsible for formation of blood vessel will fall in line and assemble over the EPCs. The stromal derived factor-1 (SDF-1) or CXCL-12 released by the stromal cells in the vicinity of tumor is also responsible for the recruitment of EPCs to the tumor site. Invasive characteristics of tumor cells and triggering intense angiogenesis are often tightly coupled processes, and it correlates with increasing degree of malignancy.

It is observed that, small number of cells within tumor gain the ability of switching the angiogenic switch and proliferate to dominate the tumor site, thereby imparting the angiogenic phenotype to the tumor. In fact, analyses of cells isolated from the explanted human tumors indicate great heterogeneity in the angiogenic powers amongst the different population to tumor cells, with some cancer cells having high angiogenic potential and some without. This indicates that, within a tumor mass, long after the tripping of angiogenic switch, the weakly angiogenic cancer cells rely on the strongly angiogenic neighboring tumor cells in order to acquire adequate vasculature.

The mechanism of angiogenic switch operation was further understood from the study of mice for an Id1 and Id3 gene mutation. The mice with $Id1^{+/-}$ and $Id3^{-/-}$ genotype, when receive the tumor transplant, fail to grow blood vessels around the transplanted tumor despite the presence of VEGF and angiopoietin, hence the tumor dies. On the other hand, mice with $Id1^{+/+}$ and $Id3^{+/+}$ genotype favor the transplanted tumor growth by facilitating growth of blood vessels. It appears that the genes, Id1 and Id3, play a major role in growth of blood vessels in the presence of VEGF and angiopoietin.

3.6.2 Suppression of Angiogenesis

Excessive angiogenesis is blocked by components secreted by the extracellular matrix like **Arrestin, Canstatin, Endorepellin, Endostatin, Anastellin, fibulin, Thrombospondin 1 and 2, tumstatin, chondromodulin and Troponin**. The best characterized of these is the thrombospondin-1 (Tsp-1). Tsp-1 interacts with the receptor on endothelial cells and halts their proliferation. In addition, it also induces the production of Fas ligand (FasL-death protein), which binds to proapoptotic Fas receptor (FasR-death receptor). Therefore, Tsp-1 induces endothelial cells to release FasL, in an autocrine fashion it will trigger the death of endothelial cells and stop further proliferation (Fig. 3.20).

Interestingly, endothelial cells that are actively proliferating and those recently stopped proliferating express Fas receptor and its expression on the membrane is suppressed once the endothelial cells have successfully formed mature capillaries and have stopped dividing. Once Tsp-1 initiates proapoptotic reaction inside the cytoplasm, it activates caspase cascade, which is further stabilized by other anti-angiogenic proteins.

The transcription of Tsp-1 is strongly induced by p53 and loss of p53 function, which is the most common feature observed in majority of tumors, leads to substantial decrease in Tsp-1 levels. This permits unchecked angiogenesis in tumor cells. The Ras oncoprotein, acting through a complex signaling cascade, acts in the opposite fashion, since it causes shutdown of TSP1 gene expression. This results in substantial increase in angiogenic power of ras transformed tumor cells.

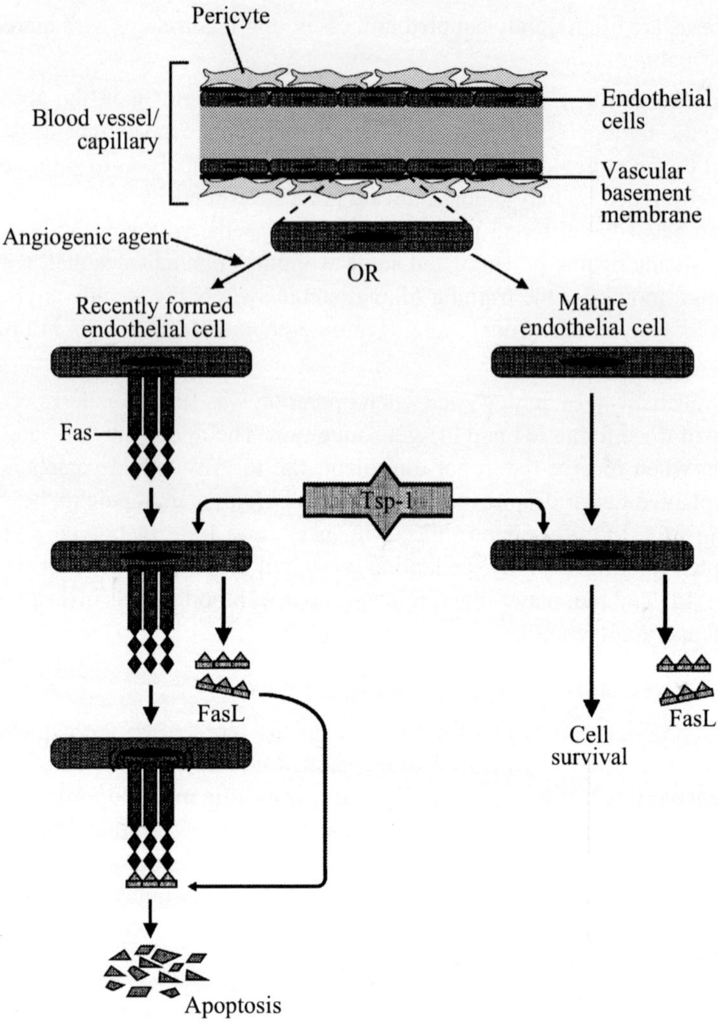

Fig. 3.20. Thrombospondin (Tsp-1) response on endothelial cells

3.6.3 Inhibition of Angiogenesis by Endogenous Factors

These are derived from extracellular matrix (ECM), which are, **Arresten, Canstatin, Endorepellin, Endostatin, Anastellin, Fibulin, Thrombospondin-1 and 2, Tumstatin, Chondromodulin I, Troponin I.**

3.6.4 Non-matrix Derived Inhibitors of Angiogenesis

Interferon-α (IFN- α); Interleukins (IL-1β, -12, -18); Platelet factor-4; Angiostatin; Antithrombin III; Vasostatin; 2-methoxyestradiol; Prolactin fragment; Plasminogen kringle 5; Prothrombin kringle 2.

3.7 INVOLVEMENT OF BLOOD VESSELS IN METASTASIS

Majority of invasive and metastatic cancers arising from epithelial tissues (carcinomas) and the cancers arising from other tissues like connective tissue and nervous tissues, often follow similar paths. Even certain hematopoietic tumors, called lymphomas, at an early phase will be localized and in later phase they may get disseminated to distant anatomical sites. This complex sequence of migration of tumor cells is called ***invasion-metastasis cascade*** as illustrated in Fig. 3.21.

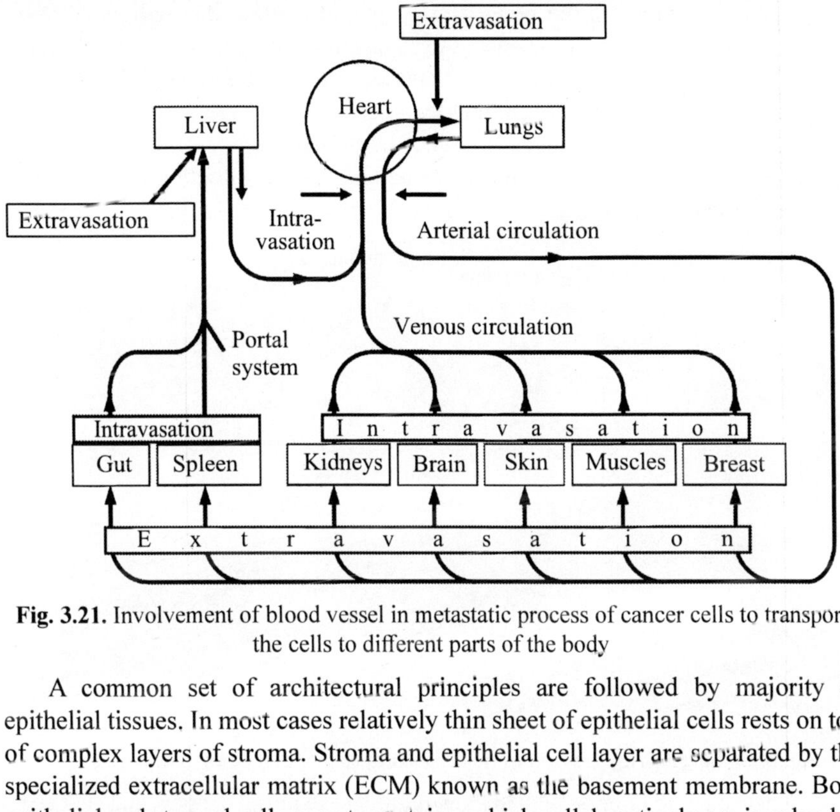

Fig. 3.21. Involvement of blood vessel in metastatic process of cancer cells to transport the cells to different parts of the body

A common set of architectural principles are followed by majority of epithelial tissues. In most cases relatively thin sheet of epithelial cells rests on top of complex layers of stroma. Stroma and epithelial cell layer are separated by the specialized extracellular matrix (ECM) known as the basement membrane. Both epithelial and stromal cells secrete proteins, which collaboratively are involved in the construction of proteinaceous meshwork called ECM.

The carcinomas originate from the epithelial cells lying on the one side of the basement membrane and at the beginning they are **benign** as long as the cells forming them remain on epithelial side. Many carcinomas, sooner or later, acquire the ability to breach the basement membrane and start migrating from epithelial side to nearby stroma resulting in invasion of that area, these migrating cells are called **malignant.** These malignant cells which have crossed over to stroma secrete angiogenic factors and stimulate angiogenesis on the stromal side of the basement membrane. The angiogenic factors diffuse through this porous barrier to endothelial cells within the stroma. Invasion through the basement membrane to stromal region gives them special ability of executing the invasion-metastasis cascade. In the stromal compartment blood and lymphatic vessels are normally present, invasive carcinoma cells get direct access to them. On establishing contact with blood vessels, invasive tumor cells get improved access to the nutrients and oxygen carried by the blood. In addition, invasive property of tumor cells enables them to move through the wall and into the lumina of blood vessels and lymphatic vessels, and this process of invasion into blood vessels is termed **intravasation**.

Once the malignant tumor cells are inside the lumen of the blood or lymphatic vessel, individual cancer cells start traveling in the direction of the flow of blood or lymph to other areas in the body. During this migration, the malignant cells are fraught with great danger because, the cancer cells will have to face different environmental conditions in other tissue spaces or in the lumen of blood vessel. An actively hostile environment in the blood possessing immune cells can attack metastasizing tumor cells. Protection to the wandering tumor cell is provided by the platelets, which surround the tumor cell and nourish them with growth factors as well as protect them from attack by immune cells (Fig. 3.22).

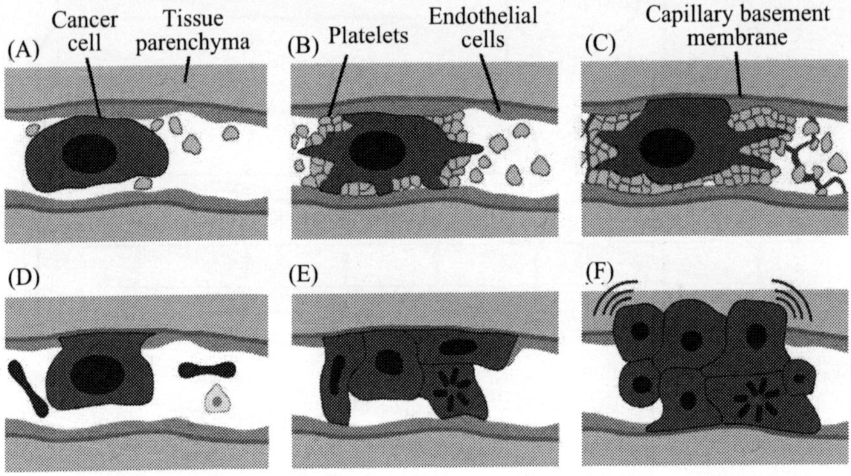

Fig. 3.22. Survival mechanism of metastasizing cancer cell in the blood vessel

The metastasizing tumor cells that overcome these initial dangers and succeed in gaining access to the larger vessels in the venous system and travel with the blood to the heart and from the heart they travel to the lungs to lodge themselves in the lungs after leaving the heart (Fig. 3.21). Unlike red and white blood cells, the malignant carcinoma cells because of their size, which is more than 20 μm in diameter are ill equipped for travel through most capillaries. The internal diameter of the capillaries is usually in the range of 3 to 8 μm, through them well adapted blood cells can pass through, because they can change the shape or deform, whereas most cancer cells are incapable of deformation.

The metastasizing tumor cells once trapped in the lungs, establish micrometastasis in the lungs. However, tumor metastasis of many different tissue types in humans are often found elsewhere in the body, indicating that metastasizing cancer cells need not always establish metastasis in the lungs, instead succeed in escaping from the lungs and travel further to other organs and establish metastasis in other regions of the body. In some cases, cancer cells trapped in the capillaries pinch off large amounts of cytoplasm to reduce their size. Such amputated or cells with reduced size may succeed in entering the narrow lung capillaries and escaping from lung to arrive in the general arterial circulation, which makes these roaming cancer cells to scatter to all tissues in the body (Fig. 3.21).

Metastasizing cancer cells traveling through arterial circulation of various tissues, must escape from the lumina of the arteries and penetrate the surrounding tissue, which is called **extravasation** (Fig. 3.21). The process of extravasation involves a complex mechanism of interaction cancer cells with the walls of the blood vessels in which they are trapped and the metastasizing cancer cells use several different strategies to extravasate. One of the strategies would be they start proliferating within the lumen of the vessel, creating micro-metastasis, which eventually destroys the adjacent vessel wall (Fig. 3.22). The micro-tumor within the blood vessel will succeed in pushing their way through the vessel wall into the new tissue space.

3.8 METASTASIS

It is the ability of cancer cells to migrate that makes task harder to eradicate them surgically or by localized irradiation. To disperse widely into different parts of the body, the metastasizing cancer cells originating from a solid tumor should be able to loosen up their adhesion from to their original neighbors and escape by burrow through other tissues until they reach a blood vessel or a lymphatic vessel. They should be able to cross the basal lamina and endothelial lining of the vessel to enter the blood circulation and exit from the circulation elsewhere in the body into the new environment, survive and proliferate to establish micro-metastasis in the new environment (Fig. 3.23). Each of these steps of metastasis

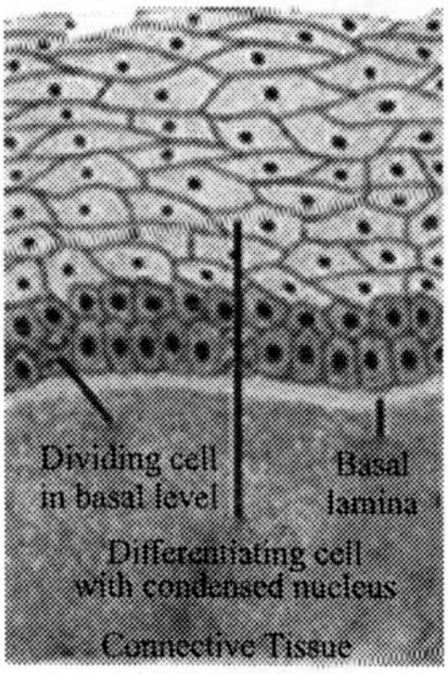

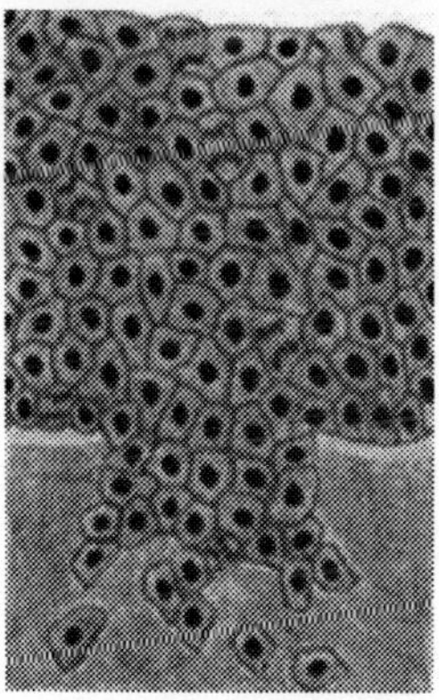

(A) Normal (B) Malignant carcinoma

Fig. 3.23. Initial process of metastasis by breaching the barrier to invade into other tissue area by crossing basal lamina

requires different properties, like loss of adhesion to neighboring cells is achieved through loss of expression of the epithelial cell adhesion molecule *E-cadherin* and the ability to burrow through tissues is obtained by the production of proteolytic enzymes (metalloproteases) that break down the extracellular matrix. The final step of metastasis that involves colonization of new environment in a new tissue is the most difficult step, where many metastasizing cells die. Therefore, large number of cells are released into the circulation by tumors, but only a few of these cells succeed in establishing metastatic colonies elsewhere.

The most dangerous manifestation of the cancer process is metastasizing cancer cells, wreaking havoc when they succeed in colonizing the new tissue sites. The metastasizing breast cancer cells leave the primary tumor mass and travel to different parts of the body through blood and lymphatic vessels to establish colonies promiscuously in many tissues like the brain, liver, bones, and lungs (Fig. 3.24). Prostate tumors often establish colonies in the bones and colon carcinomas preferentially form the new colonies in the liver.

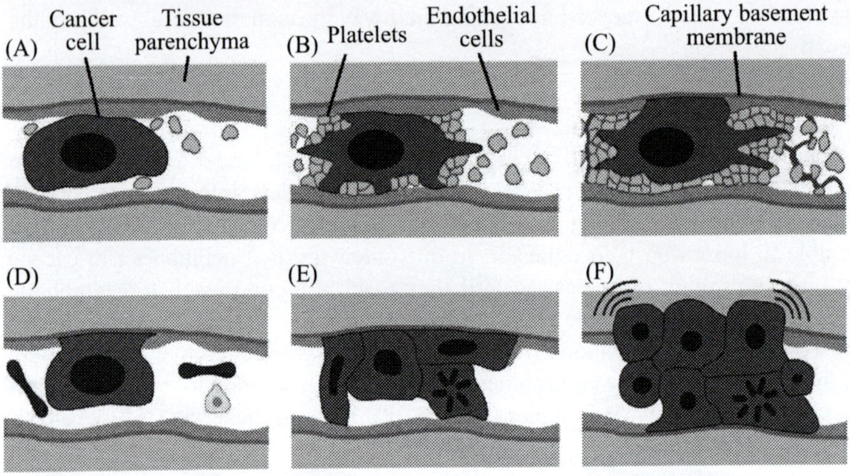

Fig. 3.24. Steps leading to extravasation of malignant tumor cells

Majority of life-threatening cancers originate from epithelial tissues giving rise to carcinomas. A common set of architectural principles is followed by epithelial tissues; in majority of cases, relatively a thin sheet of epithelial cells spread on the top of the deep complex stromal layer and in between the two extracellular matrix (ECM) exists, known as the *basement membrane*. The basement membrane consists of proteinaceous meshwork, constructed by proteins secreted by both epithelial and stromal cells in a collaborative manner.

Carcinomas originating from the epithelial side of the basement membrane and if they remain on epithelia side of the basement membrane, they are benign. Over the course of time, many carcinomas acquire malignant characteristic, due to which they will be able to break down the basement membrane. As a result, invasion of the nearby stroma by individual cancer cells or groups of cancer cells begins because these epithelial tumors have acquired this invasive ability and these masses of neoplastic cells are called malignant, which gives them the name cancer.

3.8.1 Colonization

Once the metastasizing tumor cells invade the parenchyma of a distant tissue, they may begin forming new colonies in their new found home (tissue), the process is called **colonization**. The new found home is the most challenging environment for the invaded cancer cells because it does not provide suitable environment for the cancer cells such as familiar growth factors and survival factors. Due to lack of physiological support, some of the metastasizing cells may die immediate or some may survive for an extended periods of time as single cells or as small clumps called **micro-metastases**.

Genetic evolution occurring in a micro-metastasis would provide an ability to colonize efficiently the new tissue environment. Second wave of metastatic dissemination begins from expanding micro metastasis, it also begins to seed the cancer cells throughout the body. Majority of the single cells micro-metastases are genetically identical to one another because of their common descent from the same clonal cell population. The descendent cell of new micro-metastases will have readily inherited the ability to colonize and many grow rapidly into macroscopic metastases, creating a life-threatening burden of disseminated cancer cells in the patient (Fig. 3.25).

3.8.2 E-Cadherins and Epithelial Mesenchymal Transition (EMT)

Of the many steps that lead to metastases, first step would be the acquisition of local invasiveness by the metastatic cells that involves major phenotypic changes in cancer cells within the primary tumors. Carcinoma cells derived from epithelium must shed many of their epithelial phenotypes by undergoing a drastic alteration known as **epithelial mesenchymal transition** (EMT) to detach from epithelial sheets to gain motility and invasiveness. Epithelial cells by shedding of epithelial characteristics, switch on mesenchymal transcriptional programme to transform into mesenchymal cells. Shedding off epithelial cell characteristics also involves stop expressing epithelial protein markers and start expressing mesenchymal proteins and morphology of cells also changes from typical epithelial to mesenchymal fibroblasts like in appearance.

The pathological consequence of EMT involves, significant change in the gene expression profile of cells in addition to changes in shape and acquisition of mobility. Changes observed after the epithelial-mesenchymal transition are:

Loss of

- Cytokeratin (intermediate filament) expression
- **E-cadherin** (epithelial adherence junction protein)
- Epithelial cell polarity

Acquisition of

- Fibroblast-like shape
- Motility and invasiveness

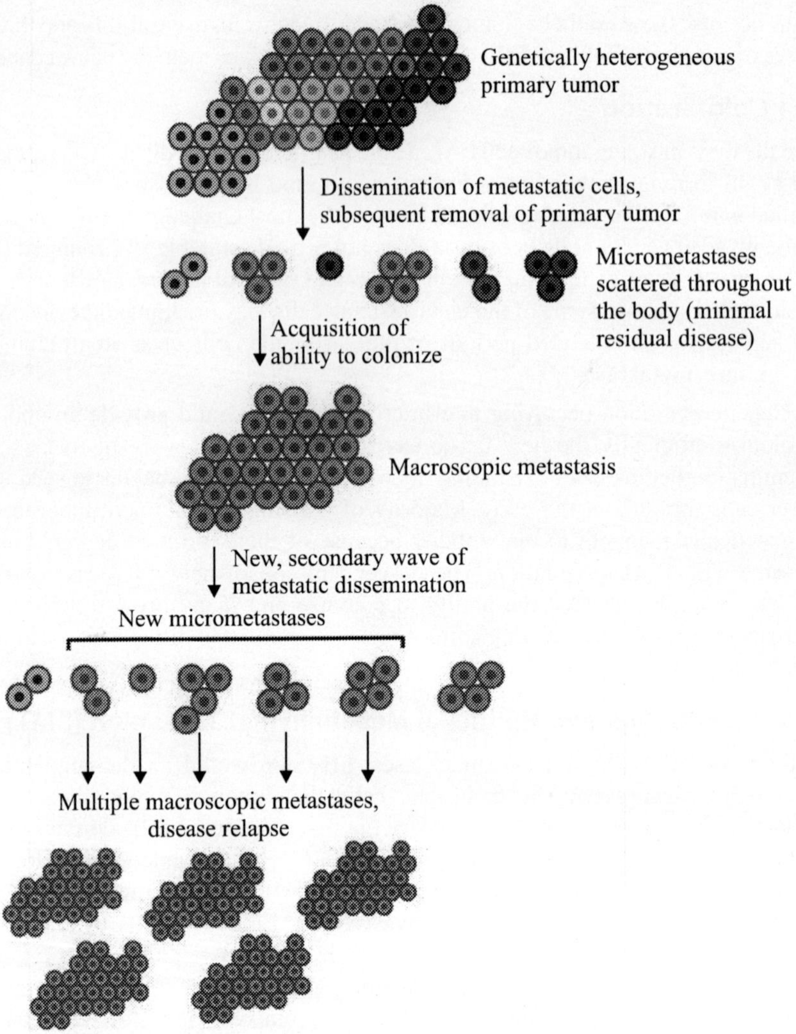

Fig. 3.25. Colonization process during metastasis

- Mesenchymal gene expression
- Expression of **N-cadherin** (mesenchymal adherence junction protein)
- Secretion of proteases like MMP-2 and MMP-9
- Expression of vimentin (intermediate filament)
- Secretion of **fibronectin**
- Expression of PDGF receptor
- Expression of αvβ6 **integrin**

Epithelial cells that have undergone EMT will repress the expression of **E-cadherin** and **cytokeratins,** the hallmark proteins expressed by the epithelial cells and mesenchymal cell protein **fibronectin** as well as an intermediate component of the cytoskeleton vimentin is induced. Fibronectin is an extracellular matrix protein, normally secreted only by mesenchymal cells such as fibroblasts and simultaneously expression of a typical fibroblast marker-**N-cadherin**-is acquired replacing E-cadherin.

In many types of invasive human cancers, CDH1 gene of E-cadherin is repressed because of promoter methylation in order to acquire malignant cell phenotype and in cancers of other organs, transcriptional repression of the gene is achieved by mutations in the reading frame. For example, 26 human breast cancer cell lines when analyzed, 8 of them had inactivation mutation of E-cadherin gene expression, 5 of them had deletion mutation in the reading frame of E-cadherin gene leading to expression of abnormal E-cadherin. In an experiment, through a plasmid vector normal E-cadherin gene, re-expressed by transfection of carcinoma cells, resulted in loss of invasiveness and metastatic dissemination characteristics of these cancer cells. From this observation expression of E-cadherin is very important in the biological behavior of epithelial cells and it facilitates cell-to-cell contacts through E-cadherins and expression of E-cadherin impedes invasiveness and hence metastasis.

In the carcinomas, the hepatocyte growth factor (HGF) promotes the replacement of E-cadherin by N-cadherin during EMT. Consequently, N-cadherin expression on the surface of the carcinoma increases the affinity of this cancer cell for the stromal cells that normally display N-cadherin. N-cadherin is also predominantly expressed by the fibroblasts in the stroma beneath the epithelial cell layer. This association facilitates invasion of carcinoma cells into stromal cell population. In the case of melanoma, same dynamics holds good, where E-cadherin is expressed by normal melanocytes, which facilitates their binding

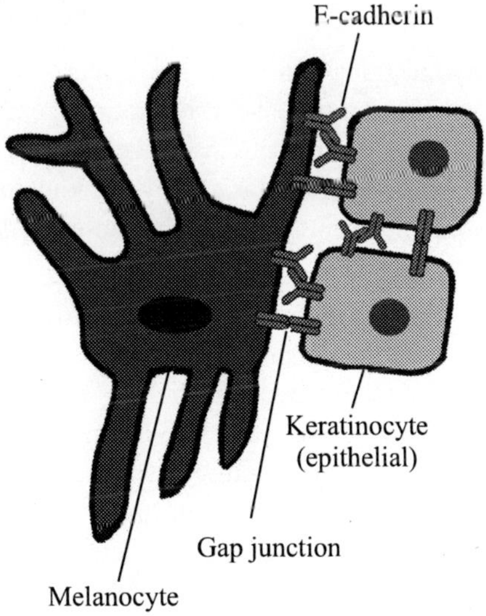

Fig. 3.26. E-cadherin expression on normal epithelial cells

to keratinocytes around them; whereas melanoma cells are the transformed cells derived from melanocytes express N-cadherin. Expression of N-cadherin by melanomas facilitates their invasion of the dermal stroma of the skin and establishes contact with fibroblasts and endothelial cells (Figs. 3.26 and 3.27). Compared to E-cadherin interaction, N-cadherin interaction seems to be weak therefore cells do not bond together and gain motility, which is one of the key features of metastasis.

Cadherin-22 is known to be expressed on hypoxic cancer cell surface, which helps it to adher together and migrate collectively as a group. The production of cadherin- 22 is triggered in metastasizing cancer cells that helps the cells to bind together, enhancing cellular movement, invasion and likely further metastasis.

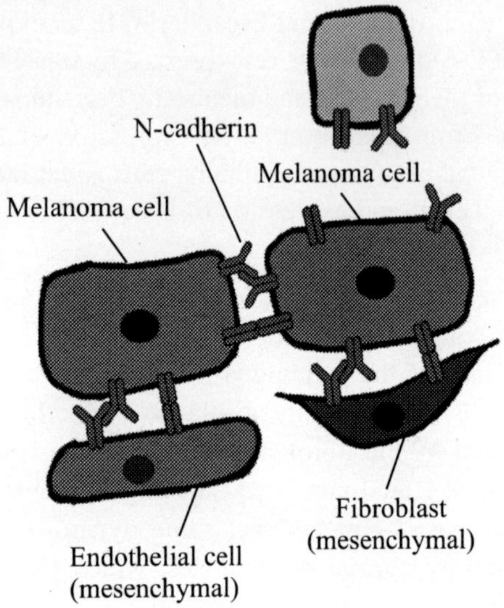

Fig. 3.27. Replacement of E-cadherin by N-cadherin in transformed metastatic cell

Epithelial-mesenchymal transition (EMT) is a temporary state acquired by malignant carcinoma cells for the purpose of migration from their origin to other areas of the body (Fig. 3.28). Once the carcinoma cells have achieved the purpose of multiple steps of invasion and metastasis, they are known to revert to a more epithelial phenotype by passing through mesenchymal-epithelial transition (MET) (Fig. 3.28).

Evidences indicate that TGF-β produced by stromal cells induces the neoplastic cells bordering the outer edges of the epithelial cell mass to undergo an EMT. Involvement of TNF-α (tumor necrosis factor – α), epidermal growth factor (EGF), hepatocyte growth factor (HGF), and IGF-1 (insulin like growth factor – 1) in EMT is also implicated. In addition, tumor associated macrophages (TAM) in the stromal environment also contribute to metastatic behavior of cancer cells by inducing secretion of CSF-1 (colony stimulating factor-1) by cancer cells, which in turn, stimulates macrophage to secrete EGF creating a positive feedback loop between these two cell types (Fig. 3.29).

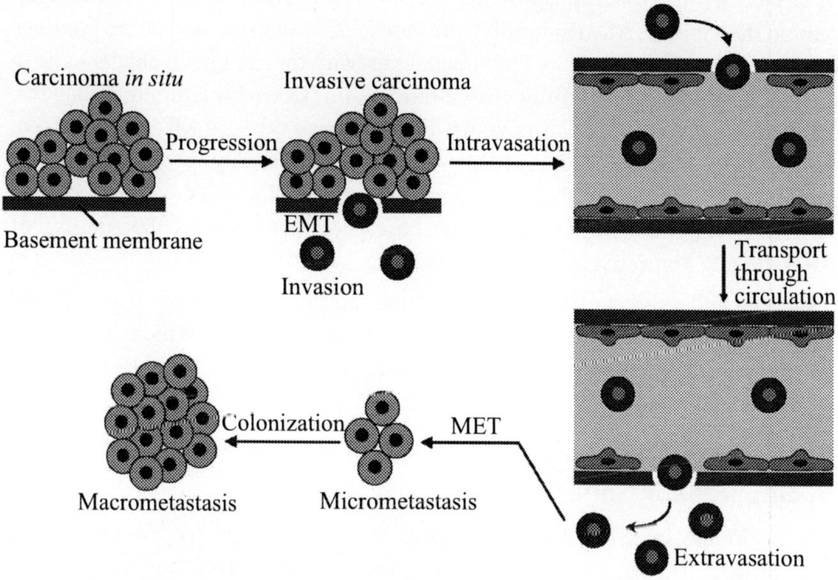

Fig. 3.28. Epithelial mesenchymal transition reversibility during metastasis

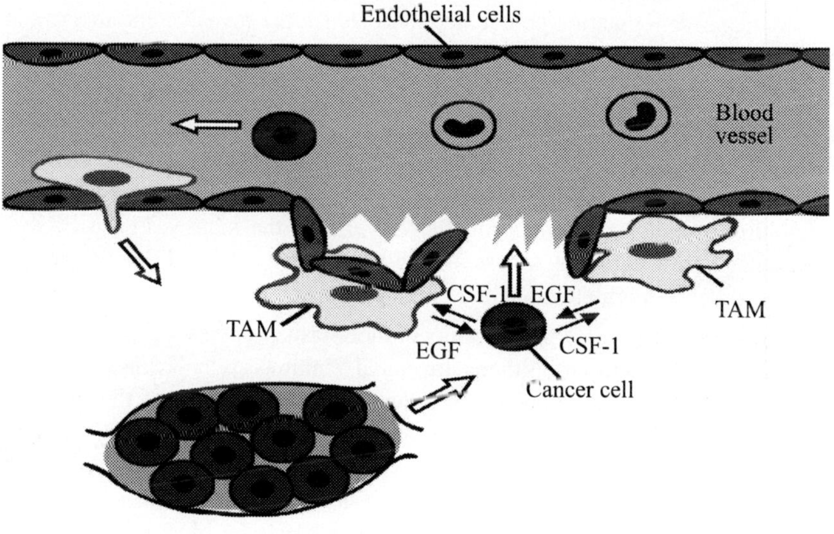

Fig. 3.29. Involvement of cytokines from another cell during metastasis

3.8.3 Invasiveness is Facilitated by Extracellular Proteases

The acquisition of epithelial-mesenchymal transition (EMT) by the cancer cells represents a complex biological behavior that helps cancer cells to acquire invasiveness and motility. Matrix metalloproteinases (MMPs) are the most important effectors, which facilitate cancer cells to excavate passageways through the extracellular matrix (ECM) during invasion. In carcinomas, all the proteases are secreted by the macrophages, mast cells and fibroblasts and stromal cells present in the vicinity. MMPs dissolve the dense ECM that surrounds and confines individual cells within tissue by creating passageway for malignant cancer cells to migrate. The MMPs successfully cleave fibronectin, tenascin, laminin, collagens, and proteoglycans of ECM components. There are two types of MMPs expressed, namely, MMP-2 and MMP-9. MMP-9, expressed largely by macrophages, fibroblasts and neutrophils, facilitates degradation of collagen IV, V, XI, and XIV, which are the major components of the basement membrane. Other targets of MMP-9 include laminin, chemokines, fibrinogen, and latent TGF-β.

Stromal cells secrete urokinase plasminogen activator (uPA), a non-MMP protease responsible for cleaving plasminogen into plasmin, which in turn, is responsible for cleaving pro-enzyme forms of other proteases leading to activation of proteases including MMP types 1, 2, 3, 9, and 14.

3.8.4 Metastatic Phenotype is Regulated by Metastasis Suppressor Genes

The steps in the invasion-metastasis cascade are promoted by the genes that encode growth factors, growth factor receptors, or signal transducing proteins. These genes have both positive regulators and negative regulators for fine tuning of the outputs. ***Metastasis suppressor genes,*** which belong to tumor suppressor genes by negative regulation counteract and balance the invasive and metastatic actions of advance malignancy.

In 1988, through in vitro experiments on mouse melanoma cells it was discovered that *NM23*- reduces the metastatic powers by suppressing the motility and invasiveness of cells. The mechanism of action of NM23 protein involves its ability to form physical complexes with the KSR protein, which serves as a scaffolding protein that brings together several of the kianses in the ERK-9 extracellular signal regulating kinases)-MAPK (mitogen activated protein kinase) cascade in order to facilitate rapid and efficient transfer of signal between them.

E-cadherin molecule is also a product of metastasis suppressor gene because it stabilizes cell-cell contacts in epithelial layer and it inhibits epithelial mesenchymal transition, thereby serves as an obstacle that blocks acquisition of the invasive cell phenotype. In invasive carcinomas through a variety of mechanisms like methylation of promoter or the gene, deletion of gene or mutation of E-cadherin gene its role is abrogated. Similarly, tissue inhibitors of metalloproteinases (TIMPs) block several steps of invasion and metastasis by binding MMPs and inactivating them in the intercellular spaces.

A membrane bound protein called KAI1/CD82 yet another tumor suppressor gene that weaves its way back and forth four times through the plasma membrane, located very close to adherins junctions plays an important role in cell-cell adhesion. Its expression is substantially repressed in many advanced lung, pancreatic, prostate, colon, and gastric carcinoma. EGF receptor signaling plays a crucial role in majority of tumors and KAI1 acts as an antagonist of EGF receptor.

KISS1 protein serves as a ligand of cell surface G-protein-coupled receptor and its ectopic expression of *KISS1* gene suppresses the metastatic tendencies in tumor cells without affecting the growth of the tumor cells in primary tumors.

The Rho guanine nucleotide dissociation inhibitor-2 (RhoGDI-2) is an inhibitor of cancer cell invasiveness and metastasis and it serves as a negative regulator of Rho proteins, which facilitates sequestering the GDP bound forms of these proteins in the cytoplasm, thereby preventing the remodeling of the actin cytoskeleton. Rho-like proteins play a key role in cell motility and invasiveness.

Breast cancer metastasis suppressor-1 (*BRMS-1*) gene expression is decreased in metastatic breast cancer and its ectopic expression in breast carcinoma and melanoma cells suppresses their metastatic tendencies without affecting their tumorigenicity. The gap-junction communication between cells is known to be increased by *BRMS-1* protein and it allows adjacent cells to exchange molecules of approximately 10^3 molecular weight. BRMS-1 protein is also involved in the nucleus for chromatin remodeling.

3.9 TELOMERES AND TELOMERASE IN CANCER

The chromosomal ends possess **telomeres,** which explains how these linear DNA molecules can stably coexist with the cell's various DNA modifying enzymes. Telomeres prevent end-to-end-fusion of chromatids of the same chromosome or the neighboring chromosome. In effect, telomeres, much like the aglets safeguarding the tips of shoelaces serve as protective shields for the chromosomal ends. When cells lose functional telomeres from their chromosomes, catastrophic events of crisis are triggered in the cell. In 1941, Barbara McClintock was the first one to report the detrimental effects of loss of telomeres in maize chromosomes. The chromosomes that have lost functional telomeres will start end-to-end fusion of chromatids and create breakage-fusion-bridge (BFB). The resulting mega-chromosome possesses two or more centromeres leading to further fragmentation of chromosome with each cycle of cell division.

The mammalian cells telomeric DNA and most of the eukaryotes are characterized by the presence of tandem repeats of hexanucleotide sequence 5′-TTAGGG-3′ in one strand, which is called the "G-rich" strand and the complementary 5′-CCCTAA-3′ "C-rich" strand. In normal human cells, several thousands of these hexanucleotide sequences are repeated in telomeric DNA resulting in 5-to 10-kilobases long stretches of such repeating sequences at the

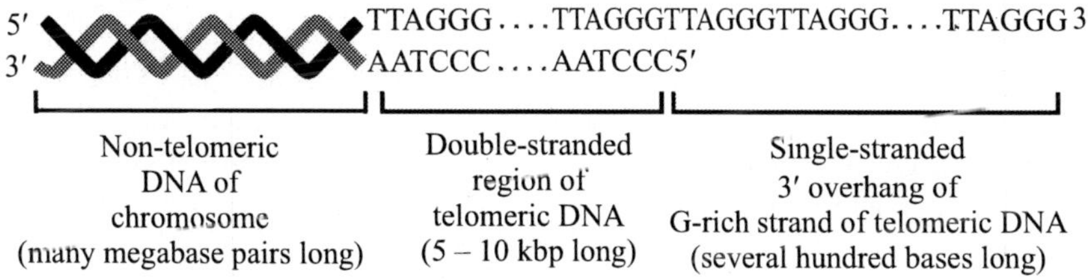

Fig. 3.30. The 3′ overhang in G-strand of telomeric DNA

ends of all chromosomes. An additional, distinctive feature exists in the telomeric DNA of mammalian cells that is a long 3′ single-strand overhang is observed in its G-rich strand, which is longer by several hundred nucleotides (Fig. 3.30).

This overhanging strand is most vulnerable for degradation by 3′ specific exonucleases; therefore, it is often found in the most unusual molecular configuration termed the **T-loop** (Fig. 3.31). The T-loop helps in protecting the ends of the single-stranded overhanging region by tucking the linear DNA molecules into a loop of double stranded region (Fig. 3.31). Several proteins are associated with the double stranded and single stranded regions of telomeric DNA constituting nucleoprotein complexes, which is called **telomere.**

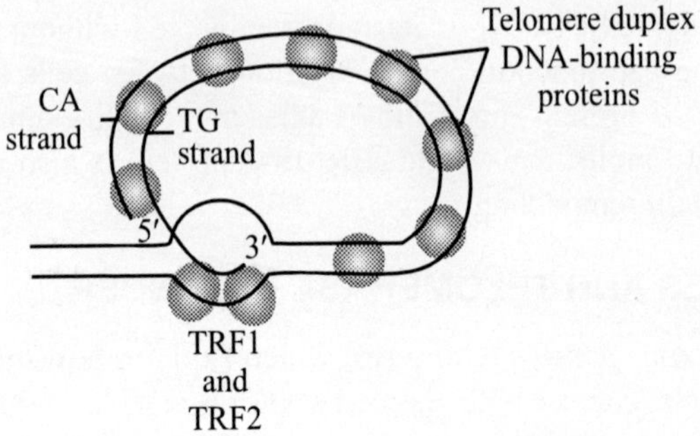

Fig. 3.31. T-loop formation at the extended G-strand 3′ end

Each time a normal cell completes a cell cycle, the telomeric DNA is shortened because of a problem associated with telomeric DNA replication. In addition to shortening of the telomeric region due to very low rate of replication of telomeric DNA, there appears to be another problem, where exonucleases within cells slowly chew on the ends of telomeric DNA, which may ultimately contribute far more to telomere erosion. For whatever reason, during each cell division of normal human cells, telomeres lose 50 to 100 base pairs of DNAs. This progressive erosion of telomeric DNA represents a simple molecular device that limits how many generations of descendent progeny a cell can spawn. Erosion of telomeric DNA down to a size that is so short that it can no longer perform its intended function of protecting the ends of the chromosomal DNA results in breakage-fusion-bridge (BFB).

To a great extent, telomere erosion can be prevented by an enzyme **telomerase**, which specifically facilitates the elongation of telomeric DNA and it is a reverse transcriptase. The striking finding is that in majority of human tumor cell samples, telomerase activity is high, whereas in normal human cells it is present at very low level. The available evidence indicates that in the early embryogenesis strong expression of the telomerase enzyme is seen, which is lost once the cells have undergone differentiation to give rise to majority of the body's tissues. The telomerase enzyme in human cells is called human telomerase reverse transcriptase (hTERT) (Fig. 3.32), which has six nucleotides present in the RNA molecule associated with it. Six nucleotides present in the RNA molecule are used

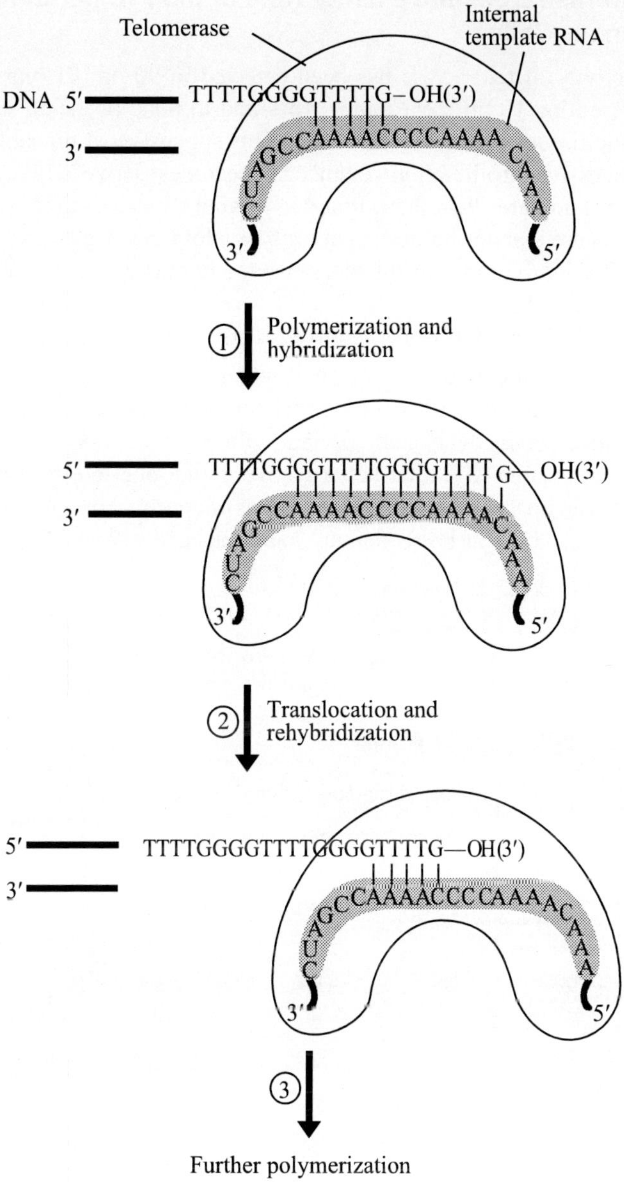

Fig. 3.32. Formation of telomeres and the action of telomerase

as complementary bases for the synthesis of telomeric DNA by utilizing telomerase (Fig. 3.32). The newly synthesized telomeric DNA attaches itself to the G-rich 3′ overhanging end of the preexisting telomeric DNA. The conventional DNA polymerases would facilitate synthesis of complementary strand of the telomeric DNA.

3.9.1 Telomerase Does have a Key Role in the Proliferation of Cancer Cells

Significant activity of telomerase has been detected in 90 of 101 human tumor samples representing 12 different tumor types and in none of the 50 samples of normal somatic tissues of 4 different tissues. This suggests that probably in cells that show excessive proliferation telomerase becomes active. Human tumors showed shorter telomeres than those found in normal surrounding cells. In tumor cells, telomeres are smaller because synthesis of telomeres begins only after the tumor cells start dividing uncontrollably. Once the telomerase is finally activated in tumor cells, its activity is stabilized the severely clipped. Telomeres prevent further erosion allowing highly proliferative cells to become immortal.

A study of human carcinomas of the esophagus, colon, and breast revealed that in each case, tumors possessing shorter telomeres are strongly associated with poor chances of recovery and survival, while the tumors possessing long telomeres are associated with a far better recovery and long-term survival. Here, once again, we can imagine that the chromosomes of cancer cells with sub-optimal telomere express hTERT at levels that are barely adequate to maintain telomeric

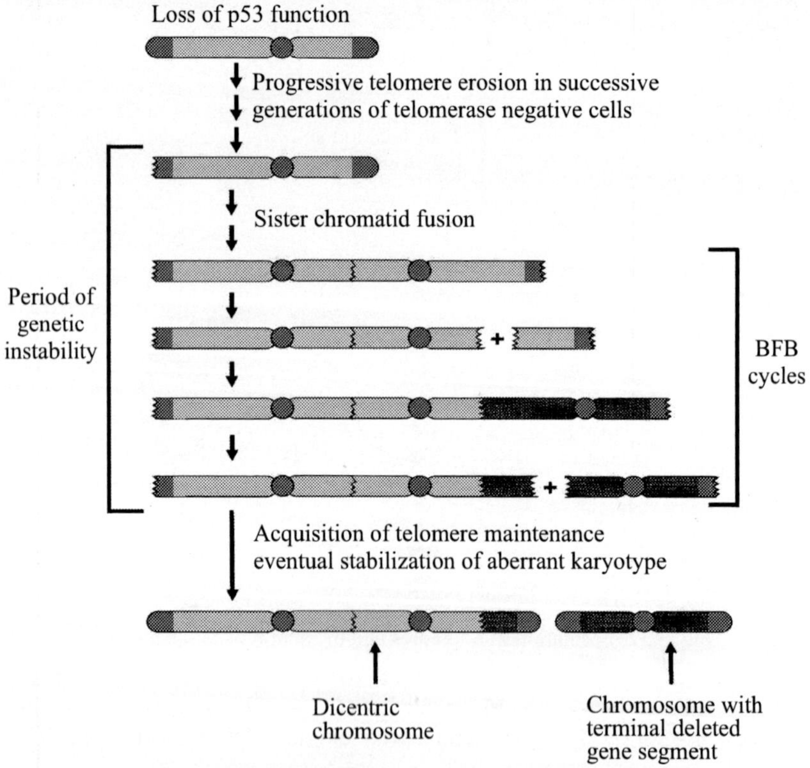

Fig. 3.33. Loss of p53 function by LOH or by spontaneous mutation of one copy of p53 and BFB formation due to loss of telomeres

DNA lengths undergo relatively frequent breakage-fusion-bridge cycles. These BFB cycles, in turn, increase the chromosomal instability that would continue throughout the tumor's life cycle to generate new set of genotypes (Fig. 3.33). Some of the new combination genotypes generated may favor more rapid proliferation and increasing aggressiveness in tumor cells and some genotypic combinations may lead to death of tumor cells. Certain human chronic inflammatory conditions are attributed to the eroded telomere and BFB cycles, which are associated with increased risks of cancer.

This is probably one of the mechanisms that explains how highly aneuploid karyotypes are acquired by many types of human tumor cells. Although not directly demonstrated, it is widely assumed that the acquired aneuploid genomic constitution confers growth advantages on these tumor cells by creating novel oncogenes through translocations caused by BFB, by increasing the dosage of growth-promoting proto-oncogenes. BFB may also favor eliminating tumor suppressor genes that were blocking cell proliferation. Hence, the BFB cycles may be responsible for favoring tumor progression because they accelerate genomic mutability and permit the pre-malignant cells to choose a multitude of novel, possibly advantageous, genotypes for further progression.

3.9.2 Maintenance of Telomeres without Telomerase by Immortalized Tumor Cells

Almost all human tumors have telomerase activity. The remaining small number of human tumors lack telomerase enzyme activity, yet the cells within this second group of tumors maintain their telomeres above some minimum length by a different mechanism in order to proliferate indefinitely. The alternate mechanism is called alternative lengthening of telomeres (ALT), which does not involve telomerase to construct and maintain the telomeres in cancer cells.

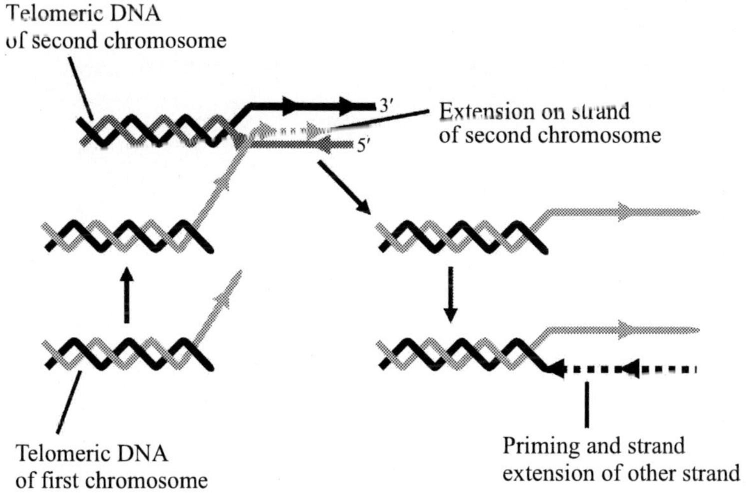

Fig. 3.34. Copy-choice mechanism adopted for alternative lengthening of telomeres

The molecular mechanism used by ALT-positive tumor cells to maintain their telomeres is by interchromosomal **copy-choice** mechanism (Fig. 3.34). Thus, the polymerase responsible for replicating DNA on one chromosome may for a short period of time utilize the sequences of second chromosome as a template for the elongation of telomeric DNA strand and jump back to the original chromosome to continue replication of this chromosome's DNA. In effect, the DNA polymerases "borrow" sequence information from the second chromosome in order to incorporate it into the newly synthesized copy of the first chromosome.

In order to proliferate in an immortalized fashion, all types of human cancer cells must develop ways to maintain their telomeres above a certain threshold length and existence of the ALT mechanism emphasizes the fact. Most human cancer cells enhance or de-repress the expression of the *hTERT* gene on priority basis and a small proportion of cancer cells activates the ALT mechanism.

The ALT state is associated preferentially with a specific subset of the tumors encountered in oncology clinics. These include, osteosarcomas and soft tissue sarcomas as well as many glioblastomas.

Exercise

1. Epigenetics has an important role in the development of cancers. Explain.
2. Explain the role of proto-oncogenes in cell function.
3. What are oncogenes? What is their role in cancer development?
4. How telomeres are maintained in cancer cells without the presence of telomerase? Explain with a diagrammatic presentation.

   OR

   What is the mechanism involved in alternate lengthening of telomeres?

   OR

   What is meant by copy-choice mechanism? Where and when does it occur?
5. Explain the role of growth factors and their receptors in the process of oncogenesis.
6. Explain the role of protein kinases and nuclear transcription factors in the development of cancer.
7. What is the mechanism of activation of oncogenes leading to tumor formation?
8. Angiogenesis is the key for cancer progression. Justify the statement.

   OR

   How does thrombospondin control the development of blood vessels.

   OR

   What is the role of hypoxia inducible factor-1 (HIF-1) is angiogenesis?

   OR

List out the anti-angiogenic factors and explain how they inhibit angiogenesis.

OR

List out the angiogenic factors and explain how they promote angiogenesis.

9. What is the role of following during metastasis:
   (a) Ecadherins
   (b) Extracellular protease
   (c) Metastasis suppressor gene
10. With reference to metastasis explain the following:
    (a) Metastasis and metastatic tropism
    (b) Epithelial mesenchymal transition
11. How telomeres are maintained in cancer cells without the presence of telomerase? Explain with a diagrammatic presentation.

OR

What is the mechanism involved in alternate lengthening of telomeres?

OR

What is meant by copy-choice mechanism? Where and when does it occur?

CHAPTER

4

Tumor Suppressor Genes (TSGs)

4.1 TUMOR SUPPRESSOR GENES AND THEIR FUNCTIONS

Research carried out between 1970s and early 1980s indicated that in addition to proto-oncogenes and oncogenes, cells growth cycle is controlled by some other genes, which suppress the cell growth and cell proliferation. In other words, they are called **antigrowth genes** or **tumor suppressor genes (TSGs).** When these genes are inactivated by mutation or lost by deletion, they are unable to prevent tumor formation. When the cell loses these genes, growth-suppressing effect in the cells is lost. Almost three decades later, it is quite evident that the tumor suppressor inactivation of genes has equally important role to play as much as activation of oncogenes for cancer pathogenesis. Indeed, for the formation of many kinds of cancers, loss of TSGs from a cell's genome is even more important than oncogene activation.

During the cancer development, in the evolving cancer cells, one or more of these growth-suppressing genes are inactivated, which accelerates proliferation of the cancer cells and achieve malignancy. However, if intact wild type TSG is transfected into a cancer cell or transferred by cell fusion technique, the proliferative and tumor forming ability of the cancer cell abruptly halts.

In a diploid cell, two copies of tumor suppressor genes exist in the homologous pair of chromosomes, both the copies of the tumor suppressor genes need to be silenced by a developing cancer cell before it becomes a full-blown cancer. Therefore, *tumor suppressor genes are considered to be dominant and the mutation that inactivates them is considered to be recessive*. On the other hand, *oncogenes are considered to be recessive, but the mutation that occurs in them to induce tumorigenesis is said to be dominant.*

TSGs and their encoded proteins block the development of cancer through different types of signals that lead to growth-inhibition and promote differentiation of cells. The first two intensively studied TSGs are Rb gene and p53 (Trp53 or TP53) gene, both play a major role in cancer pathogenesis. The Rb protein encoded by the Rb gene is responsible for regulation of cell cycle and perhaps in all human tumors, Rb gene induced growth control is disrupted. In all types of human cancers, p53 tumor suppressor gene control is also disrupted.

The remaining tumor suppressor genes discovered till date suppress cell proliferation by dispatching their products to control diverse activities in intracellular sites. These proteins involved in the growth control activity are the products of $p16^{INK4A}$, $p15^{INK4B}$, and $p19^{ARF}$ genes responsible for controlling cell proliferation and survival.

Generally, an individual may be born with one mutated allele of tumor suppressor gene and the other allele is normal. For a cancer cell to progress, it needs both copies of tumor suppressor genes being mutated or non-functional. For this reason, cancer cells have invented a mechanism of knocking off the normal tumor suppressor gene by **loss of heterozygosity (LOH)** through mitotic recombination mechanism. Even if a cell shows mutation at the rate of 10^{-6} per cell generation and the LOH at the rate of 10^{-5} to 10^{-4} per cell generation, which would be the easiest way to get rid of the remaining wild-type copy of tumor suppressor gene by a cell. Because LOH is thought to occur at a far higher frequency than compared to alteration of genes through mutations, still intact copy of a second gene loss through LOH is far more likely than through a mutation.

Several familial cancer syndromes that are known to have mutant germ-line alleles of tumor suppressor genes, transmit the gene in a recessive manner and their presence in most cells of an embryo will not be apparent. For this reason, mutant TSGs inherited in this manner will not harm normal embryonic development and the cancer phenotypes created by them will appear in a small number of cells after great delay, allowing the individual to survive through much of adulthood. This implies that a mutant oncogene or a TSG may be required for tumor formation but will not be sufficient on its own. Hence, many cells in an individual with inherited mutant TSG may undergo LOH of this gene and a small population of these cells will succeed in acquiring the additional genetic mutations that promote development of clinically detectable tumor.

4.1.1 Experiment to Prove that the Phenotype of Cancer is Recessive

Normal cell on transfection of tumor virus genome will transform that cell into cancer, which means that cellular behavior is dictated by viral oncogenes despite the presence and continuous expression of opposing cellular genes that usually performed all normal cell functions and proliferation within the virus infected cell. Because, the viral oncogenes could induce ***dominant*** phenotype in the cell and supersede the expression of cellular genes, thereby bring about transformation of cell. This suggests that cancerous cell growth is a dominant phenotype in contrast to normal (wild type) cell growth, which is therefore considered to be ***recessive***.

In order to understand the genetic status of the genes involved in cancer phenotype and normal phenotype, cell fusion experiments were performed to bring the alleles responsible for normal growth and those responsible for malignant growth to come together in one cell.

In these fusions, when cancer cell is derived from non-virus-induced tumors, i.e., rodent tumors induced through chemical carcinogenesis were used, the hybrid cells obtained from fusion were non-tumorigenic (Fig. 4.1). On the contrary, when

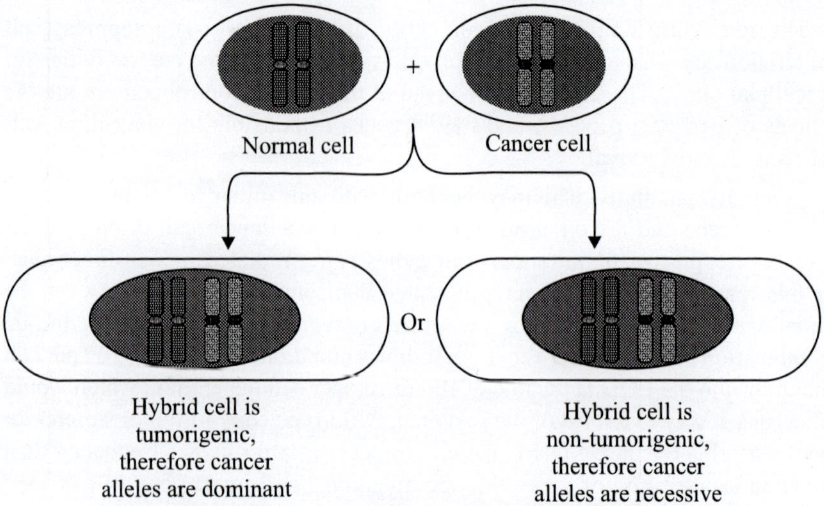

Fig. 4.1. Cell fusion technique to demonstrate dominance and recessive status of the tumorigenic phenotype

virus induced tumor cells were used the hybrid cells were tumorigenic indicating virally induced tumors are dominant (Fig. 4.1).

Since the wild-type tumor suppressor genes (TSGs) suppress the cancer cell phenotype, by mutation, these genes could be inactivated in a cell thereby promoting uncontrolled growth. The mutant, inactive alleles of tumor suppressor genes if it really did play a role in promoting the growth of cancer cells and by being recessive, it will be of no benefit by inactivating only one copy of the gene from the two copies of a tumor suppressor gene in a tumor, because the recessive mutant allele is suppressed by dominant wild type allele in this cell. Hence, for an aspiring cancer cell, it is essential that both wild type copies of a tumor suppressor would need to be inactivated. This requires two separate individual mutations, which is only possible by somatic recombination and loss of heterozygosity.

4.1.2 Inactivation of Tumor Suppressor Genes by Promoter Methylation

Promoter methylation of CpG domains of TSGs is one of the mechanisms by which the TSGs are silenced or prevented from expression. In familial cancer syndromes, more than half of the TSGs that are involved have undergone germ-line mutation are silenced by promoter methylation in sporadic cancers. For example, in familial retinoblastoma (Rb), there is a germ-line mutation in Rb gene which leads to familial retinoblastoma. In sporadic retinoblastomas, Rb gene is inactivated either by somatic mutations or by promoter methylation in the later part of the life. Many TSGs whose promoters are methylated in cancers. For example, APC in colon carcinoma, p57Kip^2-CDK inhibitor in gastric, pancreatic, hepatic and AML, p15^{INK4B} & p16^{INK4A} in various tumors, TGFβRII in colon, gastric and small cell lung carcinoma, Rb in retinoblastoma.

There are two mechanisms involved in promoter methylation for the inactivation of tumor suppressor gene function. First, there is a possibility of methylation of both copies of the tumor suppressor gene independently. Secondly possibility would be, methylation of one copy of TSG and the second may be inactivated by loss of heterozygosity (LOH) by copy choice mechanism. In majority of cancers, the second mechanism seems to quite frequently used. For example, in a study on in vitro culture of normal bronchial epithelia of the lungs of non-smokers and former smokers, in 44% of bronchial epithelial cells of former smokers the $p16^{INK4A}$ TSG was found to be methylated and not at all in the epithelial cells of non-smokers. LOH in the $p16^{INK4A}$ TSG was found to be 71 to 75% of the smoking populations and 1.5 to 1.7% of never smokers.

During the tumor formation, promoter methylation of "caretaker" genes responsible for maintaining the structural integrity of the DNA sequences in the genome may also take place simultaneously with promoter methylation of TSGs. One such gene is BRCA1, the protein products of the gene are involved in maintaining the DNA architecture in chromatin. There is evidence of involvement of mutation in BRCA1 gene in familial breast cancer syndrome and to a lesser extent, in ovarian carcinomas. It is well known that 10 to 15% of sporadic breast carcinomas carry inactive BRCA1 gene due to promoter methylation.

4.1.3 Insight into Genetics of Tumor Suppressor Genes

The important information on the biology of the tumor suppressor genes came from studying a rare childhood retinal cancer, which is called retinoblastoma. Retinoblastoma is observed in 1 in 20,000 children, the tumor arises in the photoreceptor cells of the retina. These tumors arise anytime between birth up to the age of 6 to 8 years, beyond which the disease is rarely seen. The retinoblastoma could appear in two forms: i.e., development of tumor in single eye in children born into families with no history of retinoblastoma, which is called sporadic retinoblastoma. If the affected eye is removed or treated with radiation, there is no further risk of retinoblastoma and other tumors elsewhere in the body. This type of sporadic retinoblastoma is termed unilateral retinoblastoma (Fig. 4.2).

The second form of retinoblastoma is called **familial retinoblastoma,** which is inherited by children born to parent who had suffered sporadic retinoblastoma and was cured of the disease in early life. In familial retinoblastoma, multiple foci develop in both eyes, which are called *bilateral retinoblastoma* (Fig. 4.2). Moreover, curing the retinoblastoma in children using radiation or surgery does not protect these children from developing cancers of other organs in late life like bone cancer (osteosarcomas) during adolescence and an increased susceptibility to develop yet another tumor in other regions of the body. Those who survive these tumors and grow to adulthood and reproduce will transfer the genes to the progeny and half of the progeny will develop familial retinoblastoma once again.

The inheritance of familial retinoblastoma follows typical Mendelian dominant fashion and is passed from one generation to the next immediate generation (Fig. 4.2). In sporadic retinoblastoma, the mutations occur de novo in the children

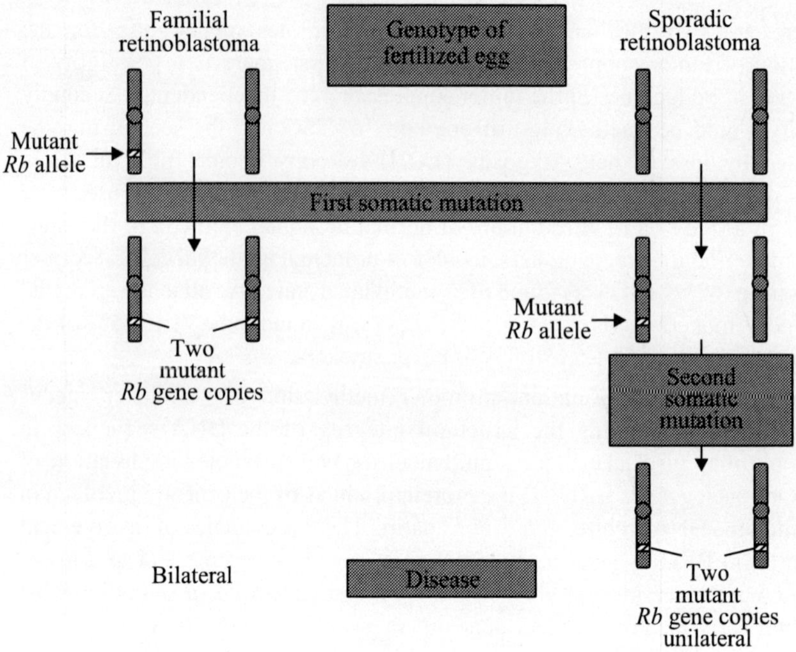

Fig. 4.2. Inheritance pattern of sporadic and familial retinoblastoma

in their adulthood during gametogenesis, with the result the children will carry cancer-causing mutant allele in their cells. This is almost identical to the familial retionoblastoma, where the mutant allele is already present in the genome, which will be transmitted to the offspring through gametes. Great majority of these de novo mutations occur in sperm rather than in eggs, because of a greater number of cell cycles to be completed by the sperm producing cell as compared to egg.

The mutation of retionoblastoma gene (Rb) is known to cause childhood retinoblastoma and the mutation results in inactivation of Rb gene, which is recessive in nature. Therefore, for the tumor development invariably both copies of the Rb gene must be mutated before a retinal cell shows uncontrolled proliferation resulting in a retinal tumor (Fig. 4.3).

For the formation of a retinoblastoma tumor in a child who has inherited a wild-type (normal) Rb gene from the parents, two successive mutations in Rb gene will be required to inactivate the two functional copies of Rb gene in a retinal cell lineage (Fig. 4.3). In half of the children born in a family of familial retinoblastoma, one of the two required Rb gene in mutated form has been passed through germ-line from a parent. This mutant Rb gene is present in all the cells of the embryo, including all the cells in the retina. Any one of these retinal cells needs one more somatic mutation to inactivate wild-type Rb allele in order to attain homozygous status where it no longer harbors any functional Rb gene copies. Once both copies of Rb gene are mutated, the cell can launch tumor development process to create a retinoblastoma.

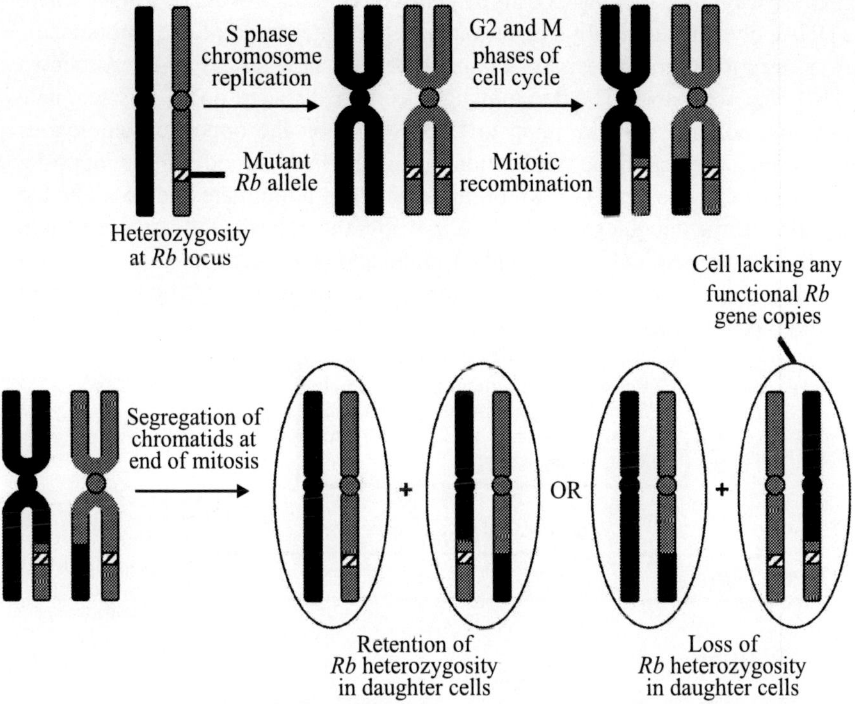

Fig. 4.3. Elimination of wild-type (normal) Rb gene copies through loss of heterozygosity

Cancer cells adopt alternative ways to silence wild-type copies of tumor suppressor genes. For this, geneticists suggested a probable mechanism as it happens with most mutational events at the rate of 10^{-6} per cell generation of inactivating first of the two Rb gene copies. As a result of this single mutation the cell will have heterozygous status for the gene with one wild-type (normal) and one mutant gene copy,that is, **Rb+/-** [+ (plus) for wild type and – (minus) for mutant allele]. In this heterozygous status of the cell the wild type Rb gene being dominant will express by suppressing the expression of the mutant Rb allele, which is recessive, thus heterozygous cell would continue to exhibit normal characteristics. Let us presume that during the active cell proliferation stage **mitotic recombination** might have taken place between chromatids of the homologs, such that the arm carrying the wild type Rb allele reciprocally exchanged the genetic segment with the arm carrying mutant Rb allele (Fig. 4.3).

As a result of this mitotic recombination event one of the cells emerging probably would have lost the remaining wild-type Rb allele, as a result its genotype would therefore be **Rb-/-**. Importantly, the frequency of mitotic recombination was found to occur at the rate of 10^{-5} to 10^{-4} per cell generation, which would be the easiest way for a cell to lose the remaining wild-type copy of the Rb gene rather than expecting the second mutational inactivation of the gene copy. This phenomenon is also called **loss of heterozygosity (LOH)** or "**allelic deletion**", frequency with which it occurs may differ in different human populations.

Other ways of achieving LOH is by **gene conversion** process (Fig. 4.4), where the DNA polymerase initially begins to read a template strand of one chromosome (lower one) for the synthesis of a complementary new strand of DNA (shown by thin line with arrow). After moving a certain distance down this template strand, the polymerase may jump to DNA strand on the opposite homologous chromosome and continue replication using a DNA strand of the opposite homologous chromosome (shown on upper side) as a template and continue the elongation of the daughter strand. After a while, the polymerase may once again jump back to the original DNA template strand and continue replication. This will result in copying a mutant allele of tumor suppressor gene resulting in replacing the wild type allele residing on the opposite homologous chromosome.

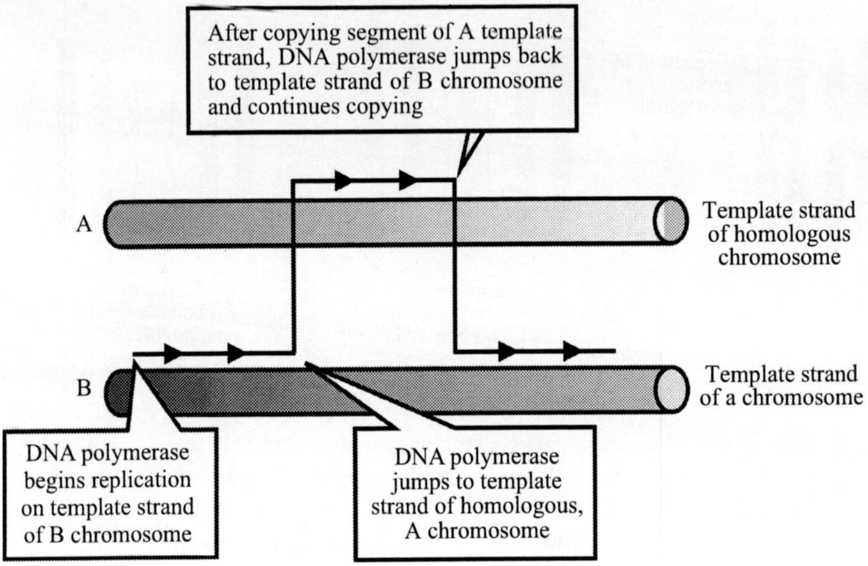

Fig. 4.4. Process involved in gene conversion

4.1.4 Loss of Heterozygosity in Rb Gene is the Most Common Feature in Tumors

Metaphase chromosome preparation from retinoblastoma patients shows interstitial deletion in the long ("q") arm of chromosome 13. The deletion involves the 3rd band of the 1st region of this chromosome, i.e., 13q14 (Fig. 4.5) resulting in loss of thousands of kilobases of genetic material.

The other way of achieving LOH is simply with a simultaneous double break in the chromatid and discarding the segment of an entire chromosomal region without replacing it with a duplicated copy from the other homologous chromosome. As a result, this chromosomal region achieves **hemizygous** status, where all the genes in this chromosomal segment are present as a single copy rather than the usual two copies per cell. With only one copy of gene on some chromosomal segments, cells can survive and this event is registered as an LOH putting a cell at a distinct

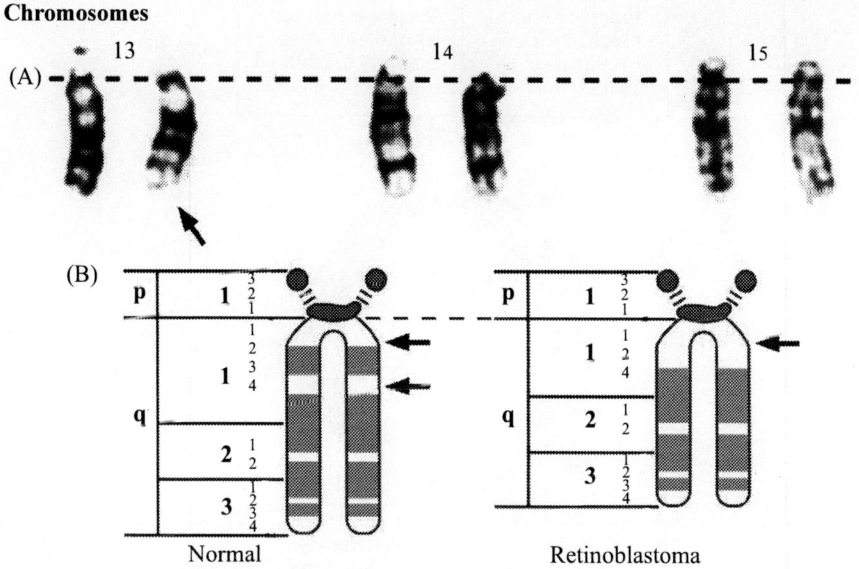

Fig. 4.5. Chromosomal localization of Rb locus

biological disadvantage. Since hemizygous status of a gene in this chromosomal region can be detected, the outcome of tumorigenesis is achieved by eliminating the remaining wild-type allele of a tumor suppressor gene.

4.2 ALTERED CELL CYCLE REGULATION AND TUMORIGENESIS

A cell that has recently been gone through the process of cell division (mitosis) has to decide at the earliest whether it should enter the second cycle of cell division for the active growth or retreat into G0 stage, which is the non-growing state in the cell cycle. This decision of cell division cycle is strongly influenced by mitotic growth factors available in the cell's surroundings. The presence of growth factors in sufficient quantity will encourage a cell to decide whether to divide or not; their absence will trigger the cell to take the decision of proceeding to G0 state.

Transforming growth factor-β (TGF-β) is a prominent anti-mitogenic factor, which influences the cell for withdrawal from the cell cycle and enter G0 state (Fig. 4.6). Withdrawal of cell from cell cycle is strongly influenced by the absence of growth factors or the presence of anti-mitogenic factor, which is often reversible. Most mammalian cells delay their entry to M phase by introducing G2 phase between M and S phases, which may last for 5 to 6 hours. In G2 phase cell prepares itself for entering M phase and cell division. The cell has devised **checkpoints** at each stage (Fig. 4.7) to see whether the cell is fit enough to enter the next stage of cell division cycle

One checkpoint at G1 phase ensures that the genome does not require repair, therefore, this checkpoint is called DNA damage checkpoint, where entrance to S

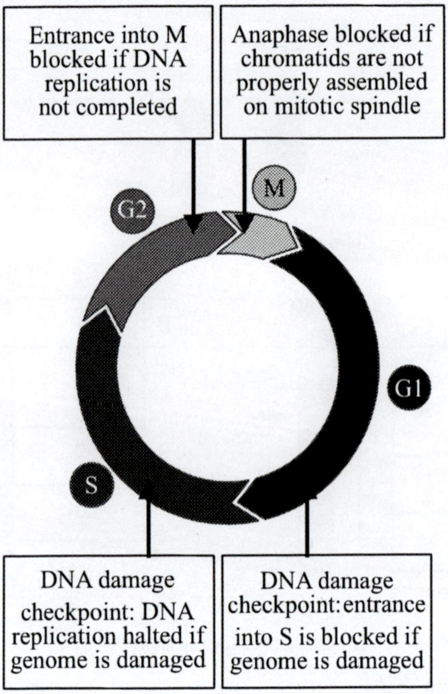

Fig. 4.6. Check points during various phases of cell cycle

phase is blocked if the DNA is damaged. DNA damage checkpoint also exists in the S phase, which halts the process of DNA replication if DNA damage exists. A third checkpoint permits the cell to proceed through G2 to M only if DNA replication is completed. During M phase, highly efficient checkpoint blocks anaphase progression as the chromatids are not properly assembled on mitotic spindle. These blocks are removed once all the chromosomes have been properly attached to the mitotic spindle.

How well these checkpoints are operative influences the formation of cancers. It is evident from studies on many types of cancers that, they succeed in inactivation of one or more of the checkpoint controls, thereby incipient cancer cells rapidly accumulate more mutant genes and altered karyotype that propel their neoplastic growth. During a specific period in the G1 phase cells make decision about growth and quiescence. Precisely at this crucial point, a cell should decide whether to stay in G1 phase or to withdraw from the active cell cycle and enter G0, or advance further into late G1 and proceed further passing through the remaining phases of the cell cycle. The transition point at which the critical decision is made is called the **restriction point** or **R point** (Fig. 4.7). In most mammalian cells studied to date, the R point occurs several hours before the G1/S phase transition.

If a cell should decide at this point to continue advancing through its growth-and-division cycle, it commits itself to proceed beyond G1 to S phase and then to complete a rigidly programmed series of events, which enables the cell to divide into two daughter cells.

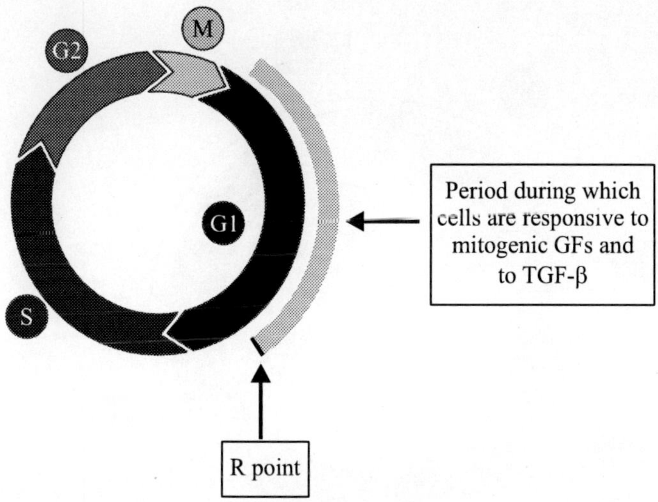

Fig. 4.7. Response to extracellular signals during the cell cycle phase

Therefore, R-point decision is the most critical determinant of whether the cell will divide or not and there is enough evidence to show that the R-point decision making is disrupted, which is crucial for the formation of most, if not all, types of cancers. Yet other decision points in late G1 may also contribute to the uncontrolled proliferation of certain cancer cells.

4.2.1 The Role of Cyclins and Cyclin Dependent Kinases (CDKs) in Cell Cycle

Cyclins are proteins, together with **cyclin dependent kinases (CDKs),** have an important role to play in cell cycle. The cyclins in association with CDKs activate the catalytic activity of **serine-threonine kinases** in contrast to the tyrosine kinases that are associated with growth factor receptors. During G1 phase of the cell cycle, **CDK4** and **CDK6** in association with a trio of related cyclins (D1, D2 and D3), which are collectively called **D-type cyclins** are in action (Fig. 4.8). In late G1 phase R point occurs from there, **E-type cyclins** (E1 and E2) associate with **CDK2** and facilitate phosphorylation of appropriate substrate required for entry of cell into S phase. As the cell enters S phase, the **A-type cyclins** (A1 and A2) replace E cyclins and partners with CDK2 and thereby enables progression of S phase of the cell cycle up to half of S phase. Remaining half of S phase is taken care of by another type of A-type cyclin, which switches the partner to CDC2 or CDK1 and associates with it, leaving behind CDK2. As the cell progresses into G2 phase, much of this phase is taken care by the A-CDC2 type cyclin and the terminal part of G2 phase as well as M phase is taken care by **B-type cyclins** (B1 and B2), which partners with CDC2 to complete the cell cycle. Finally, at the onset of M phase, the B-type cyclins partnering with CDC2 triggers many of the actual events of the cell cycle prophase, metaphase, anaphase, and telophase that together constitute the complex program of mitosis.

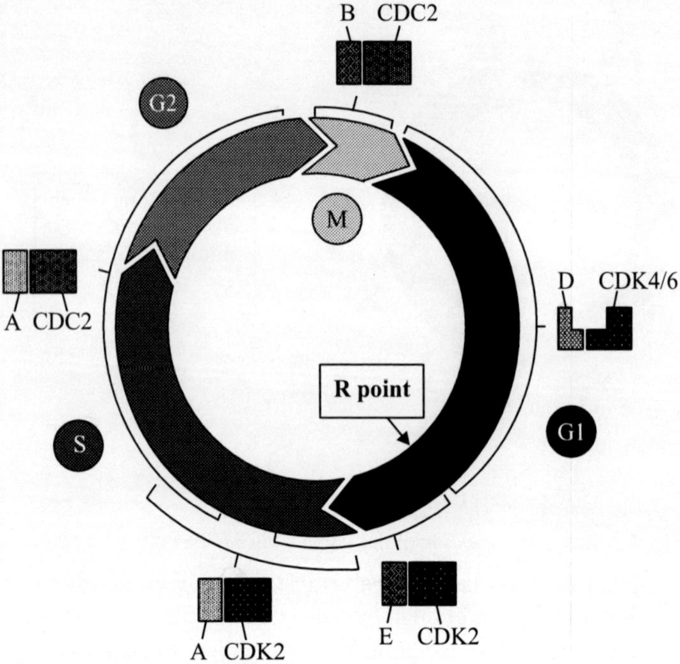

Fig. 4.8. Pairing of cyclins with cyclin dependent kinases during cell cycle

As the case with all well-regulated systems, the activities of the various cyclin-CDK complexes must be modulated to impose control on specific steps in the cell cycle. The most important way of achieving this regulation depends upon changing the levels and availability of cyclins during various phases of the cell cycle. B-type cyclin increases strongly in anticipation of mitosis, cyclin E levels rise abruptly after a cell has progressed through R-point, while the cyclin A increases in concert with the cells entrance into S phase. All these cyclins collapse as cell advances from one cell cycle phase to the next due to their rapid degradation brought about by **ubiquitin ligases**. The gradual accumulation cyclins in each phase of the cell cycle followed by their rapid destruction have an important functional consequence for the cell cycle, because it dictates that the cell cycle clock to move in only one direction and cannot inadvertently slip backward into another one. In addition to this, cells have several other layers of control that modulate the activity of the cyclins-CDK complexes and thereby regulate advance through the cell cycle.

The most important of these additional controls is imposed by CDK inhibitors or simply CdkIs. To date, seven of these proteins have been identified that antagonize the activities of cyclin-CDK complexes. A group of four of these INK4 proteins, namely, $p16^{INK4A}$, $p15^{INK4B}$, $P18^{INK4C}$ and $p19^{INK4D}$ inhibit CDK4 and 6 (Fig. 4.9). The remaining three, namely, $p21^{Cip1}$, $p27^{Kip1}$, and $p57^{Kip2}$ CDK inhibitors (Fig. 4.9), are more widely acting, capable of inhibiting all the other cyclins-CDK complexes formed at the later stage of cell cycle.

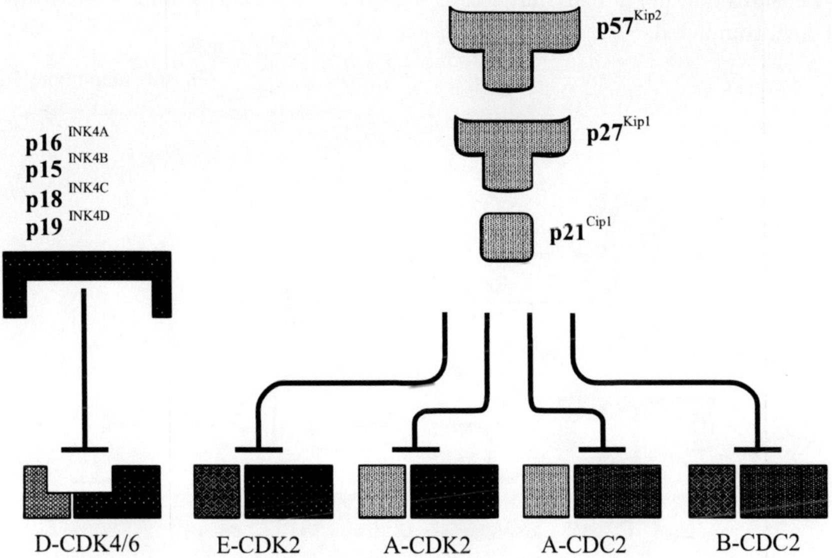

Fig. 4.9. Action of CDK inhibitors

The actions of these two classes of inhibitors are nicely illustrated by $p15^{INK4B}$ and the pair of $p21^{Cip1}$ and $p27^{Kip1}$. When TGF-β is applied to epithelial cells, it elicits several downstream responses from cells that antagonize cell proliferation. Among these are significant increases in the levels of $p15^{INK4B}$, which is the inhibitor of cyclin D-CDK4/6 complex formation and already formed complexes. In the absence of active CDK-4/6 complexes, the cell will not be able to proceed through early and mid-G1 phase of cell cycle and reach R point. The action of the D-CDK4/6 complexes is of no use once a cell has passed through R point. This may explain why the cell will not respond to growth inhibitory signal of TGF-β once a cell has passed through the R point.

$p21^{Cip1}$, a more widely acting CDK inhibitor, is also induced by TGF-β in a weak way. Far more important are the increases in the levels of $p21^{Cip1}$ that occur in response to various physiological functions. Once present in significant levels, $p21^{Cip1}$ can act through much of the cell cycle to stop the cell in its tracks. One of the prominent among these stress signals is the damage to cell's genome. As long as the genomic DNA remains in an unrepaired state, the induced $p21^{Cip1}$ will block E-CDK2, A-CDK2, A-CDC2, and B-CDC2 activities that happened to be active when this damage was first incurred; as soon as the damage is repaired, $p21^{Cip1}$ -imposed block will be relieved. Such a strategy makes special sense in G1. If a cell's genome is damaged during this period through the action of various mutagens $p21^{Cip1}$ will block the cell cycle advancement crossing the R point (by inhibition of E-CDK2) complexes until the damage is set right, ensuring that the cell does not inadvertently copy damaged DNA sequences and progresses to S phase. In addition, $p21^{Cip1}$ can inhibit the function of key component termed PCNA (proliferating-cell nuclear antigen) of the cell's DNA replication apparatus.

This ensures that the already initiated DNA synthesis is halted until DNA repair has been completed.

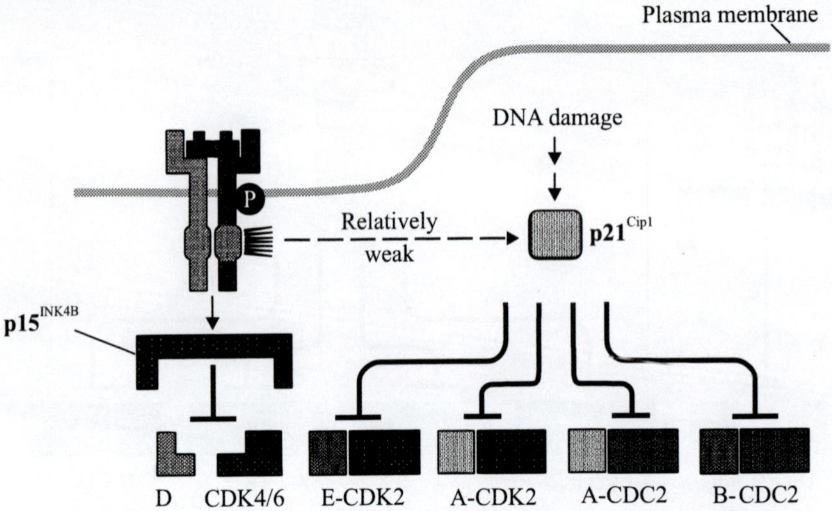

Fig. 4.10. TGF-β inhibitory signals for the regulation of CDKs activity

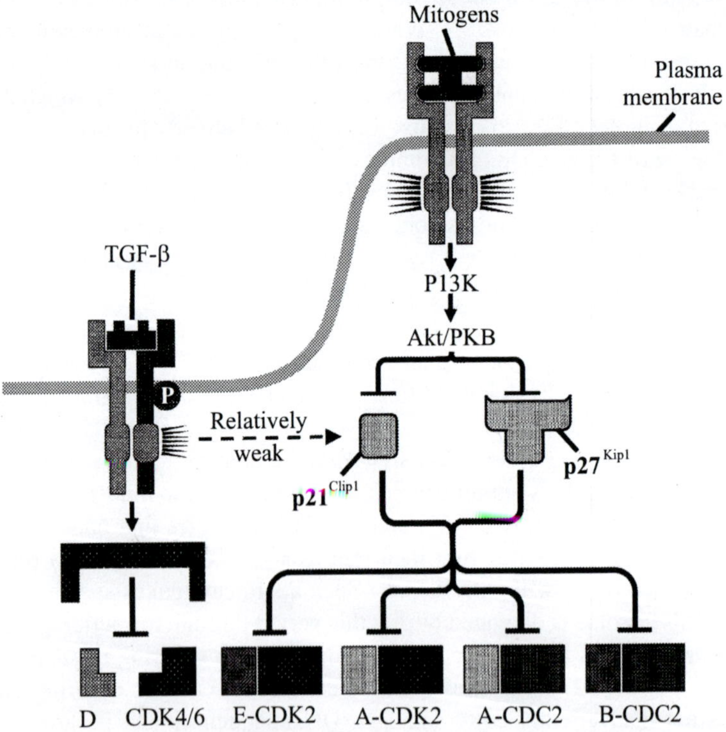

Fig. 4.11. Antimitogenic and mitogenic signals showing inhibition or release of inhibition of CDKs by proteins

While the DNA damage, and to a lesser extent, TGF-β can elicit increases in the levels of $p21^{Cip1}$ (thereby blocking cell cycle advance), mitogens act in an opposing fashion to suppress the actions of the CDK inhibitors and in this way favor cell cycle to proceed. One mechanism by which they do so depends on the phosphatidyl-inositol 3-kinase (PI3K) pathway, which is activated directly or indirectly by the mitogen that stimulates many receptor tyrosine kinases. PI3K activated by mitogen will activate an important kinase Akt/PKB downstream, which in turn, **phosphorylates $p21^{Cip1}$ molecule located in the nucleus, which leads to its export from the nucleus to the cytoplasm, where they can never engage in inhibition of CDK complexes**. Similarly, **phosphorylation of $p27^{Kip1}$**by **Akt/PKB will prevent its export from cytoplasm to the nucleus**. Taken together, these signaling responses illustrate how extracellular growth-inhibitory signals impede the advancement of cell cycle, while growth promoting signals promote its forward progress. **In high grade tumors, activated Akt/PKB is abundant and much of $p27^{Kip1}$ is now found in the cell cytoplasm**. This intracellular localization is correlated with progression of cancer to fatal endpoint.

4.2.2 Role of Rb Protein (pRb) in Cell Cycle Regulation

From several experiments it has been revealed that retinoblastoma protein (pRb) undergoes phosphorylation as the cell progresses through the cell cycle. In G0 state of the cell, pRb is not phosphorylated, which on entering G1 phase is **hypophosphorylated** on a small number of serine and threonine residues. As the cell cycle progresses through R point it is extensively phosphorylated leading to **hyperphosphorylation** on much larger number of serine-threonine residues in concert with advancement of cell cycle (Fig. 4.12).

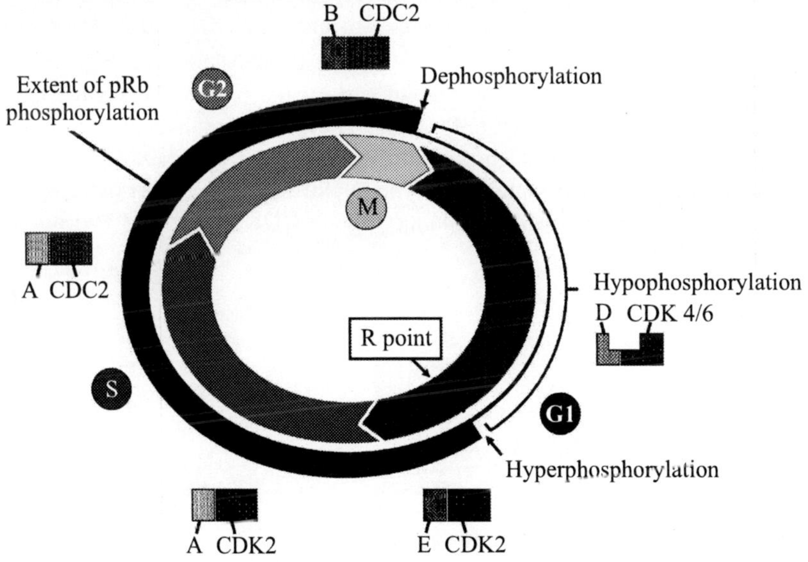

Fig. 4.12. Phosphorylation of retinoblastoma protein (pRb) during various stages of cell cycle

Once the cell has passed through the R point, during the remainder of the cell cycle pRb remains hyperphosphorylated. The phosphate groups of pRb are stripped of after the final exit of the cells through mitosis. This sets the stage for the next cell cycle through a new cycle of pRb phosphorylation.

In 1988, an important mechanism whereby a DNA tumor virus-encoded oncoprotein disruption of the cell cycle regulating circuitry was discovered. E1A oncogene of human adenovirus type 5 showed transformation of cells where E1A oncoprotein was tightly bound to pRb. Soon after this discovery, it was found that SV40 virus encoded large T oncoprotein and E7 oncoprotein of HPV were also found tightly bound to pRb in respective virus transformed cells. Within a normal cell, the Rb gene functions as a tumor suppressor gene through its product pRb protein, which inhibits cell proliferation in some fashion. Oncoproteins of DNA tumor viruses can sabotage the activities of pRb by binding to it and inactivate it.

HPV-E7 oncoprotein goes beyond simple sequestration of pRb, since it also tags pRb for ubiquitylation and thus proteolytic degradation. Another clue to the pRb function was provided by the discovery that the **oncoproteins of the DNA tumor viruses preferentially bind to the hypophosphorylated forms of pRb, i.e., forms of pRb that are present in the cell through most of the G1 phase. Viral oncoproteins target the growth inhibitory forms of pRb found in the early and mid G1 stage of mitosis and ignore those forms of pRb that are already in inactivated (hyperphosphorylated)** condition by other mechanisms.

Various lines of evidence indicate that pRb is a growth inhibitor during the early to mid-G1 phase of the cell cycle and due to hyperphosphorylation it is inactivated as the cell passes through the R-point gate and thereafter largely remains inactive until the cell cycle is completed. pRb serves as a guard of R-point gate, holding it shut, but only on hyperphosphorylation loses its growth inhibitory powers, opens the gate, and allows the cell to enter late G1 and complete the remaining phases of the cell cycle.

Since pRb is the ultimate controller of cell cycle, its phosphorylation takes place in a carefully regulated manner for which D-type cyclins in combination with their CDK4/6 kinases initiate pRb phosphorylation in the later part of G1 phase, leading to its hypophosphorylation. D-type cyclin levels are also controlled by external mitogenic signals, which collaborate with CDK4/6 partners and initiate pRb phosphorylation (Fig. 4.13).

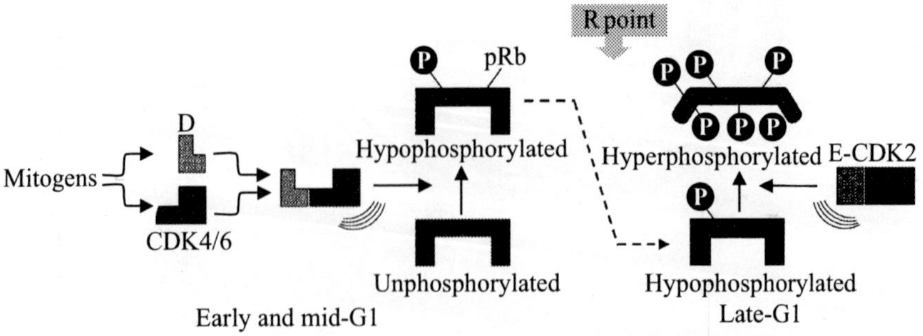

Fig. 4.13. Control of restriction point (R-point) transition by mitogens

Hypophosphorylation of pRb is necessary at the initial stage of the cell cycle but it is not sufficient for complete inactivation of pRb at the R point, which is achieved by hyperphosphorylation. For the purpose of hyperphosphorylation of pRb, E-cyclin levels start increasing steadily from the R point. **The association of E-cyclin with CDK2, its partner drives pRb phosphorylation to hyper-phosphorylated state, causing functional inactivation of pRb** (Fig. 4.14).

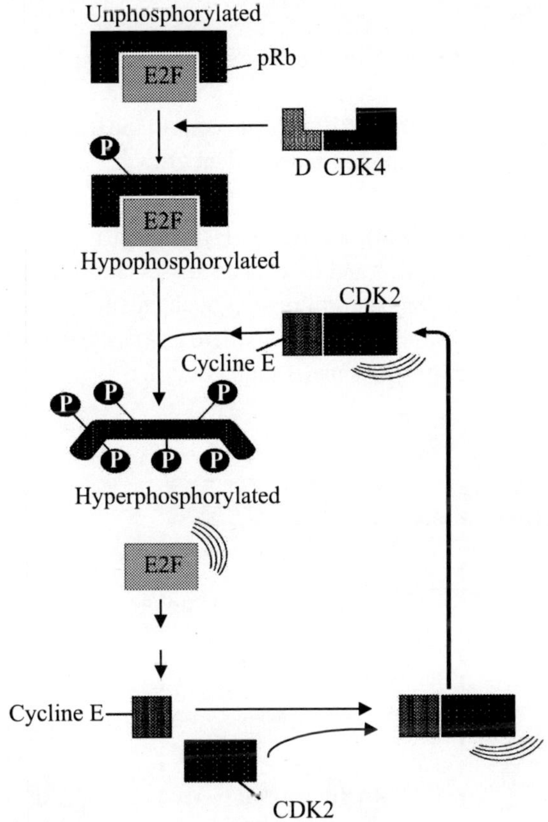

Fig. 4.14. E-CDK2 driven pRb hyperphosphorylation

The phosphorylation and functional inactivation of pRb's cousins, p107 and p130, are also under the control of cyclin D-CDK 4/6 and possibly cyclin E-CDK2.

Prior to the R point, at any time in G1 phase of cell cycle, if mitogens are withdrawn, cyclin D1 levels rapidly drop. As the cyclin D1 disappears, phosphate groups from pRb are lost by the action of a still-unidentified phosphatase, thereby pRb reverts to a state that no longer it will be a substrate for cyclin E-CDK2 complexes for phosphorylation. This indicates that **strong and continuous mitogenic signals are required during the early and mid-G1 phases of cell cycle until the R point is reached.**

As the cell passes through the R point, increased levels of E-cyclin facilitate hyperphosphorylation and functional inactivation of the pRb, followed by cyclin

A, and then by cyclin-B partnered with CDK complexes, none of which responds to extracellular signals. This is precisely what pRb does as an important regulator of cell proliferation. Rb gene mutations or promoter methylation of Rb gene or inhibition by the DNA tumor virus oncoproteins, the functions of the pRb protein will be lost from the cell. In such situation pRb protein cannot stand as the guardian of the R point gate. Moreover, in some cancers, pRb phosphorylation is deregulated, resulting in inappropriate phosphorylation and thus functional inactivation of pRb.

The activities of pRb seem to overlap with p107 and p130, where p130 is specialized to suppress cell proliferation in G0 phase, whereas p107 is most active in the late G1 and S phase. Only pRb is able to control the transition at the R-point from mitogen-dependent to mitogen-independent growth.

In hypophosphorylated state pRb and its cousins p107 and p130 bind to free E2Fs (transcription factors), as well as E2F bound to DNA. However, in hyperphosphorylated state, pRb and its cousins dissociate from E2F (Fig. 4.15). this shows the pRb regulatory control on cell cycle advancement by controlling E2F in the early and the middle part of G1, where E2Fs is responsible for binding to promoters of a number of genes under their control.

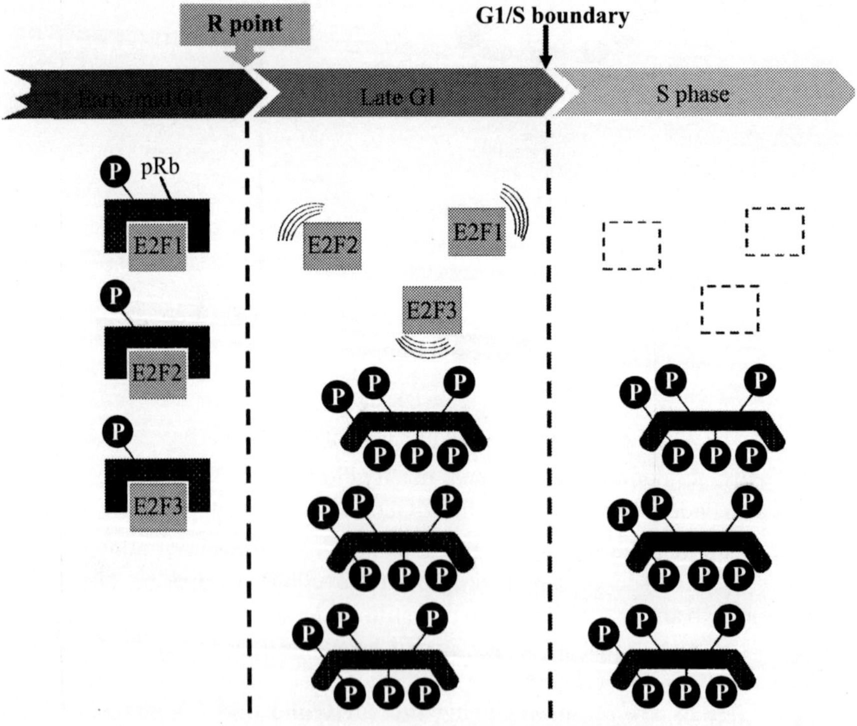

Fig. 4.15. E2Fs and their interaction with pRb

pRb and its cousins p107 and p130 are regarded as pocket proteins, which in association with E2Fs, prevent their transcription activity. With the result, genes dependent on E2F expression during much of the G1 phase of the cell cycle will remain repressed. However, on hyperphosphorylation of pocket proteins at R point in the late G1 phase, E2Fs are released from the grip of pocket proteins, permitting the E2Fs action as transcription factors for the genes under their control. The products of the genes under E2Fs action, in turn, facilitate the cell to proceed from G1 to S phase. Similarly, viral oncoproteins mimic pRb hyperphosphorylation state thereby preventing pRb from binding to E2Fs facilitating transcription of the genes under E2Fs control. E2Fs exist as 1, 2, 3, 4, 5 and 6 subunits, all of which can either bind to a DP1 or DP2 subunit of transcription factors. Once bound to DP subunits, they recognize the promoters of various genes and bind to it to initiate transcription (Fig. 4.16).

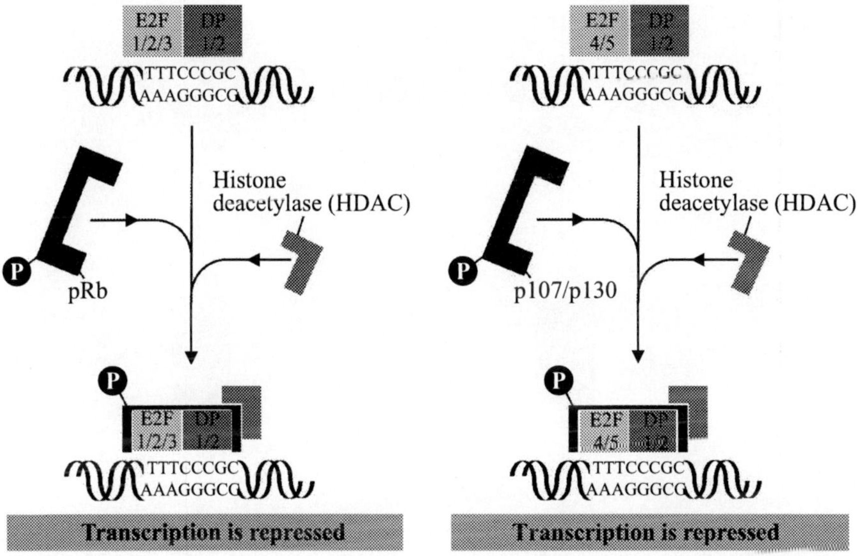

Fig. 4.16. The role of E2F in facilitating transcription by modifying histones through acetylation or deacetylation

In quiescent Go cells, for example, E2F4 and E2F5 are present in abundance and are associated largely with p130, whereas E2Fs, 1, 2 and 3 are hardly present, which are expressed largely in proliferating cells. Moreover, cells that have been genetically deprived of E2F4 and E2F5 have lost responsiveness to the growth inhibitory effects of the $p16^{INK4A}$, CDK inhibitor. Hyperphosphorylation of pRb releases its grip on E2F complexes, thereby facilitating E2Fs to attract transcription activating proteins, such as histone acetylases, which modify the histones and place them in a configuration that encourages transcription (Fig. 4.16).

Gene encoding cyclin E is the prominent activator of E2F, where inactivation of pRb leads to increases in cyclin E levels, which in turn, leads to further inactivation of pRb (Fig. 4.14).

At R point, a second positive feedback loop is simultaneously activated through the following mechanism: cyclin E-CDK2 phosphorylates $p27^{Kip1}$, and the phosphorylated $p27^{Kip1}$ is ubiquitylated and rapidly degraded (Fig. 4.17).

$p27^{Kip1}$ molecule, which normally inhibits E-CDK2 firing, destruction of $p27^{Kip1}$ liberates more amount of cyclin E-CDK2 complexes that phosphorylate $p27^{Kip1}$ thereby additional $p27^{Kip1}$ molecules are inactivated.

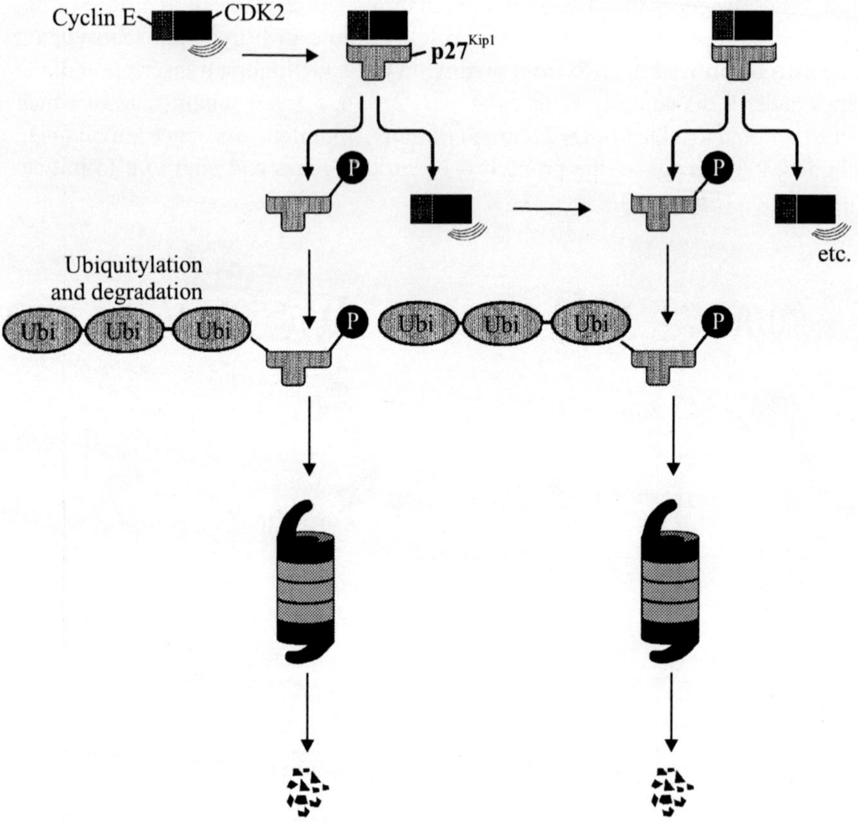

Fig. 4.17. Activation of small number of E-CDK2 leads to phosphorylation of $p27^{Kip1}$ and phosphorylated $p27^{Kip1}$ is ubiquitylated and destroyed

4.2.3 Role of myc Gene in Cell Cycle Regulation

Phosphorylation of pRb is known to be perturbed by *myc* oncoprotein thereby deregulation of control of cell cycle progression. In the normal cell, *myc* regulates the expression of severalother critical components of the cell cycle clock. When the cell expresses abnormally high levels of *myc* protein because of the presence of *myc* oncogene, it promotes uncontrolled cell division, a state like that seen in cells lacking Rb gene function (Fig. 4.18).

Myc oncoprotein targets cyclin D2 gene leading to its elevated expression resulting in hypophosphorylation of pRb. Expression of increased levels of

CDK4 gene is also driven by *myc* gene leading to formation of the cyclin D-CDK4 complexes, which causes hypophosphorylation of pRb and simultaneously, $p27^{Kip1}$ inhibitor is sequestered, thereby freeing the cyclin E-CDK2 complexes from $p27^{Kip1}$ inhibition. The expression of **Cul-1** protein is also driven by *myc*, which plays a central role in the degradation of the $p27^{Kip1}$ CDK inhibitor through ubiquitylation (Fig. 4.18).

Myc by associating with second transcription factor named Miz-1 can also function as a transcriptional repressor (Fig. 4.18). $p15^{INK4B}$ and $p21^{Cip1}$, the inhibitors CDK4/6 and CDK2 are repressed by *myc-miz* combination (Fig. 4.18). TGF-β uses $p15^{INK4B}$ and $p21^{Cip1}$ CDK inhibitors to prevent the progression through G1 phase of the cell cycle. Hence, by preventing the expression of $p15^{INK4B}$ and $p21^{Cip1}$ CDK inhibitors, *myc* confers resistance to the TGF-β growth inhibitory action. This provides a convenient environment for the cancer cells to continue proliferation under conditions that would normally prevent their proliferation. Repression of $p15^{INK4B}$ and $p21^{Cip1}$ gene expression by *myc* oncoprotein removes

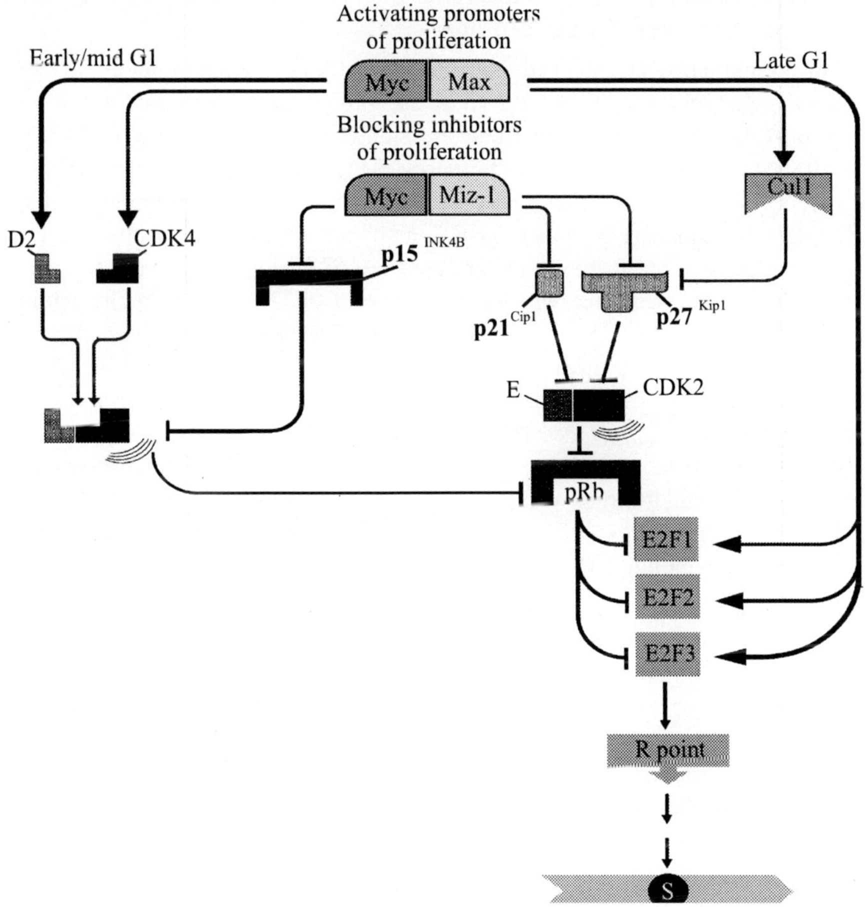

Fig. 4.18. Regulatory action of *myc* on cell cycle clock

the major obstacle of cell cycle progression. High levels of *myc* oncoprotein expressed constitutively by *myc* oncogene ensures that expression of $p15^{INK4B}$ and $p21^{Cip1}$-CDK inhibitors are strongly repressed, thereby paving the way for vigorous cell cycle advancement.

The expression of genes encoding the E2F1, E2F2 and E2F3 transcription factor proteins is also induced by *myc* oncoprotein. pRb and its two cousins, p107 and 130, negatively regulate these transcription factors. *Myc* causes the accumulation of these growth promoting factors in a cell, thereby tipping the balance in favor of cell proliferation.

4.2.4 Regulation of Cell Cycle by TGF-β

TGF-β has its own, unique receptor with serine/threonine kinase in its cytoplasmic domain to emit signals. The primary targets of these signals are Smad transcription factor family. Once phosphorylated by TGF-β receptor, Smad2 (or Smad3) protein complexes with Smad4 proteins and acts as a transcription factor. The genes encoding $p15^{INK4B}$ and to a lesser extent $p21^{Cip1}$ CDK inhibitors are the most important targets of action of TGF-β.

In normal cells, TGF-β needs to have the last word in determining whether or not the cells proliferate. In order to do so, TGF-β must ensure that *myc* does not thwart its scheme to activate the expression of the $p15^{INK4B}$ and $p21^{Cip1}$ CDK inhibitors. So, in normal cells, TGF-β suppresses the action of *myc* on the promoters of $p15^{INK4B}$ and $p21^{Cip1}$ CDK inhibitor genes by repressing the expression of the *myc* proto-oncogene (Fig. 4.19). TGF-β activated Smad3 transcription factor is capable of binding to the promoter sequence of *myc* gene. Adjacent to this sequence is another sequence, which permits binding of E2F4 or E2F5 transcription factors, that favor transcriptional repression. Smad3 ensures the shutdown of *myc* transcription by forming the tripartite complex with E2F4/5 plus 107 (Fig. 4.19), thereby eliminating growth promoting effect of the *myc* oncoprotein from the cell's regulatory circuitry. Once TGF-β has succeeded in removal of *myc* from the promoters of $p15^{INK4B}$ and $p21^{Cip1}$ CDK inhibitors, TGF-β uses its Smad3-Smad4 complexes working together with Miz-1, to activate the two promoters of $p15^{INK4B}$ and $p21^{Cip1}$ CDK inhibitors, thereby inducing expression of these critically important CDK inhibitors (Fig. 4.19).

If the cancer cells have to thrive, then they have to evade TGF-β imposed growth inhibition. More specifically, such cancer cells will depend on high levels of the *myc* oncoprotein to drive their proliferation and therefore must liberate from TGF-β induced repression of *myc* transcription. This explains why, for example, in series of 12 human breast carcinomas, *myc* expression in all 12 of these tumors was no longer responsive to TGF-β imposed shutdown even though many of TGF-β-induced responses were intact in 11 of these tumors. Similarly, when mutations lead to the formation of *myc* oncogenes, these genes acquire self-firing promoters that fire constitutively and thus are no longer responsive to TGF-β-induced repression. Once protected from the threat of this repression, the *myc* oncogenes,

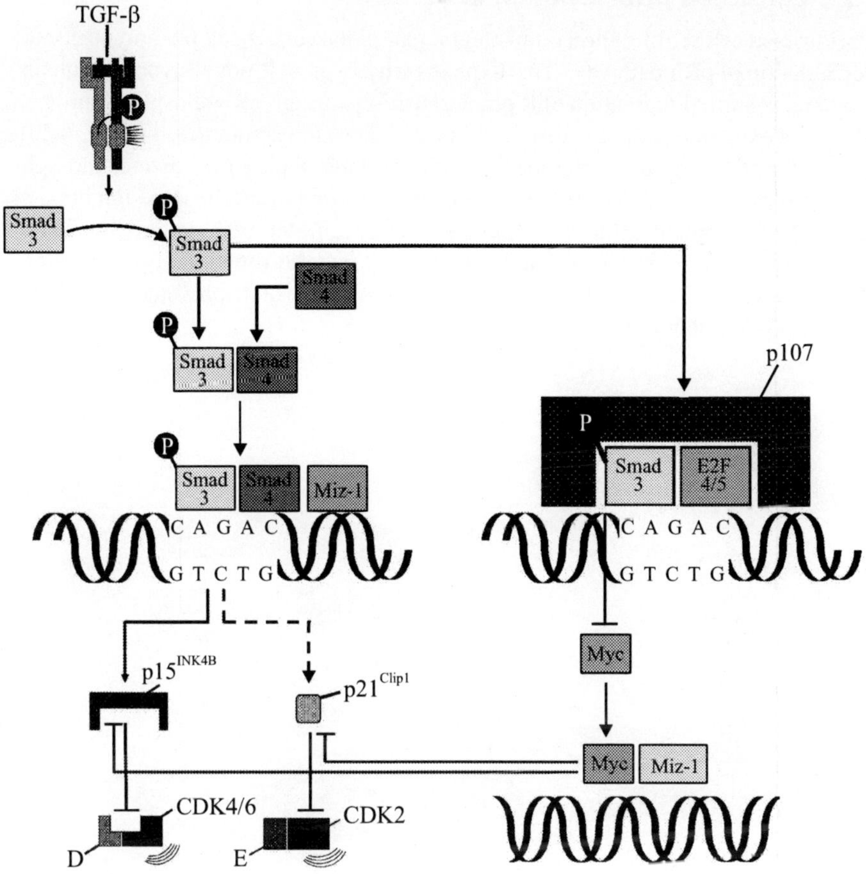

Fig. 4.19. Countervailing the action of TGF-β and Myc

more specifically, its *myc* oncoproteins hold the expression of $p15^{INK4B}$ and $p21^{Cip1}$ CDK inhibitors at a very low level and do so indefinitely.

TGF-β response can also be partially inactivated through mutations of the gene encoding the Smad3 protein, which is frequently observed in colon carcinomas. A similar partial blunting of TGF-β induced anti-mitogenic response seems to be achieved by the ***Ski oncoprotein***. This protein as well its cousin **Sno**, can bind to Smad3-Smad4 transcription factor complex and block its ability to repress *myc* transcription.

Mutation inactivated Smad4 proteins have been identified in all pancreatic carcinomas and more than quarter of all colon cancers. In the absence of Smad4, neither Smad2-Smad4 nor Smad3-Smad4 complexes can be formed, with the result no shutdown of cell proliferation. Some tcancers like colon cancers that suffer "microsatellite instability" carry mutant TGF-βII receptors. Such cells acquire the ability to evade TGF-β imposed growth inhibition.

4.2.5 Perturbed pRb Function in Cancers

Unrestricted cell proliferation is an integral part of the cancer cell phenotype due to deregulation of pRb pathway. This explains why in most if not all types of human tumor cells normal regulation of R point transition through pRb phosphorylation is likely to be disrupted. These disruptive mechanisms are summarized in Fig. 4.20. We are familiar with the direct mechanisms for deregulating the advance through the R point by inactivation of the Rb gene through mutation. In some tumors, an equivalent outcome is achieved through Rb gene promoter methylation. In others, though normal amounts of pRb are synthesized, may be functionally inactivated by viral oncoproteins, such as the HPV-E7 protein, which prevents pRb from binding and regulating E2Fs.

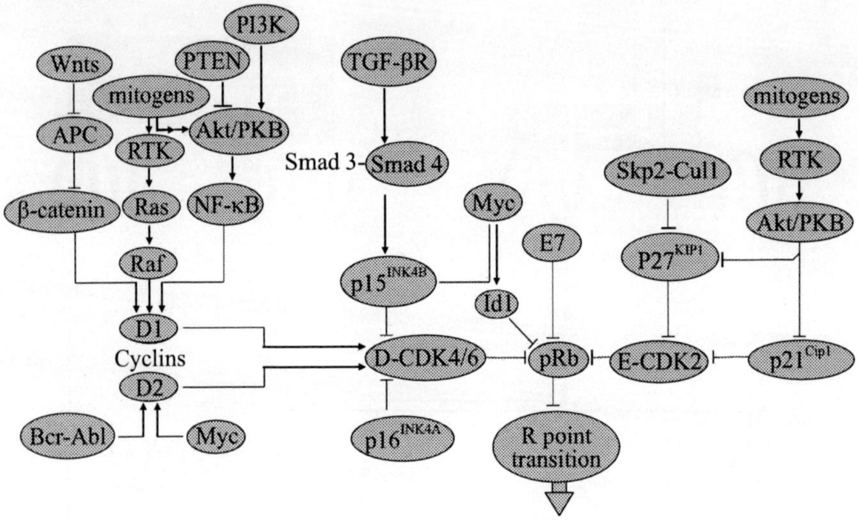

Fig. 4.20. Coordinated perturbation of the R point transition by different genes in human tumors

Yet another strategy used by cancer cells to inactivate pRb function is through enhanced expression of cyclin D1 as observed in a variety of human tumor cells. This is most widely documented in breast cancer cells, in which as many as half of tumors have been reported to show elevated levels of this protein. In these and other carcinomas, the overexpression is sometimes achieved by increasing the copy number of the cyclin D1 gene (gene amplification).

A more devious ploy frequently exploited by cancer cells is to disable the pRb machinery by shutting down expression of p16^{INK4A} tumor suppressor protein. Recall that the p16^{INK4A} protein, like its p15^{INK4B} cousins, inhibits the cyclin D-CDK4/6, which is responsible for pRb phosphorylation. When p16^{INK4A} protein is not produced, excessive cyclin D-CDK4/6 kinase activity is observed resulting in pRb phosphorylation and inappropriate inactivation of pRb, which operates without an important braking mechanism, deregulating pRb phosphorylation (Fig. 4.20). Individuals suffering from one form of familial melanoma inherit defective version of the $p16^{INK4A}$ gene, reasons unknown. In sporadic tumors (non-familial) tumors of various sorts, cancer cells resort far more frequently to another strategy to shed $p16^{INK4A}$ function; they methylate CpG sequences present in the promoters.

pRb functions are closely linked with the controls of differentiation process. Cell differentiation is a process of crucial importance to cancer pathogenesis and as such, cells throughout the body can exist in either of two alternative growth states. They may be found in a relatively undifferentiated state in which they retain the option to divide if mitogenic signals call for their proliferation; this is essentially the behavior of stem cells. The alternative is that cells leave this state and enter a more differentiated state, whereupon they give up the option of ever proliferating again and thus become post-mitotic. The opposition between cell proliferation and differentiation is seen most clearly in the formation of most types of cancer cells in which differentiation is partially or completely blocked. This would require two independent changes in the cellular control circuitry during the formation of cancer cells; one that deregulates control of proliferation and another that blocks differentiation. More specifically, signals favoring the hyperphosphorylation (and thus functional inactivation) of the three pocket proteins, namely pRb, p107 and p130, operate to block differentiation, while those that prevent pRb hyperphosphorylation favor differentiation.

Yet another line of evidence indicating coupling between differentiation and the cell cycle machinery comes from research on the *myc* protein. The *myc* protein shifts the balance between proliferation and post-mitotic differentiation in favor of proliferation. *Myc* works to increase production of the Id2 protein, and the latter acts as an antagonist of the βHLH (helix-loop-helix) transcription factors that program differentiation. The Id proteins operate as dominant negative inhibitors of the other βHLH transcription factors by forming heterodimers with βHLH transcription factors, but lack the ability to bind to DNA to bring about inhibition of βHLH induced differentiation transcription factors, thereby blocking differentiation.

In the genomes of a small number of both sporadic and familial melanomas evidence of an even more cunning strategy for destabilizing this control circuit has been found. In these cancers a **dominant point mutation in the CDK4 gene**, which makes it resistant to inhibition by family of p15, p16, p18 and $p19^{INK4}$ molecules has been observed. While these molecules are perfectly normal, they are unable to inhibit CDK4 target. Once again, this permits K4, together with its cyclin D partners, to drive the initial steps of pRb phosphorylation in a deregulated fashion. Since CDK4 mutation is a dominant one, only one copy of the gene needs to be inactivated to achieve proliferative benefit.

The most critical CDK inhibitor involved in cancer pathogenesis may well be $p27^{Kip1}$. As mentioned earlier, $p27^{Kip1}$ is largely involved in inhibiting the activity of cyclin D-CDK4 complexes. As cells exit from the cell cycle to G0 quiescent stage, rise in $p27^{Kip1}$ levels takes place. Conversely, with the re-entry of cell into the cell cycle and passing through G1 phase, $p27^{Kip1}$ levels are reduced progressively throughout early and mid-G1 and then are made to fall drastically during late G1 phase by the actions of cyclins E-CDK2 complexes. These low levels are not created by reduced transcription of the gene encoding $p27^{Kip1}$. Instead, it seems $p27^{Kip1}$ levels are reduced by the actions of the Skp2 protein, which acts together with *Cul1* and several other proteins to recognize $p27^{Kip1}$ and ubiquitylate it for destruction. Indeed, the declining levels of Skp2 explain the increase in $p27^{Kip1}$ as cells enter Go.

In the inverse relationship between $p27^{Kip1}$ levels and those of Skp2 is especially apparent in various human cancers. Thus, in mammary and oral carcinomas, as well as lymphomas, the levels of $p27^{Kip1}$ are inversely correlated with those of Skp2, with higher levels of Skp2 portending shorter patient survival. Moreover, poor patient survival is correlated with low levels of $p27^{Kip1}$ CDK inhibitor in the cells of human esophageal, breast, colorectal and lung carcinomas. In all these tumors, Skp2 seems to act as a growth promoting oncoprotein by forcing the degradation of the critical $p27^{Kip1}$ proliferation inhibitor. Notch protein, which is hyperactive in many types of human tumors, increases the expression of Skp2 gene.

It is evident that the hyperactive state of the Akt/PKB kinase in many human tumors is caused by a variety of molecular defects, including hyperactive growth factor receptors, loss of the PTEN tumor suppressor protein, and mutation in PI3K. By phosphorylating $p21^{Cip1}$ and $p27^{Kip1}$, Akt/PKB ensures the cytoplasmic localization of these two antagonists of cell cycle, thereby marginalizing their action. At the same time, Akt/PKB can suppress expression of the gene encoding $p27^{Kip1}$ by phosphorylating a transcription factor of the Fork head family, which serves to further reduce the overall concentration of $p27^{Kip1}$ in the cell.

In normal cells, levels of *myc* protein are highly dependent on extracellular mitogenic growth factors. In many cancer cells, however, the *myc* protein is produced constitutively, independent of mitogenic signals coming into the cell. It can be deduced that, many perturbations wrought by the *myc* protein are magnified in many types of human cancer cells that carry either *myc* oncogenes or the oncogenic version of its cousins, N-*myc* and L-*myc*. Among the many products induced by *myc*, the Id2 proteins may well have the greatest physiological importance. On the one hand, they can act as dominant negative inhibitors of βHLH transcription factors. On the other hand, they can bind to pRb and seem to inhibit its functioning in a way that is reminiscent of the actions of viral oncoproteins such as T, E7 and E1A. Id2 protein has been reported to be overproduced in diverse tumors including endometrial, head-and-neck, breast, pancreatic, esophageal, cervical carcinomas, neuroblastomas, and melanomas. Its expression is positively correlated with the degree of malignancy and invasiveness in many of these tumors.

The diverse genetic and biochemical strategies shown in Fig. 4.20 are all focused on overwhelming and deregulating pRb function, thereby, destroying the tight control imposed on R point transition. Darwinian selection, occurring in the microcosm of living tissues, favors the outgrowth of cells that, by hook or crook, have succeeded in inactivating the critical pRb braking system and thus deregulating the R point transition.

4.3 p53 GENE AS TUMOR SUPPRESSOR GENE

Various studies on wild type p53 gene are also referred to as Trp53 in mice. TP53 in humans showed that it functions as tumor suppressor gene and prevents cell proliferation. It was also found that a point mutation in the reading frame of p53 leads to acquisition of growth promoting powers. By 1987 it became apparent that in the genomes of a wide variety of human tumors point-mutated alleles of p53 are common. p53 gene is found to be the most frequently mutated genes among all the other genes that are mutated in human cancer cell genomes. Detailed study of p53 gene function revealed that, it prevents the appearance of abnormal cells that promote tumors rather than prevent proliferation of tumor cells. It was also found that large number of DNA viruses (SV40, adenovirus, polyoma virus, HPV, Herpes virus saimiri, Epstein-Barr virus) and at least one RNA virus (HTLV-1) has been found to specify oncoproteins that associate with p53 or perturb its function. These viral proteins also block apoptosis.

From the studies on different tumor cell genomes, frequent mutation in the p53 gene is found to be common feature suggesting that many cancer cells eliminate p53 function before they become malignant. Mutant p53 alleles sequence analysis revealed that in great majority of human tumor cell genomes the mutant p53 alleles has point mutation in their reading frames that causes **missense** mutation resulting in amino acid substitutions rather than nonsense codons (which cause premature termination of the growing polypeptide chain). Studies carried out on p53 alleles found in more than 15,000 human tumor cell genomes have revealed that, 75% of them carry missense mutations. From this, researchers concluded that the presence of a slightly altered p53 protein provides benefit to tumor cells rather than from its complete absence by outright deletion or by null alleles due to nonsense mutations of the p53 gene.

The evidence to the puzzle of how mutant p53 protein might foster tumor cell formation came from two different studies. In the first study, it was found that the mutant allele interferes with the ongoing activity of the normal wild-type p53 gene in a cell and such an allele is called ***dominant-interfering*** or ***dominant-negative*** allele. The second line of evidence came from the biochemical analysis of the p53 protein, which exists in the cell as a **homotetramer** made up of an assembly of four identical polypeptide subunits and it serves as nuclear protein.

Assume that a mutant p53 allele in a human cancer cell encodes a mutant version of p53 protein, which cannot perform normal function but has retained the ability to participate in tetramer formation. Due to co-dominant expression, if one such mutant allele was to coexist with a wild-type allele in a cell and the p53 tetramers assembled in such a cell would contain mixtures of mutant and wild type p53 protein in various proportions (Fig. 4.21).

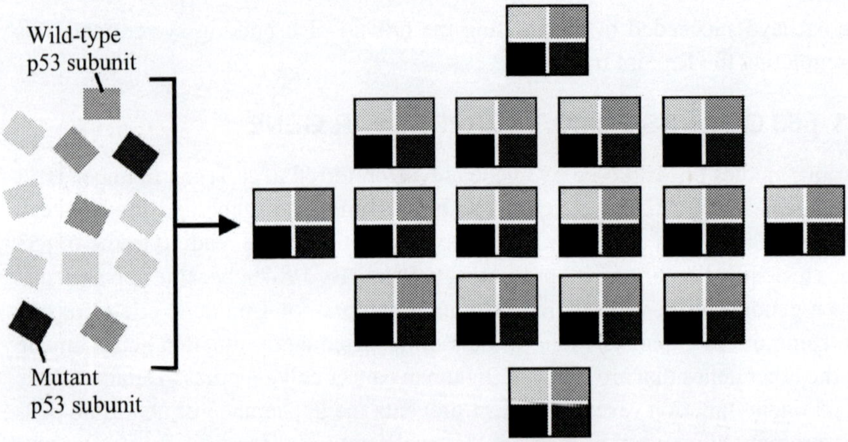

Fig. 4.21. Homotetrameric assemblage of p53 protein showing various combinations of mutant protein with wild type and assemblage of wild-type protein

In a p53 tetrameric assembled protein, the presence of a single mutant p53 protein monomer will interfere with the tetramer function. Figure 4.21 illustrates the fact that 15 out of the 16 equally possible tetrameric combinations of mutant and wild-type p53, a tetramer would contain at least one mutant p53 protein subunit. This assembly would therefore lead to lack of some or all the activity associated with a fully wild-type p53 tetramer. Consequently, only 1/16 of the p53 tetramers assembled in this heterozygous cell which would contain wild-type p53 subunits and retain full wild-type function (Fig. 4.21).

The above logic might suggest that many human tumor cells, which seem to gain advantage by shedding p53 function, will have one wild-type and one mutant p53 allele in their genome. In the great majority of human tumor cells having a mutant p53 allele would show a loss of heterozygosity (LOH) to shed the wild-type (normal) allele thereby yielding a cell with homozygous mutant p53 alleles. Thus, one copy of the p53 gene undergoes initial mutation in a tumor cell followed by elimination of the surviving wild-type copy through loss-of-heterozygosity mechanism.

Dominant-negative allele arising from initial mutation will be useful for the tumor cell than a null allele, which causes total loss of an encoded p53 protein. The elimination of the surviving wild-type p53 allele is necessary because the residual 1/16 of fully normal p53 gene function would interfere with tumor cells growth. So being most opportunistic, tumor cells jettison the remaining wild-type p53 allele in order to proliferate even better.

In normal cells, p53 protein has a short half-life of 20 minutes. p53 is a highly unstable protein, which is subjected to degradation soon after its synthesis. Agents like X-rays, ultraviolet (UV) radiation, certain chemotherapeutic drugs that cause DNA damage, inhibitors of DNA synthesis and the chemicals that disrupt microtubule components of the cytoskeleton were found to be capable of inducing rapid increases in p53 protein levels (Fig. 4.22). Increase in the level

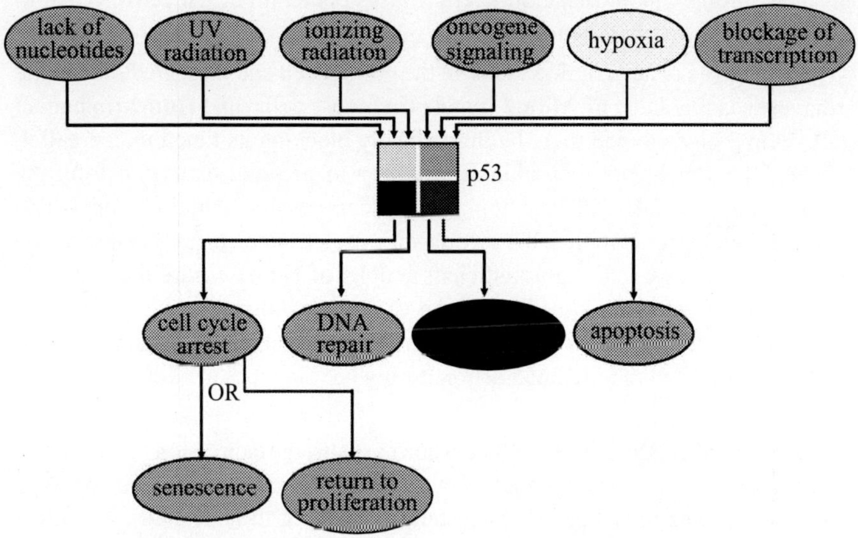

Fig. 4.22. p53-activating signals and p53's downstream effects

of p53 in cells was seen within minutes of exposing the cells to some damage causing agents, which otherwise would have shown only minimal levels of this protein with short half-life. This rapid increase in p53 protein occurred without any marked increase in transcription of the p53 gene, which was entirely due to the post-translational stabilization of the normally unstable p53 protein. In the following years, an even greater diversity of cell-physiologic signals was found to be capable of provoking increase in p53 levels. Among these were:

- Oxygen tension (hypoxia)
- *myc* expression or E1A oncoprotein expression
- expression of excessive amount of E2F1 transcription factor
- increased demethylation of chromosomal DNA
- decreased intracellular pool of ribonucleotides
- inhibition of RNA or DNA synthesis

Diverse array of surveillance systems provides signals to p53 gene. If p53 receives specific alarm signals from these monitors, it stops cell proliferation or triggers the apoptotic suicide program. For the incipient cancer cells advancing to malignancy, these pro-apoptotic and anti-proliferative signals of p53 are a major threat. Several stress signals, including hypoxia, genomic damage, and imbalance in the signaling pathways are commonly experienced by the cancer cells during many stages of tumor development (Fig. 4.22). By having partially or totally inactivated state of p53 alarm response, cancer cells can tolerate hypoxia, extensive DNA damage and altered growth-controlling circuitry. Once a tumor cell acquires resistance to these debilitating factors, the path is cleared for it and its descendents to continue their march towards a highly malignant state. At the same time, normal cells must also avoid excessive p53 activity, since it threatens to end their lives through apoptosis and thereby causes depletion of the cells needed to maintain normal bodily functions.

p53 serves as a transcription factor in the normal cell and its degradation in the normal cells is regulated by **Mdm2** protein (in mouse cells) and **Hdm2** (in human cells). Hdm2 binds to p53 there by immediately blocking its function, thereafter, facilitates the attachment of a ubiquitin moiety to p53 and exports it from the nucleus to the cytoplasm. In the cytoplasm it undergoes polyubiquitylation, which ensures its quick degradation in the cytoplasmic proteasome. In normal unstressed cells, the continuous, and highly efficient actions of Hdm2 ensure the short (20 minute) half-life of p53. Phosphorylation of amino acid residues in N-terminal domain of p53 is known to protect it from Hdm2 directed degradation as and when the normal cell required p53 action during certain types of stress for the cell survival.

Further investigation revealed that in normal cells, the expression of alternative reading frame (ARF) protein causes rapid increase in p53 levels. ARF binds to Hdm2 and inhibits its action by sequestering Hdm2 in the nucleolus. As Hdm2 is diverted from its interactions with p53, the latter escapes Hdm2 mediated ubiquitylation and resulting destruction and therefore accumulates rapidly to high levels in the cell. The enemy of an enemy is a friend: ARF can induce rapid increase in p53 levels because it kidnaps and inhibits p53's destroyer, Hdm2. In normal unstressed cells, Hdm2 must be allowed to play its normal role of keeping p53 levels very low. Otherwise, p53 will build up to intolerably high levels and ***inappropriately shut down cell proliferation or induce apoptosis.***

Figure 4.23 shows a variety of oncogenic proteins like adenovirus E1A protein, the *myc* and the Ras oncoproteins favor apoptosis by enhancing the E2F activity, which in turn , leads to increased ARF expression. This suggests that this signaling pathway has been evolved to prevent elimination of cells with other defects and overly active E2F signaling.

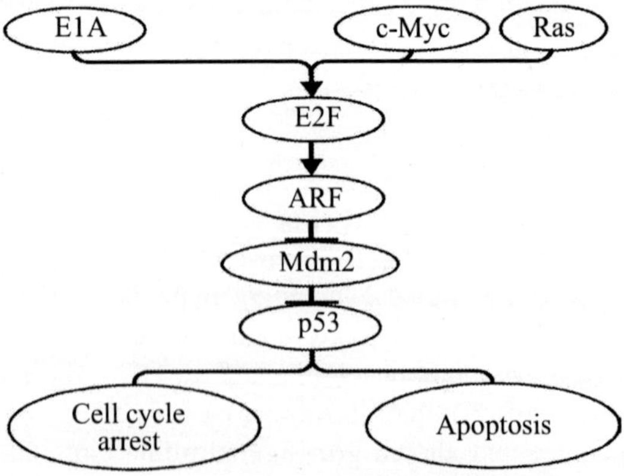

Fig. 4.23. Cascade showing influence of E2F transcription factor on ARF and its control on Mdm2/Hdm2 and the regulatory control of Mdm2/Hdm2 on p53 protein

In many human lung tumors and sarcomas, ***Hdm2 gene expression is known to be frequently amplified*** through mechanisms that remain unclear.

4.3.1 p53 Gene Inactivation Gives an Advantage to Tumor Progression

The formation of a malignant tumor involves more than half a dozen distinct steps that usually occur over a long time. An early step in the development of a cancer is activation of an oncogenc by some type of mutation. This oncogene activation may put cell at great risk of p53-induced apoptosis. The cells that have acquired oncogenic mutation will provide additional growth advantage to tumor by shedding p53 function.

Later during tumor development, a growing population of tumor cells would experience hypoxia due to the absence of adequate number of blood vessels to provide them access to oxygen. In the face of such oxygen depletion normal cells would die, whereas tumor cells may survive because of their predecessors managed to inactivate p53 gene during an early stage of tumor development.

Tumor progression involves long and multi-step process in the absence of p53-gene products, which permits the survival of cancer cells that are accumulating mutations at a faster rate. Such increased mutability would favor the activation of oncogenes and suppress the action of tumor suppressor genes, thereby enhancing the rate of evolution of pre-malignant cells to a malignant state. Loss of telomere, another catastrophe faced by evolving, pre-malignant cells, also supports the survival of such tumor cells that have lost their p53-dependent DNA damage response.

Thrombospondin-1 (TSP-1) is responsible for inhibition of formation of blood vessels, one of the important target genes whose expression is increased by p53. Consequently, in the absence of p53 function, there is reduced Tsp-1 expression, which otherwise would have prevented development of blood vessels around the clusters of cancer cells during early stages of tumor development.

Under normal circumstances, accumulation of multiple mutations in cells would not have taken place due to strict vigilance by p53 proteins, which would have promoted the cells to undergo apoptosis. But in the cancer cells, these diverse consequences of p53 inactivation permitting the cells to acquire multiple alterations accruing multiple benefits and survive explains the importance of p53 products, which is absent in most if not all types of human tumors.

4.3.2 Predisposition to a Variety of Tumors due to Inherited Mutant p53 Allele

In 1982, Li-Fraumeni identified in a group of families showing increased susceptibility to develop a variety of different tumors, like glioblastomas; leukemias; carcinomas of breast, lung, and pancreas; Wilm's tumor; and soft-tissue sarcomas. This familial cancer syndrome is named Li-Fraumeni syndrome. It was found that, many of these cases were due to mutation on human chromosome

17p13 locus, precisely where the p53 gene is located. Considering various roles that p53 plays in suppressing cancer risk in cell throughout the body, it seems reasonable that mutant germ-line alleles of this gene should predispose a person to diverse group of malignancies.

Li-Fraumeni syndrome patients carry different types of point mutations scattered across the p53 reading frame, which are transmitted through the germ-lines, with a distribution reminiscent of that shown by the somatic mutations that have been documented in more than 15,000 tumor genomes. Analysis of spectrum of germ-line mutations showed a higher frequency of G:C to A: T transitions at CpG domains, where spontaneous deamination 5-methylcytosine causing it to become thymidine.

A familial cancer syndrome in families that inherit mutant, defective forms of the Chk2 kinase behaves very much like the Li-Fraumeni syndrome has been discovered. The Chk2 kinase is responsible for phosphorylating p53, thereby saving it from destruction, and keeping the p53 alarm machinery intact. In 5% of breast cancer patients, a mutant germ-line allele of the Chk2 gene is present. This suggests that inheritance of a mutant Chk2 allele confers a measurably increased risk of developing malignancy. Yet another related cancer predisposition syndrome derives from an alteration in the promoter of the Mdm2 gene.

4.3.3 Some or All the Apoptotic Machinery is Inactivated in Cancer Cells by Various Means

In all human cancer cells anti-apoptotic strategies suggest that apoptosis is a vital anti-neoplastic mechanism found in all normal cells in order to prevent tumor progression. Two major anti-apoptotic strategies widely adopted by cancer cells are suppression of the p53 gene function by missense mutation, and silencing of ARF gene, the regulator of p53 by promoter methylation or deletion of the gene.

In many melanomas, methylation of the promoter of the APAF1 (apoptosis activation factor-1) gene, which encodes the cytosolic protein that assembles to form the apoptosome and combines with released cytochrome *c* and activates caspase 9 (Fig. 4.24). Inactivation of proapoptotic Bax gene in more than half of the colon cancers due to mutation and microsatellite instability has been observed. Enhanced expression of anti-apoptotic Bcl2 in a large number of human tumors of different tissue origin and misregulated expression of Bcl2 is found in follicular B cell lymphomas. It is observed that at least half of all human tumors show increased Bcl2 expression.

Hyperactivation of the PI3K→Akt/PKB pathway is yet another highly effective strategy adopted by cancer cells for acquiring resistance to apoptosis (Fig. 4.25). The signal emitting tyrosine kinase receptors and the Ras oncoprotein collaboratively activate PI3K resulting in increased levels of PIP3 and activation of Akt/PKB (Fig. 4.25). Inactivation of the gene encoding PTEN (phosphatase and tensin homolog deleted on chromosome 10), the phosphatase responsible for breakdown of PIP3, has a similar effect. Accumulation of PIP3 due to activation of Akt/PKB leading to phosphorylation of pro-apoptotic proteins such as Bad, caspase 9 and IκB causes

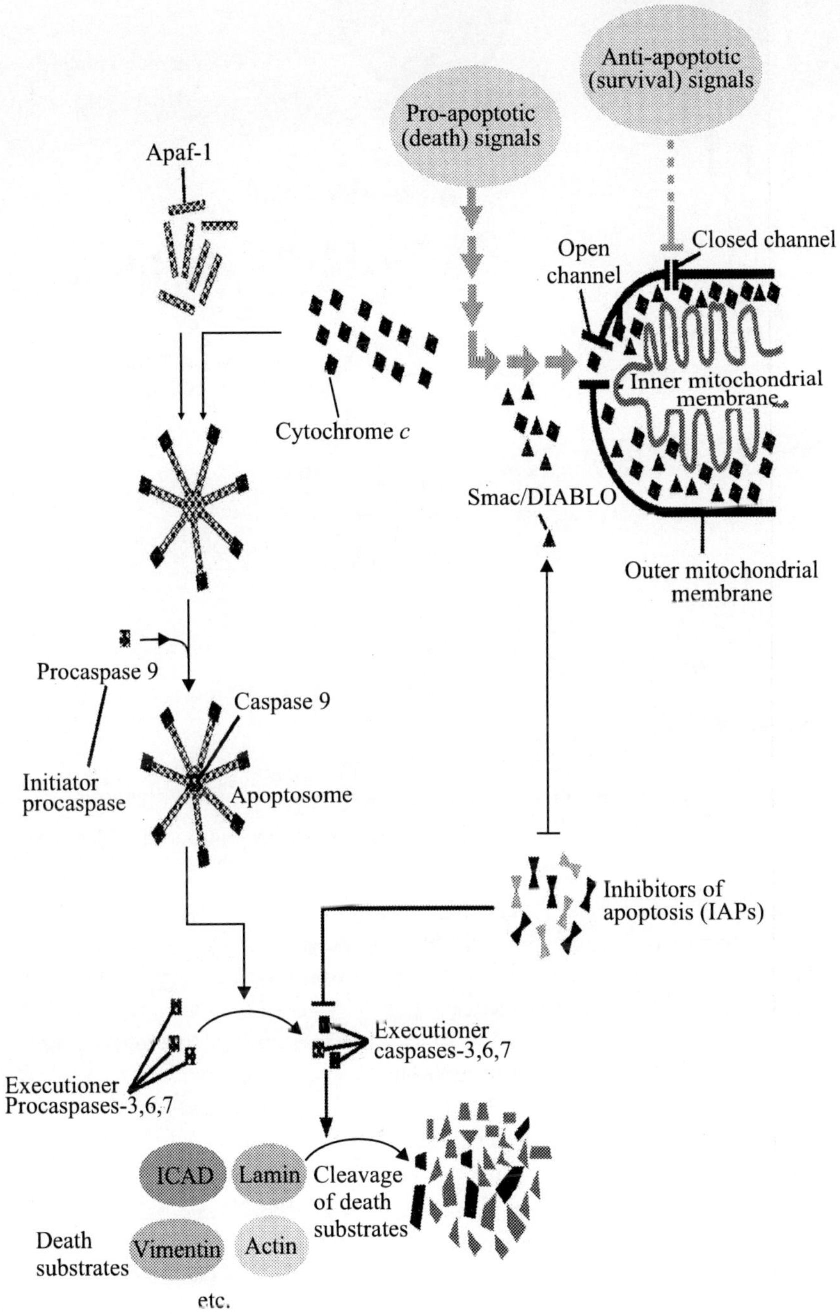

Fig. 4.24. The pro-apoptotic caspase cascade in normal cells

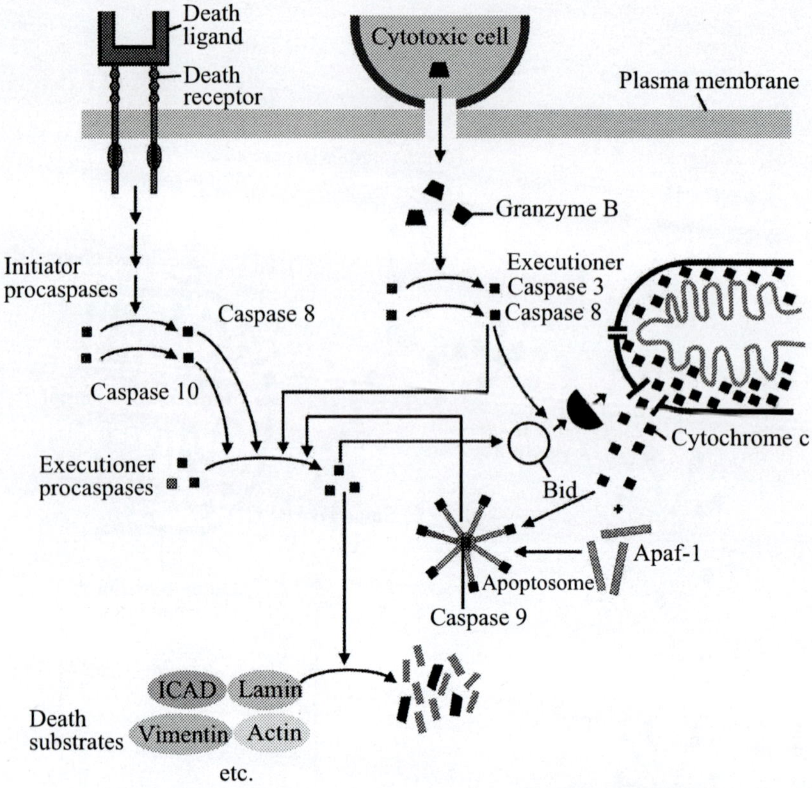

Fig. 4.25. Conversion of intrinsic and extrinsic pathways favoring apoptosis

their inhibition (Fig. 4.25). At the same time phosphorylation of Hdm2 will activate it, which is the key inhibitor of p53.

Majority of cancers have been found to resort to yet another mechanism to protect themselves from apoptosis by activating the expression of NF-κB transcription factor. In normal cells, NF-κB is usually sequestered in cytoplasm in an inactive form and in response to certain physiologic signals, it is released and transported to the nucleus, where it activates numerous target genes. Some of these genes are involved in pro-inflammatory and angiogenic functions. In addition, a good number of NF- κB target genes function as anti-apoptotic, such as IAP-1, IAP-2, XIAP, IWX-1L, TRA-1 and TRAF-2, which serve to block the intrinsic and extrinsic apoptotic signals.

In childhood neuroblastomas, amplification of the *N-myc* gene normally indicates aggressive tumor growth and short life expectancy is yet another strategy for avoiding apoptosis is evident. On its own, enhanced expression of *myc* oncogene threatens the proliferation of neuroblastoma cell since the actions of the *myc* oncogene and its cousin *N-myc* represent a double-edged sword. These oncogenes release potent mitogenic signals, but at the same time is strongly pro-apoptotic. Many neuroblastoma cells that have overexpressed *N-myc* through gene amplification seem to solve this problem by inactivating the gene encoding **caspase 8** either by **methylation** or **deletion.**

A protein called FLIP (FLICE-inhibitory protein) is deployed by some cancer cells, which on binding to the death domains of death receptors inhibits the activation of the extrinsic apoptotic cascade. This results in interference in processing and autocatalytic activation caspase-8 initiator (Fig. 4.26). Yet other

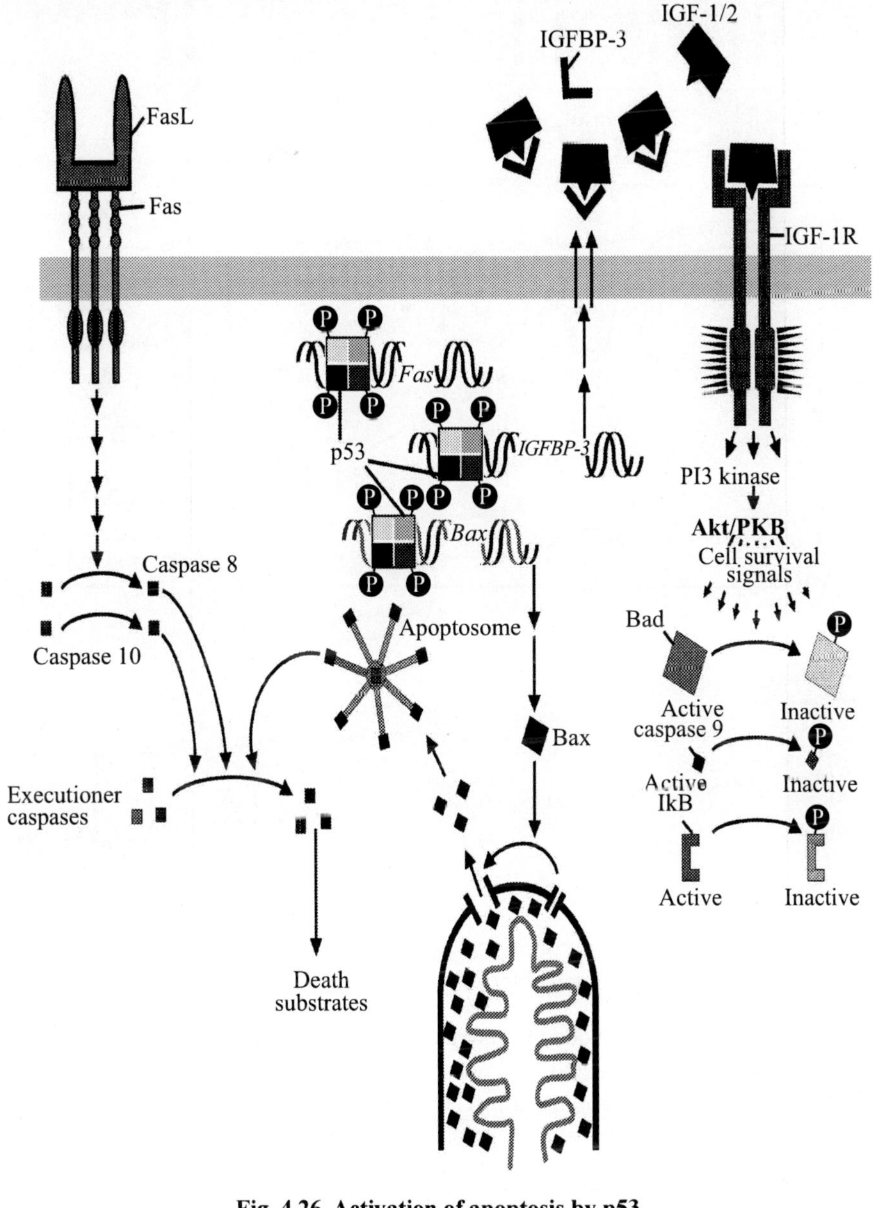

Fig. 4.26. Activation of apoptosis by p53

tumor cells adopt the strategy of suppressing the expression of their TNF receptor by promoter methylation of the TNFR-1 encoding gene.

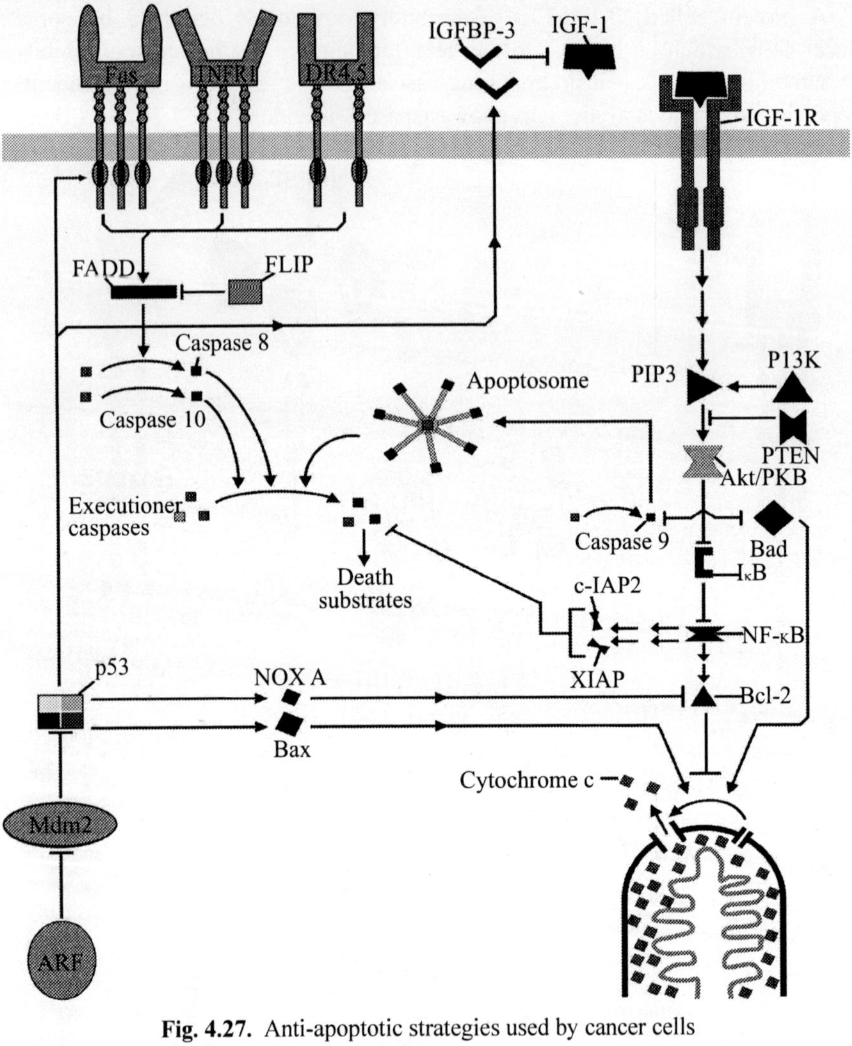

Fig. 4.27. Anti-apoptotic strategies used by cancer cells

4.4 TUMOR SUPPRESSOR GENES ENCODED PROTEINS FUNCTION IN DIVERSE WAYS

Tumor suppressor genes encoded proteins adopt diverse mechanisms to suppress the development of cancer. TSGs suppress proliferation of cells as a response to a variety of growth-inhibitory and differentiation-inducing signals. Yet other TSGs inhibit cell proliferation because of metabolic imbalances and genomic damage.

The Rb gene and p53 play a significant role in suppression of human cancer. In normal cells, Rb gene encoded Rb protein controls growth-and-division cycles, which are disrupted in almost all human tumors. The protein encoded by p53 tumor suppressor gene also plays an equally important role in preventing the development of cancers, which seems to be equally disrupted in almost all types of human cancers.

The remaining TSGs that have been discovered to date dispatch gene products that operate in different manners to suppress cell proliferation. Several proteins encoded by the TSGs such as $p16^{INK4A}$, $p15^{INK4B}$, and $p19^{ARF}$ genes included in this circuitry are responsible for controlling cell proliferation and survival.

In addition to Rb, p53, $p16^{INK4A}$, $p15^{INK4B}$, and $p19^{ARF}$ TSG genes functions discussed earlier, functions of three more tumor suppressor genes are discussed in the following section. These genes reveal the diverse mechanisms deployed by a cell to prevent runaway proliferation and itsdisruption in the malignant cancer cells.

4.4.1 Neurofibromatosis (NF1) Gene Encoded Protein is a Negative Regulator of Ras Signaling

Neurofibromatosis (NF) is another common familial cancer syndrome, on an average worldwide incidence of 1 in 3500 individuals. The characteristic of this disease is the shell sheaths around the nerves in the peripheral nervous system develop benign tumors. A subclass of this is **neurofibromas**, which progresses to become malignant. It is known as **neurofibrosarcomas.** Patients suffering from neurofibromatosis type 1 are at increased risk of developing glioblastomas (tumors of the astrocyte lineage in the brain), **pheochromocytomas** (arising from the adrenal glands), and myelogenous leukemias. These tumors involve cells from diverse embryonic lineages.

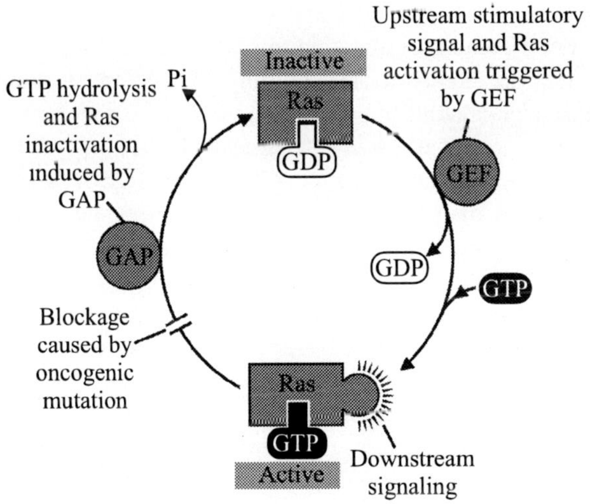

Fig. 4.28. Role of neurofibromatosis (NF1) encoded protein in regulation of GTPase activation protein

The NF1 gene was cloned in 1990 and the NF1 gene behavior is almost like that of Rb gene. As observed in retinoblastoma, inheritance of mutant, inactive alleles of the NF1 gene gets transmitted through the germ-line and acts in a dominant fashion to create disease phenotypes. At the cellular level, through loss of heterozygosity, the originally inherited heterozygous configuration of the gene (NF1+/-) is converted to a homozygous state (NF1-/-) in tumor cells. Patients suffering from neurofibromatosis, nearly, half of them do not have family history of the disease, indicating that the mutation of the allele that they carry occurs spontaneously in the germ-line especially during spermatogenesis in the fathers of afflicted patients as is the case with Rb gene.

NF1 gene is expressed widely throughout in almost all the cells of the body, especially high levels NF1 gene expression is observed in the adult peripheral and central nervous systems. Growth factor stimulation of the cells promotes degradation of NF1, because NF1 is known to interfere with Ras signaling. However, NF1 levels return to normal after 60 to 90 minutes and accumulation of NF1 protein shuts down further Ras signaling. NF1 function is absent in neuroectodermal cells, therefore, Ras proteins bound to GTP remain inactivated state for longer than normal periods of times. Same status is observed in neurofibromas in homozygous (NF1-/-) are known to have elevated levels of activated Ras and Ras effector proteins. Consequently, in the absence of NF1 function in tumor cells, they mimic the situation of functionally activated Ras proteins as though created by mutant Ras oncogene. Half normal dose of NF1 protein, which is called **haploinsufficiency** can indeed affect a cell and thus perturb the cell phenotype by affecting Ras signaling.

4.4.2 The Role of Adenomatous Polyposis Coli (APC) Tumor Suppressor Gene in Tumor Suppression

Heritable colon cancer syndrome, also known as familial adenomatous polyposis coli (FAP), is caused because of mutation in Adenomatous Polyposis Coli (APC) gene. The mutation increases the susceptibility to develop adenomatous polyps in the colon. Such adenomatous polyps by themselves are non-malignant but tend to develop into carcinomas at a low but predictable frequency. Degradation of β-catenin in normal cells is facilitated by APC protein. Inactivation of APC gene through different types of mutations like deletion or premature termination of translation of the APC protein due to appearance of nonsense codon in the reading frame. Premature APC protein will be lacking the domains that are important for β-catenin to associate with it together with axin to promote degradation of β-catenin is the predominant feature observed in colonic epithelial cells of the crypts. In 90% of sporadic colon carcinomas accumulation of β-catenin takes place, which is an indication of nonfunctioning APC gene. Inactivation of APC causes β-catenin to accumulate in precursors of enterocytes because of which they retain stem cell-like features leading to accumulation of a large number of relatively undifferentiated cells in the colonic crypt, which gives rise to adenomatous polyps (Refer to Fig. 3.14).

Hypermethylation of APC gene promoter is observed in approximately 10% of sporadic colon carcinomas, thereby inactivating the APC alleles. In some colon carcinomas, point mutation in the gene encoding β-catenin is observed resulting in mutant β-catenin molecule, which loses the amino acid residue that is normally phosphorylated before the degradation of β-catenin (Refer to Fig. 3.15). Hence, β-catenin accumulation is the precise outcome that invariably involves inactivation of APC function followed by other multiple mutations. Recent research shows that cell lacking APC function shows significant increase in chromosomal anomalies leading to ploidy (increase or decrease in number of chromosomes) due to inappropriate segregation of chromosomes during mitosis. The resulting aneuploidy arising due to chromosomal segregation defects alters the function of critical growth-promoting and growth-inhibiting genes because of increase or decrease in relative number of these genes. These chromosomal changes, in turn, favor tumorigenesis by accelerating the accumulation of advantageous genotypes in pre-malignant cells.

4.4.3 Von Hippel-Lindau Syndrome

Von Hippel-Lindau (VHL) syndrome is because of germ-line mutations of the VHL tumor suppressor gene due to which it hereditarily predisposes a person to the development of a variety of tumors. Some of the tumors listed due to VHL mutation are clear-cell carcinomas of the kidney, pheochromocytomas (tumors of adrenal gland), and hemangioblastomas (blood vessel tumors) of the central nervous system and retina. As in the case of mutant Rb alleles, the mutation in VHL alleles also acts as an autosomal dominant manner to create disease by undergoing a loss of heterozygosity (that results in a VHL negative (-/-) genotype in the tumor cells of the individuals inheriting a germ-line mutant VHL allele.

Seventy percent of sporadic non-familial kidney carcinomas express inactivated VHL gene due to promoter methylation. The main task of the protein product of VHL gene (pVHL) is to destroy the subunit of **hypoxia-inducible factor-1α (HIF-1α)** (Refer to Fig. 3.16) transcription factor. The activation of HIF-1 transcription factor influences the expression of several genes, which promote **angiogenesis** (generation of new blood vessels), **erythropoiesis** (formation of red blood cells), energy metabolism (specifically glycolysis), and glucose transport into the cells. The intention of the cell in hypoxic conditions is to induce the synthesis of proteins that enable it to survive in this extreme condition for a short while and then in the longer term to gain access to an adequate supply of oxygen by promoting vasculature. Vascular endothelial growth factor (VEGF) is one protein that is induced by **HIF-1α** and promotes the growth of new vessels in the hypoxic area of a tissue. The formation of new blood vessels is also very important for the growth of tumors, which require rich supply of oxygen and nutrients. The newly grown blood vessels provide all these to the growing tumors and facilitate evacuation of carbon dioxide, and metabolic wastes.

In the cells, pVHL exists as a complex with several other proteins and this association facilitates acquisition of ubiquitin to link it covalently to specific substrate protein, which will be destroyed through proteasome. pVHL binds to HIF-1α only when both the proline residues of HIF-1α which are critical to it are oxidized to hydroxyproline under normal oxygen tension (normoxia) and causes its destruction. Under hypoxic conditions, HIF-1α lacks these hydroxyprolines, due to which binding pVHL to HIF-1α does not occur, therefore, HIF-1α escapes degradation. Long lasting HIF-1α activates VEGF expression in both normal and neoplastic hypoxic tissues.

In some tumors having mutant VHL allele, the pVHL protein is undetectable in the individual cancer cells and in some other tumors, pVHL is inactive without affecting the levels due to more subtle changes in the protein. One such change is point mutation leading to alteration in the hydrophobic pocket of pVHL due to change in amino acid residue that recognizes and binds to hydroxyproline residues of HIF-1α. Through either mechanism, such as absence of VHL gene activity or the constitutive expression of the HIF-1 transcription factor would lead to expression of several powerful growth-promoting genes like VEGF, PDGF and TGF–α. The cell types bearing the corresponding receptors for these growth factors stimulate proliferation leading to tumor growth. In addition, tumor cells may cause increased production and accumulation of VEGF in circulation, which is responsible for stimulation of erythropoiesis in the bone marrow resulting in abnormally high number of red blood cells in Von-Hippel-Lindau patients.

Cells lacking functional pVHL are incapable of assembling fibronectin within cells and one of the key features of malignant cells is absence of fibronectin. A substantial amount of pVHL is responsible for stability and architecture of cytoplasmic microtubules (cytoskeleton) and abnormal cytoskeleton is another key feature of malignant cells.

Exercise

1. With suitable examples, highlight the role of tumor suppressor genes in normal cells.
2. Describe the experiment to demonstrate the status of tumor suppressor genes with respect to oncogenes
3. Explain how loss of heterozygosity leads to loss of function in tumor suppressor gene.

   OR

   What is the role of gene conversion in loss of heterozygosity? Explain with illustration.
4. Write notes on:

   (a) The role of retinoblastoma (Rb) gene in cell cycle regulation

   (b) The role of retinoblastoma (Rb) gene proteins in cell cycle regulation

(c) CDK inhibition and their impact on cell cycle

(d) Antagonism by viral oncoproteins on Rb proteins

5. Explain how perturbation of Rb function leads to tumorigenesis.
6. Explain the role of:

(a) TGFβ in cell cycle regulation

(b) p53 in normal cell

7. Describe how:

(a) mutant p53 gene interferes with normal p53 function;

(b) Mdm2 and ARF play their role in p53 function;

(c) apoptotic machinery is inactivated in cancer cells; and

(d) mutation in p53 gene predisposes an individual to cancer.

8. Present an account on the role of following tumor suppressor genes:

(a) Neurofibromatosis (NF1)

(b) Adénomatose Polyposies Coli (APC)

(c) Von-Hippel Lindau syndrome (VHL)

CHAPTER

5

Therapies for Cancer

5.1 CHEMOTHERAPY OF CANCER

Chemotherapy is a broad term used when the chemicals are used for the treatment of an ailment caused by microorganisms or cancerous cells. Chemotherapeutic drugs, used for the treatment of cancer, are called *anti-neoplastic* drugs and those used for controlling microbial infections are called *antibiotics* (*antibacterial chemotherapy*). In 1909, chemotherapeutic agent called arsphenamine (an arsenic compound) was discovered to treat syphilis, later followed by sulfonamides (sulfa drugs) and penicillin as antimicrobial agents.

Chemotherapeutic agents act on rapidly dividing cells and kill them by causing cytotoxicity within the cytoplasm of the cell and promote apoptosis or programmed cell death. It will also kill rapidly dividing normal cells of the bone marrow, intestinal epithelial cells, and hair follicles. One of the most common side effects of chemotherapy is immunosuppression due to myelosuppression leading to decreased production of blood cells; inflammation of the lining of the digestive tract (mucositis), and alopecia (hair loss).

Chemotherapeutic drugs are effective against "younger" tumors (i.e., more differentiated), because cell growth regulating mechanisms are usually still preserved. As the tumor growth progresses, tumor cells lose differentiation ability, growth regulation and develop resistance to chemotherapeutic agents. Usually, in solid tumors, in the central location, cell division stops, making them resistant to chemotherapy. Another problem encountered with solid tumors is the chemotherapeutic agent fails to reach the core of the tumor. This problem can be overcome by including radiation therapy and surgery together with chemotherapy called *combinatorial therapy.*

Cancer cells develop resistance to chemotherapeutic drugs by incorporating p-glycoprotein efflux pumps that facilitate removal of chemotherapeutic drug from inside the cell and send it out of the cell. Research is being carried out on these p-glycoproteins efflux pumps to work on the modalities of inhibiting these pumps to enhance the efficacy of chemotherapy.

Combined modality chemotherapy or combinatorial therapy is the modern approach where the chemotherapeutic drug together with radiation therapy or surgery is practiced with cancer treatment protocols. In combination chemotherapy, patients are treated with more than one drug with different mechanisms of action to minimize the chances of drug resistance by the cancer cells and the side effects of the drugs.

Neoadjuvant chemotherapy is a preoperative treatment protocol, to minimize the destructive effect of radiotherapy and surgery by designing a strategy to shrink the primary tumor, thereby rendering local therapy like surgery or radiotherapy more effective.

Adjuvant chemotherapy is a treatment protocol followed when there is hardly any evidence of cancer present, but there is a possibility of recurrence from the residual cancer cells. This can also help reducing the chances of developing resistance to drugs even if the tumor develops from the residual cells. Adjuvant chemotherapy is also useful in killing malignant tumor cells which have migrated to other parts of the body.

Palliative chemotherapy is given to decrease tumor load and increase the life expectancy without curative intent. For this toxicity profile needs to be studied properly.

Before chemotherapy regimens start, there is a requirement of thorough study to see whether the patient will be able of undergo treatment, for which, age and other co-morbidities need to be taken into consideration. Performance status is often taken into consideration after one cycle of treatment regimen in order to see whether a patient can be further given chemotherapy or to find out whether there is requirement of dose reduction. Because with each treatment regimen, only a fraction of the cells in a tumor dies, called *fractional kill*. To reduce the size of the tumor, repeated doses of drugs and radiation treatment must be undertaken.

5.1.1 Types of Chemotherapeutic Drugs

The chemotherapeutic drugs are divided in to six categories, namely, alkylating agents, antimetabolites, anthracyclins, plant alkaloids, topoisomerase inhibitors, and other antitumor agents. All these drugs are known to affect cells during the early phase of cell division, i.e., S phase of the cell cycle when DNA synthesis will be taking place.

There are newer chemotherapeutic drugs being introduced for cancer treatment, which do not show direct interference with DNA replication. These include monoclonal antibodies, which are also called "molecular bullets" because they target the cancer cells directly by interacting with the receptors or proteins expressed by the cancer cells. Nowadays, engineered monoclonal antibodies are available for the treatment of different types cancers, which can be linked with radionuclides or toxic drugs that are delivered directly to the cancer cells thereby avoiding systemic toxicity of the chemotherapeutic drugs. (This strategy of monoclonal antibody therapy will be discussed in detail in the later part of this chapter.) The new tyrosine kinase inhibitor monoclonal antibody, namely, imatinib (*Gleevec* or *Glivec*), which is directed against abnormality overexpressed tyrosine kinase receptor in certain types of cancers like chronic myelogenous leukemia, gastrointestinal stromal tumors, etc. These types of therapies are also called *targeted therapies.*

5.1.1.1 Alkylating agents

Alkylating agents are the compounds that can transfer alkyl groups to biologically important molecules through nucleophilic reaction and the process is called *alkylation*, which brings about remarkable changes in the behavior of the molecule in the cell due to alkylation. The changes brought about by alkylation influence various functions in the cell, such as interference in cell cycle and other metabolic activities. Alkylating agents establish covalent bonds with the amino, carboxyl, sulfhydryl, and phosphate groups of biologically important molecules thereby impairing their functions in the cell. Cisplatin and carboplatin, as well as oxaliplatin (Fig. 5.1) are bifunctional alkylating (compounds with two reactive groups) agents which react on DNA to form intra-strand and inter-strand crosslinks (Fig. 5.2). These agents alter the conformation of the double helix thereby interfering in DNA replication by preventing DNA strands separation, which is essential for DNA replication. Bifunctional alkylating agents are more potent than monofunctional analogs because of their cross-linking ability as compared to monofunctional analogs, which cannot bring about crosslinking.

The platinum atom in cisplatin [cis Pt (II)$(NH_3)_2Cl_2$] and carboplatin forms covalent bonds with organic molecules, especially DNA. Cisplatin has four functional groups of which two are amino and two are chloride bonded to centrally located platinum atom and it is a water-soluble molecule. The NH_3 is bonded to platinum through covalent linkage and it is irreversible, whereas Cl^- is bonded to platinum in a labile manner. Since Cl^- is labile it is displaced by water in the cellular environment before the molecule binds to the N7 position of guanine and adenine in DNA. The adducts formed by cisplatin of DNA comprises over 90% of the total, resulting in DNA damage, which triggers apoptosis.

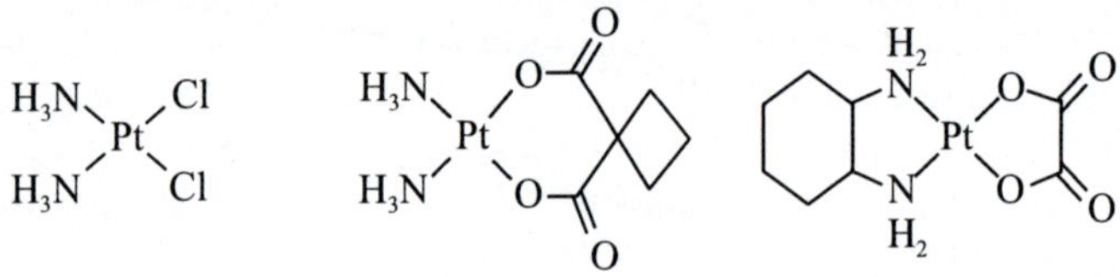

Cisplatin Carboplatin Oxaliplatin

Fig. 5.1. Platinum-based chemotherapeutics

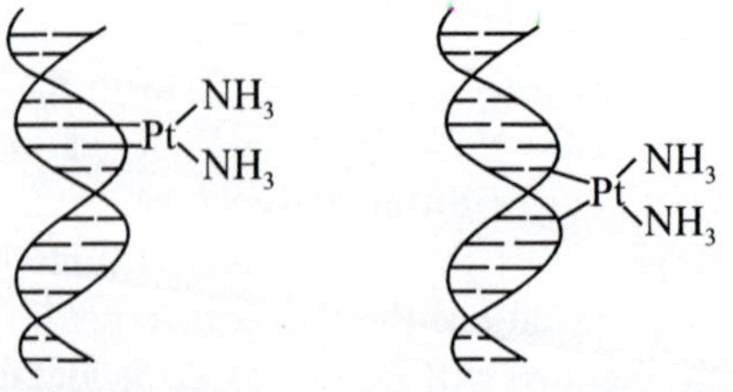

Intrastrand adduct Interstrand crosslink

Fig. 5.2. Crosslinks and adducts formed by platinum-based chemotherapeutics

(i) Nitrogen mustard: Methchlorethamine, cyclophosphamide, chlorambucil, ifosfamide, melphalan and busulfan. They form adducts with cell's DNA. The usual target of chlorambucil is the N7 position of guanine residue.

(ii) Nitrosoureas: Highly lipid soluble and is predominantly used for treatment of brain cancer. Carmustine, Semustine, Lomustine, Streptozocine for treatment of pancreatic cancer, Dacarbazine for treatment of melanoma, Temozolomidefortreatment of glioma and melanoma. Cyclophosphamide requires metabolic activation, which happens in the liver, where the liver oxidases convert it to an aldehyde, which is further converted to phosphoramide mustard, the biologically active molecule. The phosphoramide mustard reacts with DNA to form the adducts, which leads to cross-linking of DNA strands thereby interfering with DNA replication.

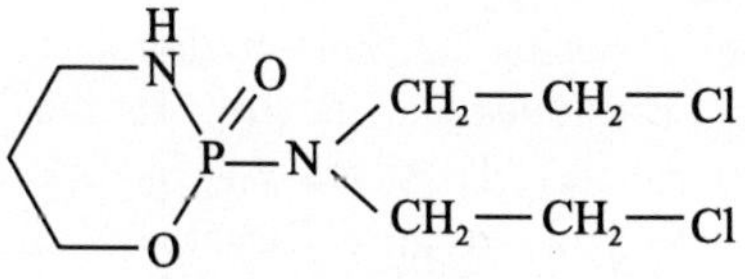

Cyclophosphamide

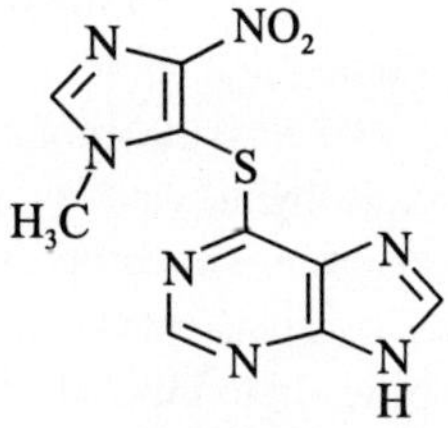

Azathioprine

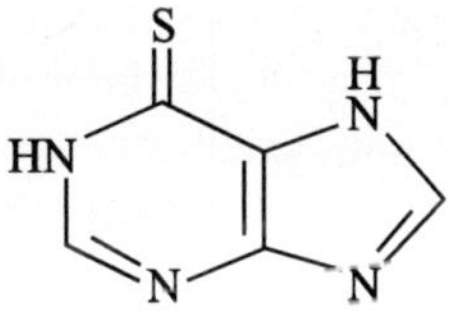

6-mercaptopurine (metabolite of Azathioprine)

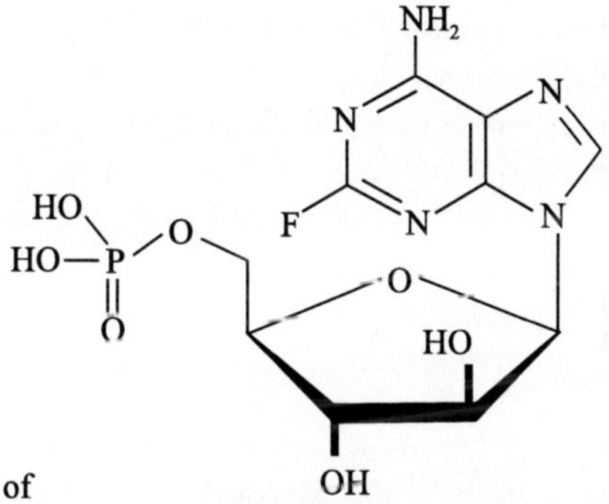

Fludarabine phosphate

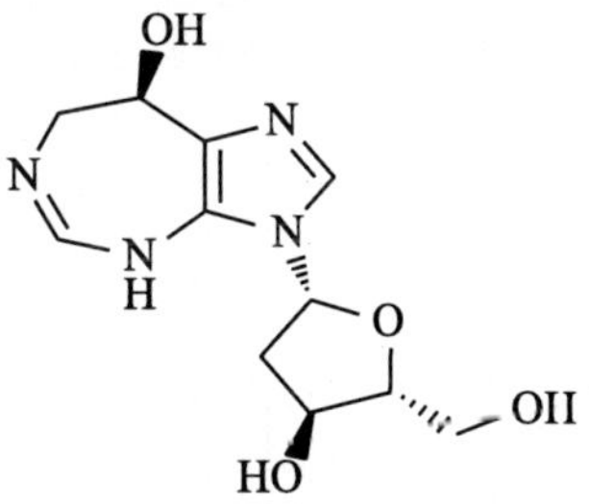

Pentostatin

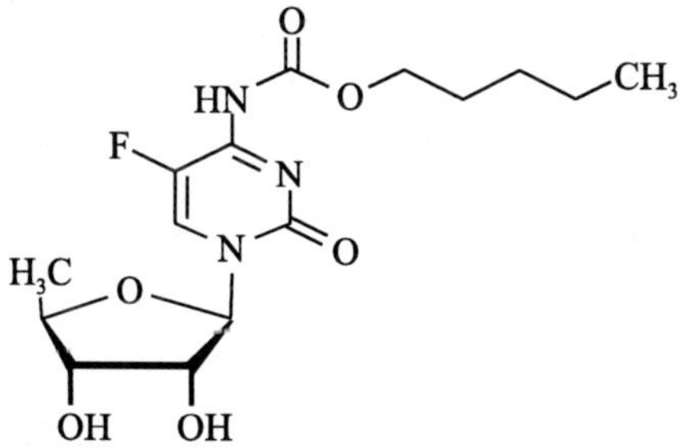

Capecitabine

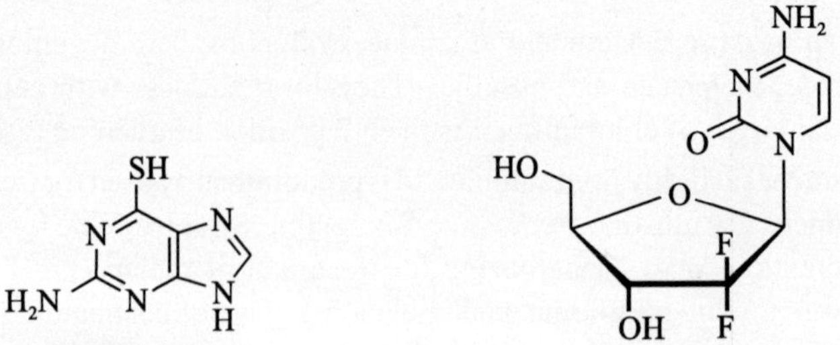

Thioguanine Gemcitabine

Fig. 5.3. Anti-cancer drugs used for chemotherapeutic purpose

5.1.1.2 Anti-metabolites

Anti-metabolites are also called **purine analogs** and therefore interfere with nucleic acid synthesis. Some examples are: azathioprine or mercaptopurine, thioguanine, fludarabine (inhibits DNA polymerase), pentostatin (inhibits adenosine deaminase), caldribine (incorporated in DNA) or pyrimidine analogs 5-fluorouracil (inhibits enzyme thymidylate synthetase), capecitabine (fluro pyrimidine), cytosine arabinoside (cytarabine)incoroporated into DNA, gemcitabine (used for the treatment of pancreatic, ovarian, cervix and lung cancer). They prevent incorporation of nitrogenous bases in to DNA during the "S" phase of the cell cycle and affect RNA synthesis also, thereby interfering with cell division. Due to their efficiency, these drugs are the most widely used cytostatic. Fluorodeoxy-uridylate (F-dUMP) is a metabolite of 5-fluorouracil, competes with the cellular dUMP for the catalytic site of thymidylate synthetase, which produces thymidylate (dTMP). F-dUMP forms a covalent complex with the thymidylate synthetase and acts as suicide inhibitor. Inhibition of thymidylate synthetase leads to depletion of dTMP and dTTP pools, which causes accumulation of dUMP and dUTP resulting in inhibition of DNA synthesis. Methotrexate yet another important antimetabolite analog of dihydrofolate, competitively inhibits dihydrofolate reductase, the enzyme required for regeneration of tetrahydrofolate, which is required in the thymidylate synthase reaction.

5.2 PLANT ALKALOIDS AND TERPENOIDS

Some plant alkaloids are capable of blocking cell division by preventing microtubule assembly or interfering with microtubule function, thereby interfering with spindle fiber formation leading to inhibition of cell division. Microtubules are an important component of cytoskeleton, which play a major role in maintenance of cell shape and size and without them the cells will be irregular in shape.

5.2.1 Agents that act on Mitotic Spindle Fibers

5.2.1.1 Vinca alkaloids

Almost all vinca alkaloids have strong affinity to specific sites on tubulin protein of microtubule and inhibits tubulin assembly thereby construction of microtubules is affected in the M phase of the cell cycle. *Vinca rosea* is commonly called

Madagascar periwinkle, which is renamed as *Catharanthus roseus*. Following are the vinca alkaloids used in the treatment of different types of cancers:

- Vincristine has been most effectively used in the treatment of leukemias, lymphomas and sarcomas.
- Vinblastine is effective against advanced testicular cancer, Hodgkin's disease, and lymphomas
- Vinorelbine is used individually or in combination with cisplatin, which is used for the treatment of non-small cell lung cancer and breast cancer.
- Vindesine is unedrgoing clinical trials for the treatment of acute lymphocytic leukemia.
- Vinflunine is a novel fluorinated vinca alkaloid, currently in phase II clinical trials for treatment of urothelial cancer and advanced bladder cancer.

5.2.1.2 Taxanes

Original name is Taxol obtained from the bark of the Pacific Yew tree, the prototype taxane or **paclitaxel** and docetaxel **(Taxotere).** Docetaxel is an artificially synthesized semi-synthetic analog of paclitaxel. Taxanes are known to enhance the stability of microtubules, in other words, they lose elasticity and contractility, thereby separation of chromosomes during anaphase is inhibited.

At present, paclitaxel is used in the treatment of breast, ovarian and non-small-cell lung cancers (NSCLC), as well as against Kaposi sarcoma. Paclitaxel triggers apoptosis by regulating the expression of pro-apoptosis proteins such as Bim, Bcl-2, Bad, $p21^{Cip}$ and TNF-α receptor, caspase-dependent and independent pathways. Docetaxel is used for the treatment of breast and ovarian cancers, head and neck carcinoma, small cell lung cancer, pancreatic and gastric cancer.

5.2.2 Podophyllotoxin

Podophyllotoxin is obtained from the American Mayapple (*Podophyllum peltatum*) and recently, Himalayan Mayapple (*Podophyllum hexandrum*) is also known to contain the same type of alkaloid. From podophyllatoxin two other cytostatic drugs can be derived, namely, **etoposide** and **teniposide.** These two derivatives interfere prior to G1 phase of cell cycle (the start of DNA replication) and at S phase of the cell cycle. The exact molecular mechanism of its action is yet to be deciphered.

5.2.3 Topoisomerase Inhibitors

Topoisomerases are responsible for maintaining the topology of DNA by preventing supercoiling of DNA during the unwinding process as DNA starts replication or transcription process. Inhibition of type I or type II topoisomerases lead to suppression of transcription and replication of DNA.

- ***Camptothecins***, namely, **irinotecan** and **topotecan** are capable of inhibiting type I topoisomerase. Topotecan is known to be effective against ovarian and small-cell lung cancers, while irinotecan is found to be effective in the treatment of colorectal cancers.

- **Amasacrine, etoposide, etoposide phosphate**, and **teniposide** are topoisomerase type II inhibitors. These are semi-synthetic derivatives obtained from epipodophyllotoxin, an alkaloid naturally found in the roots of American Mayapple (*Podophyllum peltatum*).

5.2.4 Anti-neoplastics

Doxorubicin, epirubicin **bleomycin** belong to this class. Doxorubicin is a fungal anthracycline antibiotic capable of inhibiting topoisomerase II, an enzyme that releases torsional stress on the DNA strands during DNA replication, by acting on single-strand and double strands and cut them so that the torsional stress is relaxed. Doxorubicin can easily diffuse across the cell membrane and accumulates in the cytoplasm of most cell types leading to cytotoxicity, thereby promoting apoptosis. It is primarily used for the treatment of different types of solid tumors.

(a) Epigallocatechin-3-gallate (EGCG) is a type of catechin abundantly found in green tea, which shows strong anti-proliferative and anti-tumor effects by inhibiting DNA methyltransferase activity, as well as it is capable of reactivating silenced tumor suppressor gene. EGCG shows antiproliferative effect by inhibiting the activation of transcription factors AP-1, NF-kB, and cyclin dependent kinases. EGCG prevents hyperphosphorylation of Rb protein leading to G0/G1 arrest. From several studies on head and neck, breast, and colon cancer cells, it is evident that EGCG inhibits neovascularization by blocking VEGF expression.

(b) Pomiferin is a prenylated isoflavonoid obtained from *Maclura pomifera*, which has strong antioxidant activity thereby inhibits formation of reactive oxygen species (ROS). It was found to inhibit histone deacetylase (HDAC) enzyme activity in human cancer cell lines of kidney, lung, breast, and colon cancer origin.

(c) Sulforaphane is an isothiocyanate found in vegetables Cruciferae family like broccoli, cabbage, mustard, radish, and cauliflower. It is known to inhibitor of HDAC activity in human colon, breast, and prostate cancer cell lines. Sulforaphane is known to hyper acetylate $p21^{Cip1}$ promoter and induce transcription in prostate cancer cells deficient p53 function. Higher doses of sulforaphane induce oxidative stress and promote apoptosis by inhibiting bcl2 gene and inducing tumor necrosis factor pathway.

(d) Thymoquinone is a volatile oil of black seed prevalently used in Middle East and Asian countries. The mechanism of TQ anti-cancer action is by G0/G1 arrest in colon, prostate, and skin cancer cell lines. TQ induces increased expression of cyclin-dependent kinase (CDK) inhibitors like $p16^{INK4A}$, $p21^{Cip1}$ and $p27^{Kip1}$. The growth arrest is due to suppression of transcription factor E1F1 and its positive regulator pRb. TQ induces apoptosis in cancer cell by p53 dependent or independent manner. It increases the expression of p53 gene and upregulation of pro-apoptotic Bax.

(e) Homoharringtonine, isolated from *Cephalotaxus harringtonia,* is used for the treatment of acute myelogenous leukemia and chronic myelogenous leukemia in China.

(f) **Elliptinium,** a derivative of ellipticin isolated from several species of the apocyanacea family members, is approved for the treatment of breast cancer in France.

(g) **Flavopiridol**, a derivative of natural **rohitukine** obtained from *Dysoxylum malabaricum* plant, is known to inhibit tyrosine kinase activity, thereby inhibiting the growth activity in breast and lung carcinoma cell lines.

(h) **Combrestatins**, a family of stilbenes obtained from several species of Terminalia, acts as an anti-angiogenic agent, thereby preventing angiogenesis in tumors and initiate tumor necrosis.

(i) **Roscovitine**, derivative of **olomucine** originally isolated from the seeds of radish, is known to inhibit CDKs, thereby inhibiting cell cycle progression.

(j) **Bruceatin,** obtained from a tree *Brucea antidysenterica,* shows significant inhibitory activity against leukemia, lymphoma, and myeloma cell lines by down- regulation of *myc* oncoprotein.

(k) **Thapsigargin,** obtained from *Thapsia garganica,* induces apoptosis in prostate cancer cell lines. It inhibits angiogenesis and induces tumor necrosis.

(l) **Pervilleines**, isolated from *Erythroxylum pervillei,* inhibits multidrug resistance (MDR) activity in tumors and is currently being developed for pre-clinical trials.

(m) **Quercetin,** a flavonoid, affects tumor growth by blocking cell cycle at G0/ G1 interface, by inhibiting CDKs.

(n) **Epothilones** are a class of microtubule stabilizing compounds with extreme cytotoxicity and their mode of action is like Taxol. Epothilone was first isolated from a soil bacterium *Sporangium cellulosum,* which is found to be active against Taxol resistant cancer cell lines. At present several epothilone derivatives like Epothilone B, Dehydelone and Sagopilone are being subjected for advanced clinical trials.

(o) **Laulimalide**, isolated from marine sponge *Cacospongia mycofijiensis,* is known to stabilize microtubules as paclitaxel does and at nanomolar concentration, inhibits cell proliferation.

5.3 RADIATION THERAPY

Radiation therapy, in practice for quite a long time, is used for shrinking the tumors and to kill cancer cells where high-energy radiation like X-rays, gamma rays and charged particles are used during the treatment. To deliver radiation to the cancer area **external-beam radiation therapy** may be used in which case the radiation is delivered by a machine or by **internal-beam radiation therapy**, which is also called **brachytherapy** by implanting a capsule containing radioactive material to deliver the radiation inside the body near the solid tumor. **Systemic radiation therapy** is another type of radiation therapy used for treatment of various types of blood cancers, where radioactive iodine is administered intravenously, that kills cancer cells circulating in the blood.

Some type of radiation therapy is given to cancer patients during their treatment and the mechanism of action of radiation on cancer cells involves direct DNA damage or through free radicals generated in the cell's cytoplasm, which in turn, cause DNA damage leading to inhibition of cell division or death. During radiation therapy, normal cells also suffer from some amount of damage and die.

The main intention of radiation therapy is to kill cancer cells successfully and to eliminate a tumor completely or to prevent cancer recurrence, or both. Radiation therapy may be given alone or in combination with surgery, chemotherapy, or both, which is called combinatorial therapy. Radiation therapy may also be given as palliative therapy to relieve symptoms and reduce the sufferings in a cancer patient.

Radiation oncologist and the doctors treat the cancer patients based on the information available on potential damage to normal cells and the amount of radiation tolerated by normal tissue. A course of radiation therapy is planned, which begins with simulation. This information is crucial to decide on which region, how much of radiation and the duration of radiation is to be given.

During simulation, detailed scanned images of a patient's tumor, its location and the areas surrounded by normal tissue are obtained using sophisticated instruments like computed tomography (CT), magnetic resonance imaging (MRI), positron emission tomography (PET) and ultrasound. During CT scanning, computer linked to an X-ray machine generates large number of serial section images of the target organ where the tumor is situated. By studying the images generated by the CT scans, the treatment plan for radiation therapy is decided.

During simulation and daily treatments, the radiation oncologist ensures that the patient is positioned in the same position every day in relation to the machine delivering the radiation or while the imaging is being done. To prevent patient mobility and to stay still in one position until the treatment is over, body molds, head masks or other devices are constructed for an individual patient. For precise patient positioning, temporary marking on the skin to focus the radiation to that area is done.

After the simulation, the radiation oncologist maps the exact area that requires the total dose of radiation to be delivered at the tumor site without significant harm to normal tissues around the tumor and the safest angles (paths) for radiation to be delivered to minimize the damage to the normal tissues are calculated by physicist and the person with knowledge on dosimetry.

The technician working with the radiation oncologist plans the exact radiation treatment by using a sophisticated computer and after getting approval from the radiation oncologist, will start the treatment. On weekly basis after the first cycle of treatment, assessment of blood parameters and the tumor images are undertaken to see to it that the treatments carried out is as planned.

The unit of measurement of radiation is gray (Gy), which is a measure of the amount of radiation energy absorbed by 1 kg of human tissue. To kill different types of cancers depending on the location and depth in the body radiation dose may differ.

For the radiation treatment, entire tumor area and a small area of normal tissue surrounding the tumor is selected. There are two reasons for treating the normal tissue around the tumor:

(1) as the treatment is in progress, due to breathing movements, location of a tumor may change as the organs within the body move normally with respiratory movement; and

(2) to prevent to a great extent tumor recurrence from cancer cells that might have spread to the normal tissue adjacent to the tumor due to micro metastasis.

Many factors are taken into consideration by radiation oncologist before the radiation treatment starts. These factors includes: cancer phenotype, its size, its location in the body and the depth to which radiation needs to travel passing through the normal tissue area, proximity to organs sensitive to radiation, age and medical history, co-morbidities if any. Radioactive cobalt is used for delivering high energy radiation of X-rays or gamma rays through high linear energy transfer (LET) device called linear accelerator or LINAC.

5.3.1 External Beam Radiation Therapy (EBRT)

Linear accelerator or LINAC is the machine used for delivering external-beam radiation therapy, which generates high energy photon beams of X-rays or gamma rays by using high voltage electric current. A photon consists of high amount of energy, which can vary. For example, gamma rays have the highest energy photons, followed by the X-rays. A fast-moving subatomic particle of high-energy radiation are generated by LINAC, which is used for the cancer treatment.

EBRTis given to the cancer patient for a particular duration on daily basis for four weeks. Depending on the tumor characteristics and the factors mentioned above, the number of treatment sessions and the total radiation dose will vary.

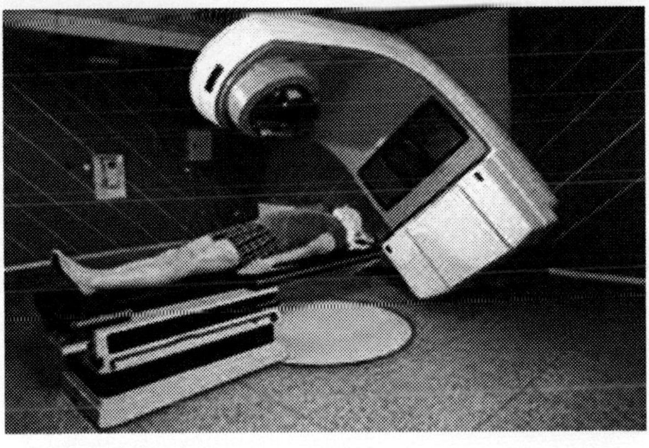

Fig. 5.4. External beam radiation therapy instrument

3-dimensional conform radiation therapy **(3D-CRT) is** one among the commonest of external-beam radiation therapy administered to cancer patients. 3D-CRT can deliver radiation precisely to tumor target using highly sophisticated computer software. Other methods of external-beam radiation therapies include, **intensity modulated radiation therapy (IMRT), image-guided radiation therapy (IGRT),** stereotactic radiosurgery (SRS), stereotactic body radiation therapy (SBRT), proton therapy, and **electron beam radiation therapy** are used in cancer treatment.

5.3.1.1 Intensity modulated radiation therapy (IMRT)

To deliver appropriate dose of radiation, IMRT uses a device called collimator, which delivers hundreds of tiny radiation beams by orienting the radiation in the required manner. The collimators are designed in such way that they can be stationary or can be moved during the treatment to achieve the required angle or distance for dose and intensity modulations of radiation to different areas of a tumor and to reach the appropriate site during the treatment sessions.

Unlike other types of radiation therapy, inbuilt computer program is used for IMRT to calculate the required number of beams and angles of the radiation treatment to different areas of the tumor and the surrounding tissue.

The advantage of IMRT is the focused radiation dose can be increased to the tumor areas that requires the most and reduce exposure of the surrounding normal tissue to radiation. Compared with 3D-CRT, using IMRT is used for the treatment of cancers pertaining to head and neck with reduced damage to the salivary glands, which otherwise, causes dry mouth or xerostomia when radiation therapy is done through 3D-CRT.

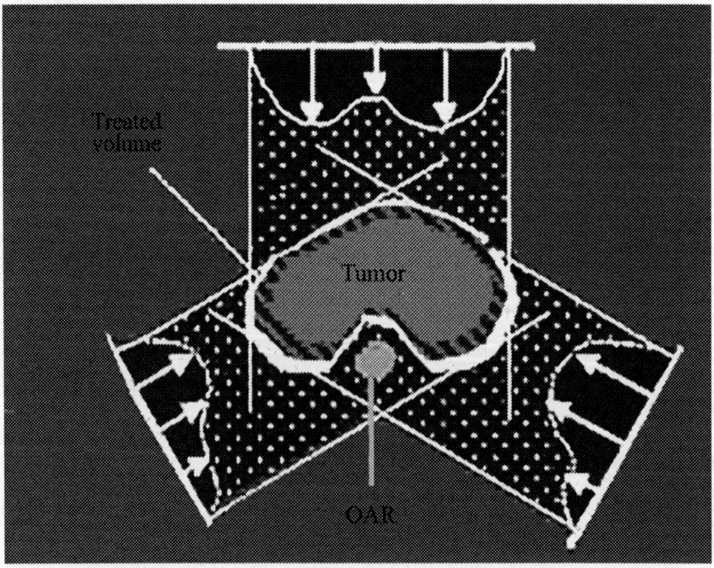

Fig. 5.5. Intensity modulated radiation therapy

5.3.1.2 Image-guided radiation therapy (IGRT)

In IGRT, images generated from CT or MRI or PET scans are used for the radiation treatment by processing the images using computer software tumor size and location are precisely identified and the patient is precisely positioned for successive radiation treatment so that the damage to normal tissue during the treatment is minimized.

Tomotherapy is one type of IGRT and the machine used for the radiation treatment is combination of CT scanner and external-beam radiation therapy machine (Fig. 5.6). The tomotherapy machine can deliver radiation and at same time can take the image of the target treatment area of the tumor by rotating and orienting the machine around the patient in the same manner as a normal CT scanner does.

Images of the patient's tumor are captured by the tomotherapy machines just like the way CT scanner does and provides sectional view of the tumor to arrive at three-dimensional treatment plans. Radiation beams are precisely targeted to the tumor and the normal tissue is spared from radiation damage.

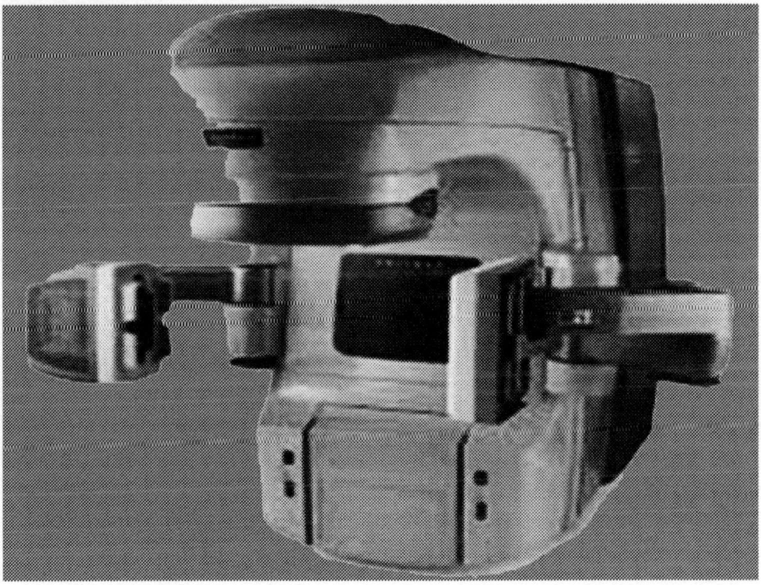

Fig. 5.6. Device used for image guided radiation therapy

5.3.1.3 Stereotactic radiosurgery (SRS)

Stereotactic radiosurgery (SRS) uses device or machine which involves extremely accurate image-guided targeting tumor with high doses of radiation and prevents damage to normal tissue by accurately positioning the patient. SRS is used for treating only small tumors in restricted area with properly defined borders. SRS is mostly used in the treatment of neurological tumors of brain and spinal cord origin and for the treatment of some brain metastases, where, in addition to SRS whole-brain radiation therapy is carried out. SRS for brain tumor requires the use of a head frame (Fig. 5.7) to position the patient's head during the treatment to ensure that the high dose of radiation is delivered accurately to the tumor.

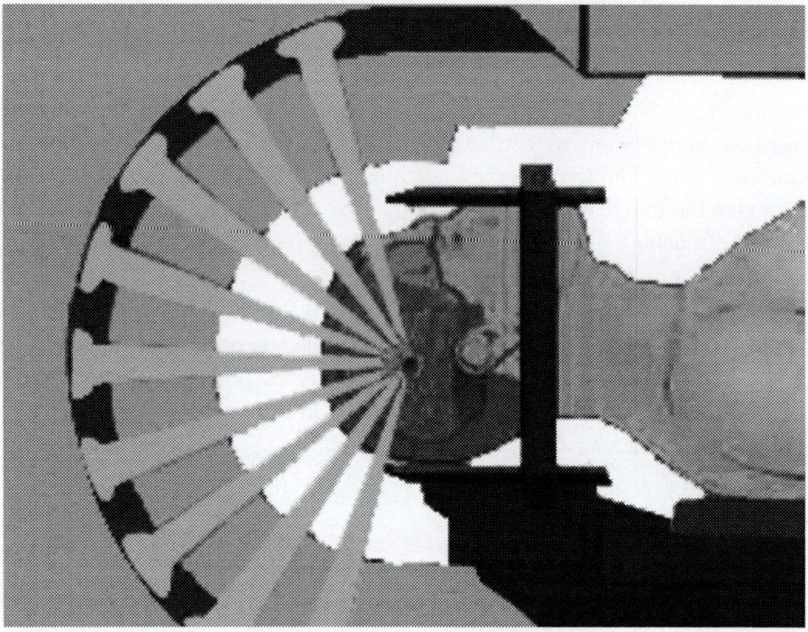

Fig. 5.7. Stereotactic radiation therapy

5.3.1.4 Stereotactic body radiation therapy (SBRT)

Compared to 3D-CRT, SBRT is administered using smaller radiation fields and higher doses of radiation in fewer sessions. SBRT is used for the treatment of tumors in organs other than the brain and spinal cord. Tumors of other organs other than the brain and spinal cord show movement within the body with normal respiratory motion, therefore accurate targeting becomes difficult as compared to tumors within the brain or spine. SBRT is usually follows short spurts of higher dose of radiation on isolated small tumors in the brain, lung, and liver. Many doctors refer to it as CyberKnife®.

5.3.1.5 Proton therapy

It is a modified version of external-beam radiation therapy, where proton beams like the photon beams are used to target the tumors. Protons are positively charged particles, which deposit energy in the living tissue in a different way from that of photons of X-rays and gamma-rays, that deposit energy in small packets all along their path through the tissue (Fig. 5.8a), whereas much of their energy energy deposited by protons is at the end of their path, which is called the Bragg peak (Fig. 5.8b), therefore, along the way least amount of energy is lost. It is the most expensive therapy reported because of focused delivery of higher doses of radiation to a tumor site, thereby reduces the exposure of normal tissue to radiation.

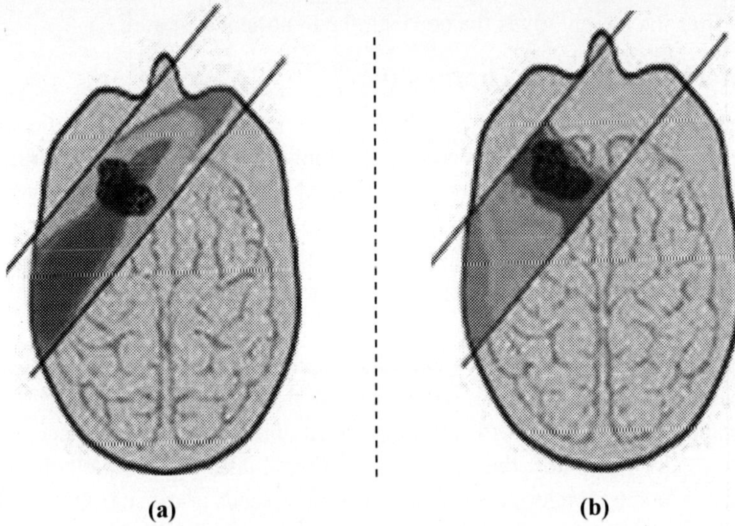

Fig. 5.8. Comparison of radiation dosage distribution in (a) X-ray and (b) proton beam therapy

5.3.1.6 Electron beam radiation therapy (EBRT)

Electron beam radiation therapy is used for the treatment of superficial tumors of skin origin. Electron beams cannot travel deep into the tissues therefore it cannot be used for the treatment of tumors deep within the body.

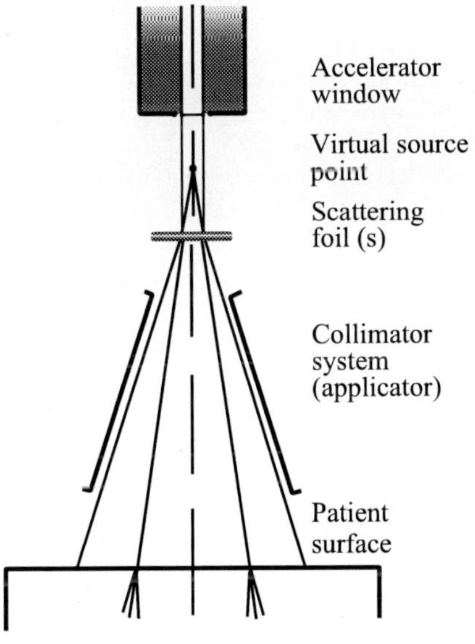

Fig. 5.9. Modality of electron beam radiation therapy

Doctor discusses these different methods of radiation therapy with patients and explains in detail the consequences to be borne by the patient post-radiation therapy. Patient also goes through a counseling session before the treatment begins and only after the patient gives the consent, the treatment is started.

5.3.2 Internal Radiation Therapy (IRT)

For internal radiation therapy (brachytherapy) radiation source (radioactive materials) is kept inside or on the body in a proximity to the tumor. For **interstitial brachytherapy,** the radiation source is implanted within the tumor tissue stroma, provided the tumor is easily accessible. For **intracavitary brachytherapy** radiation source is implantd within a body cavity, such as the chest or the abdominal cavity at a proximity to tumor. **Episcleral brachytherapy** is used for the treatment of melanoma inside the eye, where the radiation source is attached to the eye.

For brachytherapy, radioactive isotopes are encapsulated, therefore, they are called seeds, which are placed in patient's body using needles, catheters. As the radio isotope decays naturally, the radiation given off kills the nearby cancer cells. For a few weeks or months, the therapy is continued until the complete decay of the isotope, which no longer gives off radiation. The seeds or capsule are harmless because they are made up of biodegradable material. They undergo degradation within the body if they are left in the body.

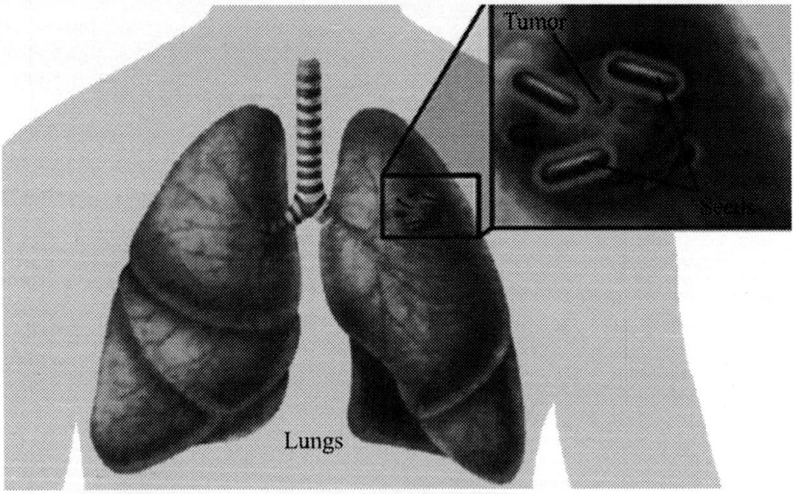

Fig. 5.10. Radioactive source is implanted as seed or capsule at the site of tumor for internal beam radiation therapy

Brachytherapy may be used for delivering higher doses of radiation to some cancers with minimal damage to normal tissue when compared to external-beam radiation therapy.

Brachytherapy can be given at two dosage levels, low-dose, or high-dose treatment:

- In low-dose treatment, over a period of several days, cancer cells receive continuous low-dose radiation from the implanted radioactive source.
- In high-dose treatment, depending on the tumor size, one or more treatment sessions are held through a robotic machine attached to delivery tubes inserted into the body such that the radioactive source is placed near a tumor. The source is then removed once the treatment session is over. MammoSite® system is an example of a high-dose treatment used for the treatment of breast cancer patients who have undergone breast conservation surgery.

5.3.2.1 Systemic radiation therapy

In systemic radiation therapy, radioactive substance is administered through intravenous route, like radioactive iodine or a radioactively labeled monoclonal antibody. Radioactive iodine (^{131}I) is commonly used for the treatment of thyroid cancer, which is a type of systemic radiation therapy. Because of strong affinity of thyroglobulin to iodine, radioactive iodine is taken up easily by thyroid cells.

For the treatment of some other types of cancer, systemic radiation therapy in the form of monoclonal antibody conjugated to radioactive source is used to deliver the radiation at the target site. These targeted monoclonal antibodies are called magic bullets, which are directed against a predominant receptor expressed by the cancer cells alone. The monoclonal antibody conjugated to radioactive source on administration through intravenous route travels through the blood, precisely locates the tumor and binds to it and kills tumor cells without any damage to the normal cells. Two of the US-FDA approved radioactive monoclonal antibodies used for the cancer treatment are as follows:

- The drug ibritumomab tiuxitan **Y^{90} (Zevalin®)** has been approved for the treatment of certain types of B-cell non-Hodgkin lymphoma (NHL). The monoclonal antibody is directed against the protein receptor expressed only on the membrane of the abnormal B lymphocytes.
- The combination drug regimen of iodine (I^{131})- tositumomab **(Bexar®)** has been approved for the treatment of certain types of NHL.

Some systemic radiopharmaceuticals have been used for palliative purpose to relieve pain from bone metastases such as **Samarium-153-lexidronam (Quadramet®)** and **Strontium-89 chloride (Metastron®)**.

In certain cancer treatments, chemotherapy in combination with radiation therapy are given at the same time, which is called chemoradiation or radio chemotherapy, that may kill more cancer cells but also cause more side effects.

The US-FDA approved monoclonal antibody ***cetuximab (Erbitux),*** meant for binding to epidermal growth factor receptor (EGFR) thereby inhibiting the signal transduction process of the receptor. This, in turn, causes hypoxia, affects DNA repair and cell proliferation. This treatment is predominantly used for the cancers associated with head and neck.

The outcome of radiotherapy is influenced by three main biological factors of tumor microenvironment: the extent of hypoxia tolerance; the ability of the surviving cells to repopulate within a treatment time of 6 – 7 weeks; and the radio resistance developed by the tumor cells.

Two aspects of the tumor microenvironment, hypoxia, and vasculature development, are known to influence considerably the response of tumors to ionizing radiation because both are crucial targets to improve the response of the tumor to radiation therapy. In normal tissues hypoxia hardly occurs and it is not tolerated, therefore for the tumors, it is an attractive tumor-specific target for improving the response to ionizing radiation.

There is evidence to prove that hypoxia is the most common feature of malignant solid tumors. Tumor cells can tolerate oxygen concentration of less than 0.02% (0.15 mm Hg), which provides them adaptability to resist killing by ionizing radiation by a factor of 2-3. Hypoxic cells suppress cell division and are difficult to reach by drugs because of poor vasculature, rendering them resistant to intravenously administered chemotherapeutic drugs. In order to make cancer cells susceptible to radiation and chemotherapeutic treatment, hypoxic tumor cells can be radio-sensitized with oxygen mimicking agents such as ***nimorazole*** or by specifically targeting the hypoxic tumor cells with a cytotoxic drug such as ***tirapazamine,*** which gets activated in hypoxic condition. Alternatively, oxygen delivery to the hypoxic tumor site can be enhanced by using drugs such as ***efaproxiral,*** which attracts oxygen towards it and reduces oxygen binding to hemoglobin.

To quantify hypoxia, assays have been developed, where positron emission tomography (PET) tracers are used for imaging hypoxic sites, which does not require invasive approach. These tracers are mainly derived from **2-nitroimidazole**, such as **^{18}F-fluoromisonidazole** (^{18}F-FMISO) and **^{18}F-azomycin arabinoside.** Another tracer that specifically accumulates in a hypoxic microenvironment is **^{64}Cu-methyl-thiosemicarbazone.** At oxygen pressure below 10 mm Hg, the nitroreducatases facilitate binding of 2-nitroimidazoles irreversibly to cellular macromolecules through bioreduction process.

Imaging of tumor cell proliferation can be successfully carried out using **^{18}F-fluorothymidine (^{18}F-FLT),** which is retained inside the cell by thymidine kinase-1 and is specifically active during DNA synthesis, therefore, serves as an S-phase marker.

5.4 TARGETED THERAPIES

Targeted therapies are used for blocking essential biochemical pathways or mutant proteins produced by the tumor cells that are required for tumor cell growth and survival. These targeted drugs can arrest tumor progression by inducing cytotoxicity and it is individual-specific treatment. In 76% of patients with chronic myelogenous leukemia, the BCR-ABL kinase inhibitor **imatinib,** rapidly induces complete cytotoxic response.

Sipuleucel-T is an autologous (self) dendritic cell vaccine, pulsed with prostatic antigens, that stimulates T cells having specificity to prostate acid phosphatase (PAP) antigen, which is overexpressed in prostate carcinoma, has been recently approved by the US Food and Drug Administration (FDA) for the treatment of metastatic, castration-resistant prostate cancer.

Ipilimumab is a monoclonal antibody developed against cytotoxic T lymphocyte-associated antigen 4 (CTLA-4). The monoclonal antibody blocks T cell inhibitory signal by binding to CTLA-4 receptor on T cells, thereby enhancing T cell response for tumor destruction.

5.4.1 Strategies that Target DNA Repair Pathway

Synthetic lethal strategies is the term coined for the therapy, which involves gene interaction whereby inhibiting the functions of a gene results in cytotoxicity only when another important mutated gene is involved. For example, synthetic lethal strategy has been explored for developing poly (ADP-ribose) polymerase (PARP) gene inhibitors in tumors with BRCA1/2 mutations. PARPs are enzymes involved in base excision repair for the repair of DNA single strand breaks. By inhibiting base excision repair, accumulation of single strand breaks takes place leading to double strand breaks, which is normally repaired through homologous recombination pathways. Familial inherited breast cancers are known to have defects in DNA repair mechanism due to mutation in the gene that is involved in DNA repair. The synthetic lethal strategy takes advantage of this characteristic DNA repair defect caused by mutations in tumors. The familial breast cancer patient's germ-line mutation in either of the tumor suppressor gene BRCA1 or BRCA2 has been observed and they acquire a somatic mutation in the other BRCA1/2 allele later in life. This results in a tumor that has deficiency in homologous recombination and double-strand repair. On the contrary, the normal cells in the same patient do not carry the homozygous BRCA1/2 mutated genotype and retain the homologous recombination DNA repair pathway. Tumors cells without BRCA1/2 function when treated with PARP inhibitors show impaired homologous recombination and base excision repair pathways leading to cytotoxicity and death. On the contrary, healthy normal cells treated with PARP inhibitors show functional homologous recombination pathway, therefore, are viable. In phase I trial **Olaparib** a newly developed drug that inhibits PARP on administration showed anti-tumor effect in BRCA1 or BRCA2 deficient tumors.

5.4.2 Inhibitors of DNA Methylation

Hypermethylation of tumor suppressor genes is an important mechanism adopted by the tumor cells for progression and metastasis therefore drugs that interfere with DNA methylation are supposed to show anti-cancer effects. Generally, DNA methylation takes place at CpG domains involving methylation of 5th position of cytosine. Two 5′-modified analogs of deoxycytidine, **5′-azacytidine (5-aza-C)** and **5-aza-2′-deoxycytidine**, have been used to target DNA methyltransferases, which form covalent link with DNA methyltransferases and act as competitive inhibitors of methyl transferees leading to significant demethylation after several rounds of replication. These drugs can incorporate in DNA and bring about instability like anti-metabolite chemotherapeutic agents. Since both drugs 5-aza-C (azacytidine; Vidaza™) and 5-aza-2′-deoxycytidine (decitabine) showed anti-leukemic effects in clinical trials, they have been approved by US-FDA for the treatment of leukemia but were not found to be successful against solid tumors.

5.4.3 Telomerase Inhibitors

Tumor-specific expression of telomerase in majority of cancers is known to play a significant role in the cancer cells by facilitating them to divide indefinitely suggest that it can be used as a valuable molecular target for new cancer therapies. The catalytic protein component of the telomerase enzyme has an RNA component within it, which serves as a template for the synthesis of telomeres. Several different strategies, targeting either the RNA molecule with antisense oligonucleotides or with ribozymes have been explored in pre-clinical studies to target hTERT. Antisense oligonucleotides are complementary part of the target RNA, hybridize by Watson- Crick complementary base pairing with it, thereby inhibiting the function directly or trigger degradation by recruiting RNases. For the inhibition of telomerase action, reverse transcriptase inhibitors against the catalytic domain of hTERT and nucleoside analogs have also been investigated. **BIBR1532** is a synthetic small molecule inhibitor that directly binds hTERT non-competitively and brings about telomere-driven senescence. **Telomestatin is** a **G-quadruplex** binding molecule that prevents interaction between the telomerase enzyme and the 3' primer of the DNA have also been developed. The components of mistletoe and epigallo catechin of green tea have been found to be inhibitors of telomerase. **Imetelstat (GRN163L; Geron)** an anti-telomerase drug candidate is going through phase II clinical trials**.** Imetelstat is an antisense **13-mer oligonucleotide** binds directly to the template region of the RNA component of human telomerase (hTERT), which lies in the catalytic site of hTERT and brings about competitive inhibition of telomerase enzyme activity.

5.4.4 Drugs against Epidermal Growth Factor Receptor (EGFR)

Epidermal growth factor receptor (EGFR) is encoded by ErbB2 gene, a member of the tyrosine kinase family, is overexpressed in majority of cancers and is known to facilitate cell transformation. This suggests that ErbB2 has a crucial role in cancers. Several smallmolecules like **Iressa™ (gefitinib), Tarceva™ (eriotinib), Tykerb™ (lapatinib)** directed against the tyrosine kinase activity of EGFR family members have been developed. Currently, Iressa and Tarceva have been approved by UD-FDA for the treatment of advanced non-small-cell lung cancer and Tykerb has been approved for the treatment of breast cancer.

A different approach using monoclonal antibody **Herceptin™ (trastuzumab)** targeted against extracellular domain of the EGFR, on binding to EGFR receptor, enhances its degradation, inhibition of angiogenesis and antibody-mediated cellular cytotoxicity (ADCC) response. In 1998 Herceptin™ was approved by

US-FDA for treatment of metastatic breast cancer. **Erbitux™ (cetuximab)** and **Vectibix™ (Panitumomab,** ABX-EGF) are other types of monoclonal antibodies developed to target EGFR and have been approved for the treatment of colorectal cancer. Patients having K-ras mutation in the genome do not respond to these two drugs favorably.

5.4.5 Strategies against Raf

The drugs targeting the serine/threonine kinase Raf, one of the main effectors of RAS, is in the pipeline. **Nexavar™ (sorafenib)**, a multi-kinase inhibitor that targets the ATP-binding site of Raf was approved for treatment of advanced renal cell carcinoma and hepatocarcinoma. In patients who received Nexavar™ at well tolerated oral dose showed reduction in downstream MAPK phosphorylation, also inhibition of several receptor tyrosine kinases, namely, VEGFR1, -2 and -3, PDGFRb, c-kit and RET.

Another Raf inhibitor recently approved by the US-FDA for the treatment of melanoma is **Zelboraf™** (vemurafenib; PLX4032), which brought about 81% regression of melanoma having B-Raf mutation. This suggests that combination treatment is more effective for durable response.

5.4.6 Imatinib (Glevec™) (Tyrosine Kinase Inhibitor)

Imatinib (Glevec™), yet another tyrosine kinase inhibitor approved by US-FDA, has been successfully used for the treatment of chronic myelogenous leukemia (CML), which results in 96% remission in early-stage patients. The half-life of drug is approximately 15 hours and it was originally optimized for inhibiting PDGF-R tyrosine kinase activity but later it was found that, it inhibits **ABL** and **c-kit** as well. **Glevec binds** to the **ATP-binding pocket** of the **catalytic domain** of tyrosine kinase.

Effectiveness of Glevec decreases as the disease progresses. In advanced phase of the disease 53% response is observed and in accelerated phase 30% response is seen. 78% of the late-stage patients and 9% of early-stage patients showed relapse. In majority of the cases of relapse, the mechanism relies on enhancement of the kinase activity due to amplification Bcr-Abl fusion protein facilitated by translocation between chromosome 9 and 22 and further point mutation of the Bcr-Abl fusion gene. This clearly indicates how cancer cell develops drug resistance by multiple mutations to maintain the cancer phenotype.

Ibrutinib and **idelalisib** used in the targeted treatment of chronic lymphocytic leukemia. Both drugs are so called "small molecules" known to inhibit **tyrosine kinase** or **serine threonine kinase** signal transduction pathway. Both the drugs in clinical trials have proved to prolong the life of patients beyond 2 years without any side effect, whereas other conventional treatment of chronic lymphatic leukemia patients to prolong the life only up to 2 years.

5.4.7 Cyclin-dependent Kinase (CDK) Inhibitors

CDKs are serene-threonine kinases which facilitate phosphorylation of key regulatory proteins during cell cycle. In majority of cancers, CDKs are overexpressed or amplified, therefore, they could be used as potential molecular targets for cancer therapies. A flavonoid called **flavopiridol** is a semi-synthetic molecule, competitively inhibits all CDKs by binding to their ATP binding site and brings about **cell cycle arrest at G1/S** and G2/M phases. D1 and D3 gene of CDK family are also affected by it through interference in transcriptional control of gene expression.

Preclinical trials have shown that CDK inhibitors act synergistically with cytotoxic drugs such as cisplatin, 5-fluorouracil, possibly because cell cycle arrested cells are more sensitive to CDK inhibitors. Currently, clinical trials are in progress for the CDK inhibitors like, UCN-01, CYC202 (R-Roscovitine, Cyclacel Ltd), PD0332991 (Pfizer: a selective inhibitor of CDKs 4/6), AT-7519 (Astex), and BMS-387032 (Sunesi) are some examples.

5.4.8 Histone Deacetylases Inhibitors

Histone-modifying enzymes like histone deacetylase (HDAC) generally repress gene transcription are the potential target for the development of new cancer drugs because they are aberrantly recruited in some cancers like leukemias. Using inhibitors of HDACs, genes involved in growth, differentiation or apoptosis that were silenced in cancers can be reactivated, which provides an opportunity for treating such cancers. Several classes of drugs such as short-chain fatty acid **sodium n-butyrate, hydroxamic acids** such as SAHA; cyclic peptides such as **romidepsin (formerly FK-228);** and **benzamide derivatives** such as **entinostat** capable of binding to the catalytic site of HDACs and block its binding to the substrates like acetylated lysine of histone proteins are being investigated in clinical trials. In general, these drugs are orally administered, well tolerated seem to have no side effects on normal cells. **Romidepsin (FK-228)** and SAHA (Vorinostat; Zolinza™) have been approved by the US-FDA for clinical use.

5.4.9 Inhibitors of Mitotic Spindle

Some alkaloids of plant origin are known to inhibit microtubules and spindle formation. Tubulin proteins of microtubules are stabilized by paclitaxel/taxol, whereas tubulin assembly in microtubules is inhibited by the Vinca alkaloids, vinblastine and vincristine. These drugs activate the mitotic checkpoint by preventing the attachment of chromosome pairs to the spindle fibers. Consequently, the cell fails to divide and apoptosis is the result. KSP, an ATP-dependent microtubule-motor protein required for spindle pole separation, is being tried as a molecular target for the development of cancer therapies. A small-molecule **ispinesib** (cytokinetics) inhibits KSP and prevents mitotic spindle pole separation leading to chronic mitotic checkpoint activation and is being tested in multiple phase I and Phase-II trials.

5.4.10 Strategies for Correction of p53 Mutation

To rectify the default of mutated gene, gene therapy is one of the approaches for rectifying p53 mutation. Retroviruses are commonly used for gene therapies and some of them have proved to be successful in several pre-clinical trials of anti-tumor activity. But there is always a risk of incorporation of retroviral genome into the host genome and bring about insertional mutagenesis. Therefore, adenoviruses, being DNA viruses, are retained in the cell as extrachromosomal bodies or plasmids without causing damage to the host genome are being tried. Advantages of using adenoviruses is that, they can carry large amount of foreign DNA and through coxsackievirus and adenovirus receptor (CAR) can infect varieties of cell types with high efficiency. Replication (replicon) defective adenoviruses have been popularly used as vectors. **Advexin**™ (Introgen therapeutics, **Genedicine**™, Shenzhen SiBono Gene Tech co. Ltd) is a replicon defective adenoviral vector that carries the normal human p53 gene controlled by a cytomegalovirus (CMV) promoter. Due to safety and low toxicity, Advexin has been used as gene therapy for mutant p53 to treat individual with Li-Fraumeni syndrome. In China, Genedicine has been approved by drug licencing authority and is the world's first commercial gene therapy for cancer.

Adenoviruses with replicative ability are being tried as another strategy for cancer therapeutics. Wild-type adenoviruses can replicate in cells by interfering with the RB and p53 pathways and inactivate p53 and RB gene functions. Cancer cells with p53 mutations can be selectively killed by Onyx 015, a replication selective adenovirus, which has a deletion in the E1B gene because of which it can only replicate within cancer cells having inactive p53 pathway and kill it. The E1A protein product of the Onyx 015 virus binds to RB protein and inactivates it, as a result, inducing G1-S phase transition of the cell cycle, thereby allowing for viral replication and cell destruction. E1A mutant Onyx 015 adenovirus triggers a p53 response of growth arrest resulting in the interference of viral replication in normal cells. Encouraging results are obtained in Phase I and II clinical trials because of selective replication minimal side effects of Onyx 015 adenovirus

Small molecules capable of restoring wild-type p53 gene function by interfering with mutant p53 gene products have been investigated. Many missense mutations of p53, results in production of abnormal protein with aberrant conformation. These abnormal proteins interfere with normal p53 protein and inhibit its DNA-binding function. Consequently, MDM2, the p53 inhibitor and target genes essential for apoptosis are not induced. Tumors carrying such p53 mutations are more likely to be resistant to conventional chemo and radiation therapies, because these drugs pro-apoptotic. Reactivation of p53 mutant using a short synthetic peptide **CDB3** has been shown to stabilize the structure of several p53 mutants and to restore their transcriptional function. CDB3 acts as a chaperone protein that facilitates the refolding of the mutant p53 protein and restores its function of DNA binding and transcriptional regulation. Similarly, **PRIMA-1**, restores wild-type p53 conformation and DNA binding in mutant p53 proteins. PRIMA-1 showed low toxicity in phase-I clinical trials, hence has entered phase-II trials.

5.4.11 Strategies to Activate Endogenous p53

In almost all tumors, even though, normal p53 is expressed, its function is impaired by mutant p53 protein due to dominant interference by mutant protein leading to an altered p53 pathway. Amplified expression of the p53 inhibitor MDM2 leads to impaired regulation and p53 inactivation. In virus induced cancers, viral proteins inactivate p53 function by directly interacting with it and p53 mutation is not seen. In order to activate wild-type p53 protein, a drug molecule called **nutlins** developed as inhibitor of the p53-MDM2 interaction, has shown promising results as inhibitor in pre-clinical trials. These results show successful activation of p53 like the biological responses in cancer cells containing normal p53, which showed inhibition of tumor growth by 90% in animal models.

5.4.12 Strategies for Suppression of Endogenous p53

It is evident that p53 plays an important role in promoting cancer cells to apoptosis as well as the success of chemo- and radiation therapy is dependent on normal p53 functions. Side effects of chemo- and radiation therapy are also governed by P53. DNA damage caused by chemotherapeutic agents and radiation triggers enhanced expression of p53 in the cells of hematopoietic organs and intestinal epithelia, leading to p53 induced apoptosis, which is the mechanism behind the side-effects. Therefore, temporary, and reversible suppression of p53 in normal cells is an alternative approach to alleviate the side-effects of conventional therapies and in subjects with lost p53 function, conventional therapies will not work. A novel compound **Pifithrin** is known to inhibit p53 gene transcription.

5.4.13 Induction of Apoptosis through Pro-apoptotic Drugs

Inducing apoptosis successfully in cancer cells is an important strategy, which could be successfully achieved through conventional chemotherapies by indirect means. It has been possible to design the molecules that play a positive role in the apoptotic pathways as direct apoptotic inducers. At the same time, endogenous inhibitors should be blocked to promote apoptosis. Unlike other chemotherapeutic drugs, which are mutagenic and leukemogenic, these anti-apoptotic drugs are non-mutagenic. Moreover, the induction of apoptosis in normal cells by the drug has little effect as they are expected to trigger apoptosis to the same extent in tumor cells. Some of the strategies adopted to promote apoptosis through pro-apoptotic drugs are as follows:

5.4.13.1 Direct and indirect activation of caspases

Caspases comprise a large family of over 13 members. Selective activation of caspases is the most obvious apoptotic target in cancer cells, but selectively activating them has been a problem thus far. Three aspartate residues can successfully inhibit Procaspase-3 a pro-enzyme of a key effector caspase, called the "safety-catch", which facilitates intramolecular interaction. The activation of caspases by indirect methods holds promise in cancer treatment. Endogenous **caspase inhibitor XIAP** is overexpressed in many cancers and it is a good candidate for molecular therapy, because active site of caspase-3 and caspase-7 are directly blocked by one domain of XIAP while another distinct domain of it inhibits caspase-9. A class of **polyphenylureas,** known to relieve the inhibition of caspase-3 and caspase-7 but not caspase-9, has been identified, which binds to the XIAP domain that blocks the active site of caspase-3 and caspase-7 and show minimum toxicity for normal cells, thereby promoting apoptosis in XIAP active cancer cells. This was the first example of relieving of caspases inhibition that could induce tumor cell apoptosis.

5.4.13.2 Regulation of Bcl-2 family of anti-apoptotic proteins

The proteins of Bcl-2 family are anti-apoptotic, which are another target for the design of pro-apoptotic drugs for cancer therapy. Three main strategies have been used to achieve success in this direction by (a) application of antisense RNA, (b) inhibition of protein function and protein-protein interactions of anti-apoptotic molecules, and (c) drugs that stimulate the activity of pro-apoptotic molecules. Apoptosis in majority of tumors is inhibited by the overexpression of BCl-2, inhibition of BCl-2 expression by using antisense RNA is one of the strategies to develop a new cancer drug. **G-3139 (oblimersen sodium, Genasense™)** is an 18-mer modified antisense oligonucleotide, complementary to the first six codons of start site on the Bcl-2 mRNA downstream of, upon hybridization of antisense oligonucleotide with mRNA, inhibition of translation occurs and degradation of mRNA takes place. This alters the balance of pro- and anti-apoptotic factors in favor of apoptosis. Currently, G-3139 is being tested for its compatibility and toxicity in combination with other chemotherapeutic drugs.

Structural studies of Bcl-2 molecule have revealed that pro-apoptotic Bcl-2 family members bind to hydrophobic groove of BH3 region. Small molecule like ABT-737 by Abbott Laboratories that binds to pro-apoptotic molecules Bcl-2/ Bcl-x_L and inhibit them by interfering with protein-protein interactions, which is essential to induce apoptosis have been identified. The action of BH3 proteins is mimicked by small molecule inhibitors. They are also called BH3 mimetics. ABT-737 is administered intravenously and ABT-263 is administered orally, bind to BCL-2, Bcl-XL and Bcl-w anti-apoptotic protein with high affinity and inhibit their pro-apoptotic action. Two other small molecules, AT-101 (**Ascenta**) and GX15-070 (**Gemin X**) are in Phase-I or II clinical trials also bind to anti-apoptotic Bcl-2 molecules.

Subaroylanilide hydroxamic acid (SAHA) promotes apoptosis by increasing the activity of a pro-apoptotic factor instead of inhibiting an anti-apoptotic factor. SAHA is a **HDAC inhibitor** and therefore induces the expression of epigenetically suppressed pro-apoptotic genes. Pro-apoptotic proteins BID expression is facilitated by SAHA, which in turn, activates another pro-apoptotic protein BAX that translocates itself into mitochondria and facilitates the release of cytochrome c, which is one of the apoptotic factors. For treatment of non-Hodgkin's lymphoma **SAHA (Vorinostat)** has been given approval.

5.4.13.3 Drugs that target TRAIL and its receptor

Tumor necrosis factor-related apoptosis-inducing ligand (TRAIL) is supposed to activate apoptosis through the death receptors TR1 (TRAILR-1, DR4) and TR2 (TRAILR-2, DR5, TRICK2, KILLER), which belong to TNFR super-family. Two other membrane-bound receptors TR3 and TR4 are homologous to extracellular domain of TR1 and Apo 2 ligand (TRAIL/Apo2L) are also bound by TRAIL and initiate apoptosis through engagement of its death receptors. TRAIL is not capable of inducing apoptosis in normal cells but selectively induces apoptosis of a variety of tumor cells and transformed cells, therefore has garnered intense interest as a promising agent for cancer therapy. TRAIL is expressed on T-cells and natural killer cell of the immune system, thereby help in tumor surveillance and suppression of tumor metastasis. Some tumors with mismatch-repair-deficiency evade TRAIL-induced apoptosis and acquire TRAIL resistance through different mechanisms. Death receptors are the members of the TNF receptor family, they can signal apoptosis independently of the p53 tumor-suppressor gene. In combinatorial chemo- and radiotherapy, TRAIL treatment enhances TRAIL sensitivity or reverses TRAIL resistance by altering downstream regulatory effectors. Efforts to identify agents that activate death receptors or block specific effectors that inhibit death receptors may improve cancer therapeutics design. Recent insights into the apoptosis-signaling pathways stimulated by TRAIL by administration of recombinant human TRAIL ligand has exhibited promising anti-tumor activity in animal models and phase-I trials have been initiated for the treatment of solid tumors. Non-human primates did not show toxicity without extraneous amino acid residues associated with TRAIL. Agonistic monoclonal antibody directed against extracellular domain of TRAIL receptor has been in use for the treatment of several cancers.

5.4.14 Inhibitors of Wnt Pathway

Wnt pathway plays a major role in several cancers, particularly colorectal cancer. β-catenin, one of the molecular components of this pathway is responsible for the maintenance of stem cell-like characteristics by cancer cells. Therefore, many molecules of Wnt pathway are an excellent targets for the cancer therapeutics. One strategy that has been investigated is by preventing the protein-protein interaction between β-catenin and the Tcf transcription factor, which is the endpoint effect of Wnt signaling that occurs downstream of the APC degradation complex. The trimolecular complex of APC, axin, and GSK3β is very crucial for inactivation β-catenin by phosphorylation. Mutations leading to inactivation of APC, axin, and GSK3β, and the mutations that cause activation of β-catenin result in inappropriate β-catenin-Tcf complexes formation leading to cell retaining stem cell characteristics and cell proliferation. It is observed that differentiation of colorectal cancer cells into epithelial villi can be brought about by inhibition of Tcf is proof enough to support this approach. At present, three natural compounds are undergoing phase 1 trials as β-catenin-Tcf interaction inhibitors.

5.4.15 Inhibitors of Hh (Hedgehog) Pathway

Cyclopamine is a steroidal alkaloid isolated from wild corn lilies shows Hh pathway inhibition by suppressing the activity of **Smoothened**, a transmembrane protein, resulting in repression of transcription of target genes. In medulloblastoma cell lines, cyclopamine inhibited the growth of medulloblastoma cells by interfering with the regulation of genes involved in differentiation. Cyclopamine also suppresses the expression of neurofilament nestin, a neuronal stem cell marker, whereas expression of the neuroD, a marker of neuronal differentiation was increased.

HhAntag-691, a small molecule designed as inhibitor of Smoothened, has shown promising results in a transgenic mouse model by suppressing the expression of several genes associated with the Hh pathway leading to decreased tumor growth and increased apoptosis.

In a phase-I clinical trial, advanced basal-cell carcinoma patients were administered orally active small molecule **Vismodegib** (GDC-0449), an inhibitor of smoothened showed anti-tumor activity.

5.4.16 Therapies for Leukemia and Differentiation Process of Cells

Therapies directed against the maturation and differentiation process of cells such that by altering gene regulation a malignant phenotype is changed to a benign phenotype by suppression of growth and induction of apoptosis. The therapy directed against differentiation process for the treatment of acute promyelocytic leukemia (APL), a subtype of AML, has been a great success of the last few decades. Treatment of deadly leukemia with all-trans retinoic acid (ATRA) transformed it into one of the most treatable forms of cancer has been a great achievement. Severe leukemic patients were given combinatorial therapy of retinoic acid along with chemotherapy showed complete remission with 80% survival for 5 years. Treatment with retinoic acid alone causes retinoic acid syndrome in 10-15% of patients but administration in combination with chemotherapy reduces the side-effect. Administration of high concentration retinoic acid facilitates its binding to the ligand-binding domain of the RARα-PML fusion protein, resulting in a conformational change that induces the exchange of the HDAC-co-repressor complex for a co-activating complex. The differentiation specific transcription factor, C/EBP, is expressed as a result of retinoid treatment, which overcomes the blockage of differentiation process. Prevention of homodimerization of the fusion proteins is another strategy for a new therapy to inhibit differentiation.

5.4.17 Strategies for Restoration of Metastasis Suppressors

Like the alternatives that are being worked out to reactivate tumor suppressor genes; several therapies are also being developed to reactivate metastasis suppressor genes. NM23, one among the metastasis suppressor genes, shows suppressed expression due to mutations in the coding region of the gene, being a rare phenomenon, but a common feature in cancer cells. Therefore, reactivation of major metastasis suppressor genes expression through drug candidates may be useful in cancer therapy. The promoter of the NM23 gene is regulated by glucocorticoid response pathway. A progesterone and glucocorticoid agonist, called **Medroxyprogesterone acetate (MPA),** was found to be successful in inducing expression of the **NM23** promoter and currently, MPA is going through phase-II trials either with or without chemotherapeutic intervention in metastatic breast cancer patients. In pre-clinical trials, administration of recombinant metastasis suppressor proteins and gene therapy are being investigated as an alternative for reactivating metastasis suppressor gene.

5.4.18 Anti-angiogenic Therapy and Targeting Vasculature

Since most of the solid tumors gain the ability to induce the formation of blood vessels around them, anti-angiogenic therapy to prevent neovasculature is yet another approach for cancer therapy as an alternative to targeting the tumor cells directly. In anti-angiogenic therapy, drugs are designed to interfere with endothelial cells response or pro-angiogenic signals or the activity of the inducers that is essential for the tumor's survival. Overall, the anti-angiogenic drugs act as cytostatic rather than cytotoxic agents therefore would require long-term continuous administration in combination with other cancer therapeutics.

Some of the natural and native to the body anti-angiogenesis inhibitors like **angiostatin** and **endostatin** are being tried as anti-angiogenic therapies because, they have the advantage of being reasonably well tolerated without toxic side effects. Both these natural anti-angiogenic agents are biologically active only on endothelial cells that are actively proliferating during neoangiogenesis in vivo, but are not active in vitro. Moreover, these proteins are known to remain in blood circulation for longer time, so that the exposure of tumor vasculature to their anti-angiogenic effects is increased. Already vascularized small tumors when treated with angiostatin and endostatin, angiostatin reduced the size of tumors by 50% and endostatin caused the reduction of tumor by 80%. Relatively little effect was seen when large well-established tumors were treated with either of them, but when both were used together it caused 75% reduction in the mass of such tumors.

Yet another class of natural angiogenesis antagonist is the **Interferon** α and β **(IFN** α **and** β**)** have proven to inhibit synthesis of **basic fibroblast growth factor (bFGF)** and **interleukin-8 (IL-8)**, both are strong promoters of angiogenesis. Administration of IFNα has proven to be useful in causing the regression of some hemangiomas (endothelial cell tumors) as well as Kaposi's sarcoma, which are also of endothelial origin.

One of the strategies of anti-angiogenic therapy involves targeting pro-angiogenic factors such as vascular endothelial growth factor (VEGF). **Avastin™ (bevasizumab),** a recombinant human monoclonal antibody, has been in use for quite some time that recognizes all VEGF isoforms, used for the treatment of several different types of cancers but the drug failed in the treatment of breast cancer. The reason for this lies in the angiogenic switch, which differs in breast cancer. This proves that inhibition of just one pro-angiogenic factor does not have an effect.

Some synthetic low-molecular weight anti-angiogenic compounds have been found, first of these is **fumagillin,** compound of fungal origin and its derivative, **TNP-470**. These two compounds were found to inhibit the endothelial cells proliferation both in vitro and in vivo. Synthetic compound such as **SU5416** is known to **inhibit VEGF-R2 tyrosine kinase** receptor and **SU6668** is known to **inhibit PDGF-tyrosine kinase** receptor. SU5416 was successful in blocking the expression of angiogenic switch in 90% of the early stage, dysplastic tumors, thereby holding them to a small size and in non-invasive state. However, SU5416 has no effect on later stage, well established tumors. SU6668 had more potent effect on large tumors of late stage and it reduced their size by about half and prevented vascularization. Importantly, the only cells that express PDGF-R are pericytes and smooth muscle cells, which seem to be the targets of SU6668. Combination treatment using SU5416 and SU6668 proved to be highly effective and potent way of targeting at various stages of tumor formation, due to simultaneous inhibition of both VEGF and PDGF receptors successfully prevented activation of angiogenic switch. This drug combination showed 90% inhibition of further expansion of small, already established angiogenic tumors and caused 80% regression of large tumors, like the drug **Glevec**, another PDGF-R inhibitor.

Significantly, these combination drugs virtually did not show any toxic effects on normal tissue surrounding the neoplastic islets, confirming that recently formed capillaries within a tumor are far more vulnerable to disruption than the well-established vessels within normal tissues. These observations indicate that the most effective ways of inhibiting angiogenesis and thus blocking tumor progression are likely to depend on targeting several of the cell types that construct the tumor-associated vasculature.

Sunitinib and Sorafenib were developed to target VEGFR tyrosine kinase inhibitors and their mode of action involves inhibition of autophosphorylation of receptor. Sunitinib targets VEGFR as well as PDGFR, KIT and FLT3. Sorafenib targets VEGFR, PDGFR, KIT, FIT3 and Raf kinase.

Administration of recombinant human endogenous inhibitor **endostatin** as an anti-angiogenic strategy has not shown expected results. Drug molecules that are antagonistic to **integrins αvβ3** and **αvβ5** block endothelial integrin-ECM interactions and specifically induce apoptosis of neovasculature with limited effect on mature vessels. Two candidate drugs as integrin inhibitors have entered clinical trials, namely, **Vitaxin™** a humanized monoclonal antibody against αvβ3 and **Celengitide** a synthetic cyclic peptide antagonist that mimics the Arg-gly-Asp "ligand" sequence and inhibits αvβ3 and αvβ5 integrins.

Thalidomide has proved to be an excellent drug for the treatment of multiple myeloma. It inhibits angiogenic stimulus induced by bFGF or VEGF. However, thalidomide is not recommended to be administered to pregnant women because it is teratogenic.

During other cancer therapies anti-angiogenic effects may be seen as "side-effects". Cancer therapies targeted at oncogene products often affect angiogenesis. Like, Herceptin™, the monoclonal antibody directed against ErbB2 derived HER-2 receptor does cause anti-angiogenic effects by inhibiting pro-angiogenic factors like TGF-α and angiopoietin-1 prduction by tumor cells and up-regulation of anti-angiogenic factors like thrombospondin-1.

5.4.18.1 Targeting the vasculature

Targeting neovasculature is another alternative therapeutic approach designed to destroy the neovasculature around the young tumor in order to deprive the oxygen and nutrition to tumor and suppress the tumor growth. **Combrestatin,** an alkaloid extracted from African plant, is found to be anti-neovasculature agent. It inhibits neovasculature by binding to tubulin and disrupts the cytoskeleton. Neovasculature requires participation of cytoskeleton to maintain architecture of endothelial cells compared to the stable mature vasculature which has a support of basement membrane. During the formation of new blood vessels, loss of architecture of the endothelial cells impedes blood flow leading to vascular collapse, which deprives oxygen and nutrients supply to the tumor, triggering necrosis at the core of the tumor.

Nanoparticle based therapies have also been developed against neovasculature. The details of which are given in the section "nanoparticles in cancer therapeutics".

5.5 IMMUNE THERAPY OF CANCER

Successful suppression of tumors by immunological route requires activation of multiple immune defense mechanisms that include cytokine and chemokines of the immune system like, IL-12, IFN-γ, IFN-γ, phagocytes, APCs, and cytotoxic effector cells. Immunotherapy to cancer patients through immunological approaches has held a great promise for the next decades to come. There are five ways in which immune therapy against cancer has been worked out. Which are as follows:

1. Nonspecific stimulation of the immune system as cancer therapeutics.
2. Active immunization against tumors.
3. Adoptive cellular therapy as cancer therapeutics.
4. Passive therapy with anti-tumor antibodies as cancer therapeutics.
5. Cytokines as cancer therapeutics.

5.5.1 Cancer Therapeutics through Nonspecific Stimulation of the Immune System

In this therapy, adjuvants like Bacille Calmette-Guerin (BCG) containing attenuated mycobacterium are used for the treatment of cancer patients by injecting the adjuvant at the site of tumor, provided the tumor is easily accessible. This type of non-specific immunotherapy has been in practice for many years. This treatment causes severe inflammation at the site of tumor leading to infiltration of tumor by macrophages and destruction of tumor cells by cytotoxic response.

5.5.2 Active Immunization against Tumors (Tumor Vaccination)

The requirement of stimulation of an effective immune response against cancer is by breaking immune tolerance of tumors through presenting tumor antigens to the immune cells in a way that will activate high levels of effector pathways capable of suppressing tumor growth for a prolonged time. To achieve this goal, a variety of strategies are currently being developed, which are being investigated both in preclinical and in clinical trials.

At present it is evident that there are two barriers that need to be tackled to induce the immune response against tumor. First one is to engage the antigen presenting cells (APCs) mainly dendritic cells (DCs) with tumor antigens, which on antigen uptake get activated and travel to the nearest draining lymph node to further activate naïve $CD4^+$ T cells. The strategy involves use of oligonucleotide sequences resembling bacterial DNA having CpG motifs. For the treatment of hematological malignancies, stimulation with CpG motifs and exposure to co-stimulatory molecules like CD40 ligands to facilitate cancer cells to present intrinsic tumor antigens to immune cells.

In B cell lymphoma patients, patients are immunized with defined tumor antigens made of idiotypic epitope of the immunoglobulin expressed by their lymphoma cells. Patients immunized with idiotypic protein mixed with adjuvant or pulsed with dendritic cells showed tumor regressions. Such a type of treatment of B cell lymphoma requires individual specific treatment because of variation in idiotypic proteins expressed by each patient, which involves preparation of a different vaccine for each patient.

The MAGE-like antigen expressed by tumor cells of melanoma can also be used to develop common vaccines. Melanoma patients with HLA-A1 haplotype express MAGE-1 on their tumor cells, when injected with autologous blood monocytes pulsed with MAGE-1 encoded peptide showed minimum CTL response and tumor regression was not observed. Twelve patients of HLA-A1 haplotype having most advanced melanoma were given subcutaneous injection of MAGE-3 encoded antigenic peptide in the absence of adjuvant, showed tumor regression in 3 patients, but without CTL response.

The relative frequency of cytotoxic T lymphocyte precursors' (CTLps) response to MAGE-3 peptide presented by HLA-A1 is found to be 3×10^{-7} of the blood $CD8^+$ cells.

In another trial, a large number of patients were injected with melanoma differentiation antigenic peptides together with either incomplete Freud's adjuvant or granulocyte-macrophage colony stimulating factor (GM-CSF). Tumor regressions were observed in a few patients with enhanced delayed type hypersensitivity reactions in patients who were given GM-CSF.

E7 gene encoded tumor-specific antigenic peptide of the human papilloma virus type 16 coupled to palmitic acid was administered to 12 cervical cancer patients. Two out of seven patients showed higher IFN-γ production in the peripheral blood mononuclear cells (PBMC) post vaccination.

For stimulation of full-scale CTL effector and memory response against tumors, synthetic vaccines have been designed to provide both antigenic and accessory signals. These signals involve innate immunity receptors such as CD40 or Fc receptors or toll-like receptors (TLRs) on DCs. In most cancers, triggering of these receptors is precisely lacking, therefore, despite the concrete evidence of extensive natural processing of tumor antigens and a considerable level of natural cross-priming of antigens, very poor CTL response is observed.

5.5.3 Dendritic Cells Vaccination as Tumor Therapeutics

Several clinical trials were conducted with mature dendritic cells pulsed with MAGE, Melan-A, tyrosinase, HER-2/neu or MUC1 peptides intravenously transferred to breast cancer, ovarian cancer, or melanoma patients. Several of them showed good $CD4^+$ T cell response against the peptides presented by HLA class II and $CD8^+$ T cell response against peptides presented by HLA class I. On vaccination of sixteen metastatic melanoma patients with mature monocyte derived dendritic cells stimulated with keyhole limpet hemocyanin (KLH) antigen and simultaneously expressing melanoma differentiation antigen or MAGE genes product on HLA class-I and class-II showed good $CD4^+$ T cell response (Fig. 5.11).

Injecting the killed or irradiated tumor cells together with nonspecific adjuvants induce active immunization against a particular tumor. Memory T cells expanded by such immunization would hopefully limit the growth of already established tumors. Unfortunately, methods adopted so far for active immunization are unsuccessful, probably because tumor cell vaccines do not effectively activate specific T cell responses.

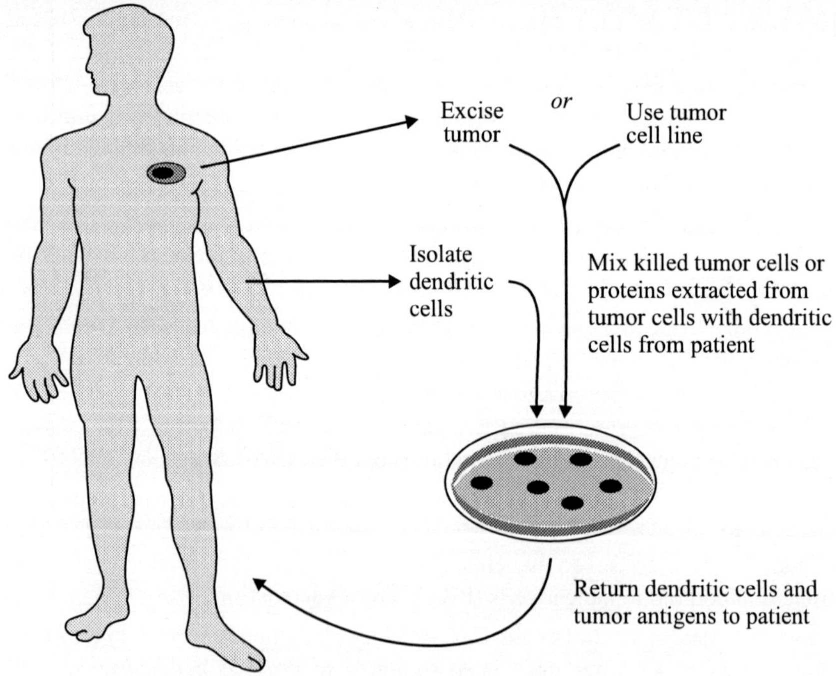

Fig. 5.11. Dendritic cell vaccination as tumor therapeutics

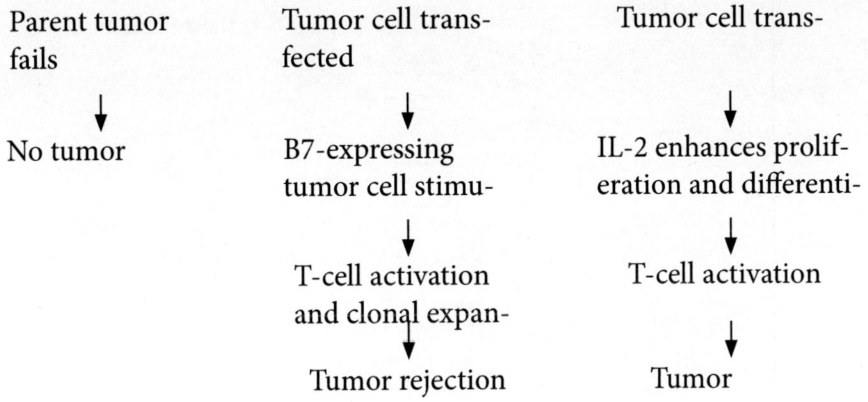

Fig. 5.12. Schematic representation of mechanism involved in tumor cell destruction by transfection of co-stimulation molecule B7 or by IL-2 gene into tumor cells makes them more prone to destruction by T-cells (cytotoxic)

Recent experiments demonstrated that when animal tumor cells are transfected with exogenous genes that code for either cytokines or co-stimulatory molecules and these cells were transferred back to the host from which they were derived (ex vivo approach) showed significant reduction in tumors or complete disappearance of tumors (Figs.5.12 and 5.13).

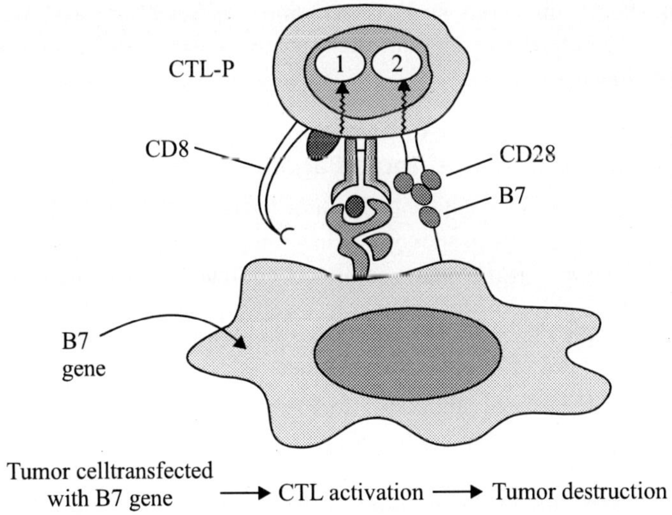

Fig. 5.13. Expression of co-stimulatory molecule by genetically engineered tumor cells to make it vulnerable for immune attack by T cells

For example, rodent tumor cells transfected with any of the genes encoding cytokines like IL-2, IL-4, IFN-γ, or granulocyte macrophage colony stimulating factor (GM-CSF) when injected back into the same animals from which it was harvested, tumors rejection or regression was observed. Eosinophils and

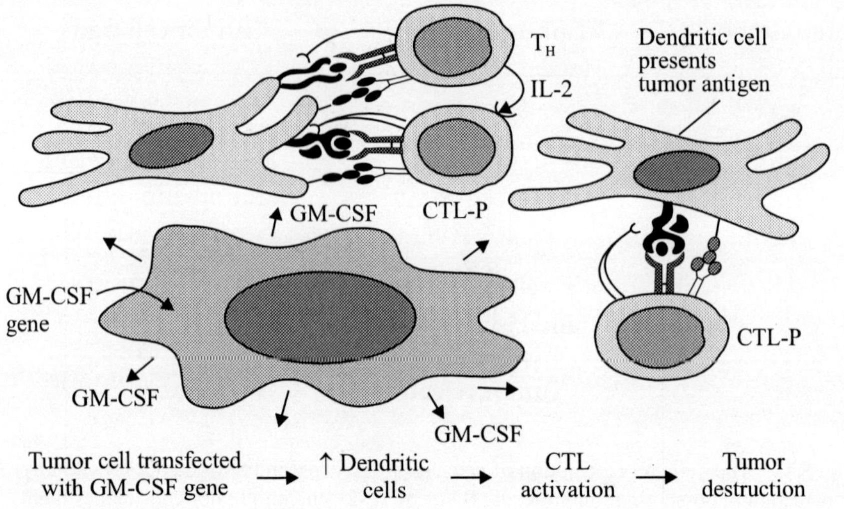

Fig. 5.14. Tumor cells transfected with GM-CSF gene express the cytokine to enhance immune response against the tumor

macrophage accumulate around IL-4 producing tumors, macrophages will be seen infiltrating in large numbers around IFN-γ secreting tumors, and IL-2 producing tumors are generally surrounded by massive lymphocytic infiltrates. The tumors surrounded by inflammatory cells recruited by different cytokines may involve in different effector functions such as activation of T cells against the tumor antigens. Accordingly, active immunization against cancer can be carried out in the following manner.

5.5.4 Enhancement of Anti-tumor Immunity by Monoclonal Antibody Treatment Directed against T-cell Receptors

From several experiments conducted in tumor bearing mice, it has been proved that, maintenance of T cells in active state in a tumor bearing mice induces potent anti-tumor immunity. On the premises of this approach, two novel monoclonal antibody treatment protocols for enhancing T cell-mediated anti-tumor immunity in the tumor-bearing host have been developed. In one approach, inhibitory receptor of T cells, namely, cytotoxic T lymphocytic antigen-4 (CTLA4) receptor is blocked by monoclonal antibody (mAb). CTLA4 of T lymphocytes on interaction with B7.2 expressed by antigen presenting cells (APC) leads to suppression T cell activity or causes T cell anergy. On the contrary, interaction of CD28 receptor expressed by the T cell with B7.1 expressed by APCs leads to T cell activation. By using monoclonal antibody directed against CTLA4, CTLA4 signal generation can be blocked and prevent T cells anergic state thereby, keeping the T cells in active state is possible by the interaction CD28 of T cells with B7.1 of APC. This was demonstrated by administering anti-CTLA4 monoclonal antibodies to tumor-bearing mice led to induction of a potent anti-tumor immunity, because of blocking the CTLA4 inhibitory pathway, which favored T cell activation pathway.

In an alternative second approach, monoclonal antibodies directed against 4-1BB were used activate tumor reactive T cells. 4-1BB is the T lymphocyte specific receptor expressed on their membrane to interact with co-stimulatory molecule 4-1BB ligand (4-1BBL) expressed by APC during antigen presentation by APC. Tumors were rejected in tumor-bearing mice given anti-4-1BB mAb, presumably because of the second signal necessary for T cell activation provided by 4-1BB-4-1BBL interaction was not there, in addition to CD28 and B7.1 interaction.

5.5.5 Adoptive Therapy Using Tumor Antigens as Targets

Many potential tumor rejection antigens have been characterized utilizing CTLs reactive against melanoma. Some of these melanoma antigens are considered to be tumor specific, such as MAGE-1, MAGE-3, NA17A, mutated cyclin dependent kinase (CDK4), and mutated β-catenin. Some other melanoma antigens are associated with monocyte differentiation antigens, such as tyrosinase, MART-1/MelanA, gp100 and gp75. In addition to melanomas, MAGE-1, 2 or 3 antigens are expressed by significant percentage of glioma cell lines, breast tumors, non-small cell lung carcinomas and head or neck carcinomas. These shared antigens have been exploited for clinical therapeutics.

5.5.6 Adoptive Cellular Transfer (ACT) Therapy

In this ex vivo immunotherapy, tumor infiltrating immune cells showing anti-tumor reactivity harvested from the cancer patients are genetically modified in vitro and introduced back into a tumor-bearing host through intravenous route. Two treatment approaches have been tested, in clinical trials: a) lymphokine activated killer (LAK) cell therapy, and b) tumor infiltrating lymphocyte (TIL) therapy.

5.5.6.1 Lymphokine activated killer (LAK) cell therapy

NK cells or CTLs isolated from the peripheral blood of cancer patients are cultured in vitro for the generation of LAK cells under the influence of IL-2. While they are growing in the culture, they are pulsed with host tumor homogenate. NK cells and CTLs get activated under the influence of IL-2 and become lymphokine activated killer (LAK) cells. The LAK cells are transferred back to the cancer patients through intravenous route. LAK cells are predominantly derived from NK cells and autologous LAK cells adoptive therapy in combination with in vivo administration of IL-2 or chemotherapeutic agent has shown positive response in mice, with significant reduction of solid tumors. LAK cell therapy clinical trials in humans have so far been largely restricted to advance stages of metastatic tumors, responses were found to be highly variable from patient to patient.

5.5.6.2 Tumor infiltrating lymphocyte (TIL) therapy

Inflammatory infiltrates obtained from surgical resection specimens of the solid tumors, usually contain mononuclear cells from which LAK cells are derived. This approach is used for enrichment of TILs as tumor-specific killer cells against the tumor. TILs include activated NK cells and CTLs, but the specificity of the mixed population of cells is not really established (Rosenberg et al., 1987). Immunotherapy based on the adoptive transfer of TILs is found to be the best approach for the treatment of patients with metastatic melanoma. In a recent study of 93 patients with stage IV melanoma were treated with the adoptive transfer of autologous TILs together with administration of IL-2 following host conditioning regimens. 20 of the 93 patients showed complete regression of tumor and 19 among these 20 have ongoing complete regression with a minimum follow-up of 57 months. Indeed, some of these patients who underwent adoptive TIL immunotherapy, have been alive and disease free for more than 8 years and are probably cured of metastatic melanoma. Thus, ACT therapy with autologous TILs is capable of mediating durable complete remission in patients with metastatic melanoma.

5.5.6.3 Chimeric antigen receptor (CAR)-T cell therapy

This immunotherapy has been approved by US-FDA **Tisagenlecleucel (Kymriah™)** in 2017 to treat **Acute lymphoblastic leukemia (ALL) (B-cell lymphoma)** where T cells harvested from ALL patient are genetically modified in vitro to express **chimeric antigen receptor (CAR)** on T cells, which is capable of recognizing CD19 receptor overexpressed by B cells in ALL patients. Car-T cells are living drugs built by transducing autologous T cells (host T cells or self T cells) from cancer patients with CARs that fuse an extracellular antibody fragment scFv to a transmembrane segment followed by the cytoplasmic signaling domain CD3ζ of the TCR complex. Genetically modified CAR-T cells are transfused back into ALL patients through intravenous route. These CAR-T cells on recognizing the CD19 receptor on B cells in vivo in the patient, will bind to the CD19 receptor and cause instantaneous killing of abnormal B cells. This therapy has been found to be successful only against ALL but not against other types of cancers of other tissue origin and other hematopoietic tissue origin cancers.

5.5.7 Passive Therapy with Anti-tumor Antibodies

In this therapeutic approach, antibodies that recognize tumor antigens expressed on tumor cell surface are coupled with toxic agents bind to tumor antigens and selectively kill tumor cells. Such antibodies are also called immunotoxins. Different types of these anti-tumor antibody therapies against tumors are described below.

5.5.7.1 Radionuclides or cytotoxic drugs coupled anti-tumor antibodies (Immunoconjugates or Immunotoxins)

Anti-tumor antibodies coupled with radioisotopes and cytotoxic drugs have all been tried for immunotherapy of cancer in humans and experimental animal models. In this approach anti-neoplastic drugs or cytocidal radioisotopes are covalently attached to anti-tumor monoclonal antibodies. Covalently linked radio isotope inflicts the damage locally to the tumor cells when the antibody binds to the suitable antigen on the tumor cell surface, whereas anti-neoplastic drugs are taken up by tumor cells through endocytic pathway and delivered to appropriate intracellular site of action.

Calicheamicin-based immunoconjugates **(Gemtuzumabozogamycin-Mylotarg-humanized mAb-Wyeth Caltech Group)**, clinically approved in 2000 for the treatment of acute myeloid leukemia (AML), and it is the first monoclonal antibody drug conjugate or biopharmaceutical to have been approved by US-FDA. Calicheamicin induces double strand breaks in DNA, leading to potent cytotoxicity and the drug is attached to humanized IgG4mAb through lysine residues and the mAB is meant for CD33 receptor antigen on myeloid cells (transformed cells) of AML patients. One of the distinguishing features of this immunoconjugate drug is that within 30 minutes of administration, it binds to target antigen (CD33 receptor) and saturates it. This immunoconjugate is now in phase I trial of Lewis antigen on breast carcinoma, colon carcinoma, lung cancer, ovarian cancer and the prostate cancer has been targeted with the Hu3S193-N-acetyl calicheamicin immunoconjugate. With similar approach, **doxorubicin** and **auristatin** immunoconjugate antibodies have been produced. Anti-CD74-doxorubicin mAb conjugate is under clinical trial for the treatment of non-Hodgkin's lymphoma.

Toxin and radionuclide conjugated monoclonal antibodies with specificities for TAA's on melanomas and carcinomas have been tried in humans. In addition, antibody conjugates specific for CD19, CD22 and CD30 receptors have been used for treating lymphomas. Adult T cell leukemias are treated with antibodies against IL-2Rα (interleukin-2, receptor α) because the T cell leukemias usually over express IL-2Rα. Anti IL-2R antibodies are conjugated with diphtheria toxin and the radionuclide **yttrium 90**, which are used to treat T cell lymphomas. In general, very small percentage of patient's show decreased burden of tumor; hence the efficacy of this procedure is limited.

Ibritumomab tuixetan-^{90}Y (Zevalin, murine mAb, by Biogen IDEC, approved in 2002), **I^{131}-tositumomab** (Bexar, murine mAb-Corixa/GlaxoSmithKline, approves in 2003) is CD20 positive B cell non-Hodgkin's lymphoma and rituximab-refractory follicular hon-Hodgkin's lymphoma. **Rituximab (Rituxan)** is another mAb against CD20 along with chemotherapeutic agents; toxin and radionuclide-conjugated antibodies. Another example of mAbs is for tumor antigen HER-2/neu, this receptor is overexpressed in breast cancers, adenocarcinomas of ovary, prostate, lung, and gastrointestinal tract. **Trastuzumab (Herceptin)** in combination with Navelbine, Taxotere, Platinol, Gemzar, Taxol is directed against HER-2/neu.

5.5.7.2 Anti-idiotypic antibodies and monoclonal anti-idiotypic antibodies

Using anti-idiotypic monoclonal antibodies for the treatment of B cell lymphomas that express on their surface mIgM immunoglobulins as B cell receptor (BCR) with specific idiotypes or Fab regions has been one of the approaches. An idiotype refers to Fab region of the antibody, which is highly specific to an antibody not only expressed as BCR on the surface of B cells stimulated by tumor antigens but also found in the antibody produced by the B cells stimulated against neoplastic cells. Anti-idiotype antibodies are produced in rabbits by immunizing them with the human B cell lymphoma cells and care was taken that the immunoglobulins in the serum reactive against all other human immunoglobulins were depleted. The modality involved in this therapy is complement-mediated lysis or antibody dependent cell mediated toxicity (ADCC) to kill the lymphoma cells. Success of this approach is very limited, because surface immunoglobulin expression as mIgM (BCR) is not specific only to malignant B cell lymphomas alone. Selective proliferation of non-immunoglobulin expressing B cell lymphomas can occur. Moreover, during immunoglobulin gene expression, there is high degree of mutations known to occur, which could result in the selective proliferation of B cell lymphomas with changed idiotypes no longer recognized by the anti-idiotypic antibody. Furthermore, since rabbit antibodies on injection to the B cell lymphoma patients trigger development of antibodies against rabbit immunoglobulins because species difference and it could to interfere with the efficiency of the rabbit anti-tumor antibodies.

Levy et al., were successful in producing mouse monoclonal **anti-idiotypic** antibody specific for B cell lymphoma idiotype and on injecting this anti-idiotype antibody was to the patient suffering from terminal B cell lymphoma showing metastasis in liver, spleen, bone marrow and peripheral blood showed complements-mediated lysis of the lymphoma cells without harming other cells. The patient underwent treatment with monoclonal anti-idiotypic antibody four times and at present has been in complete remission.

5.5.7.3 Heteroconjugate antibodies

An antibody having specificity to a tumor antigen is covalently linked with another antibody having specificity to a surface protein receptor of cytotoxic effector cells, such as NK cells or CTLs is targeted against tumor cells. Therefore, this approach is called heteroconjugate, which can promote binding of these effector cells to tumor cells. A heteroconjugate antibody consists of an anti-CD3 antibody linked to an antibody against tumor cell specific antigen has been used to enhance CTL mediated lysis of the target cell. Because of this feature, the anti-CD3 antibody not only helps in bringing the CTL into contact with the target tumor cells but it also facilitates activation of the CTL against the tumor cells. For the treatment of melanomas, anti-CD3 antibodies linked to melanocyte stimulating hormone enhances destruction of human melanoma cells by CTLs in vitro. These types of antibody therapies have so far been tried only in experimental animal studies (Figs. 5.15 and 5.16).

Monoclonal antibodies conjugated to bacterial toxins can also be used as tumor-specific **immunotoxins**. In this case monoclonal antibodies against tumor specific or tumor-associated antigens are linked to a toxin of bacterial origin like diphtheria toxin. Immunotoxins prepared in this manner against a variety of cancers, such as melanomas, colorectal cancers, metastatic breast cancers, different types of lymphomas and leukemias have been evaluated in phase I and

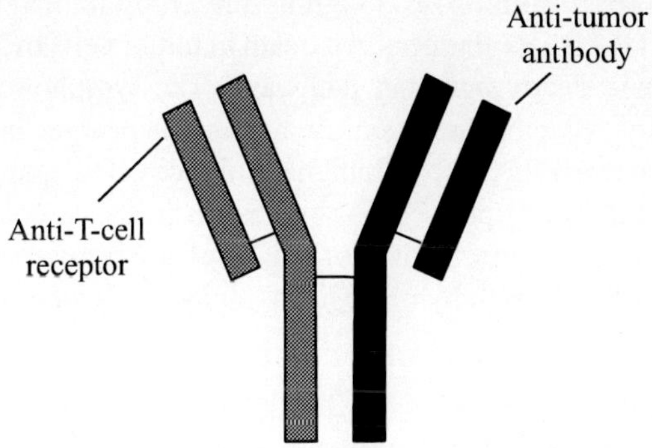

Fig. 5.15. Structure of a typical heteroconjugate monoclonal antibody

phase II trials. In eight separate trials 12-75% of leukemia and lymphoma patients there was complete remission. In contrast, the clinical response in patients with larger tumor was not favorable.

Ep-CAM (epithelial cell adhesion molecule; alternatively known as epithelial glycoprotein-2, EGP-2/GA 733-2) is overexpressed in numerous cancers, like colorectal, pancreatic, and non-small cell lung cancer. A monoclonal antibody, **Edrecolomab,** recognizes Ep-CAM, has gone through extensive clinical trials shows significant efficacy in colorectal carcinoma treatment.

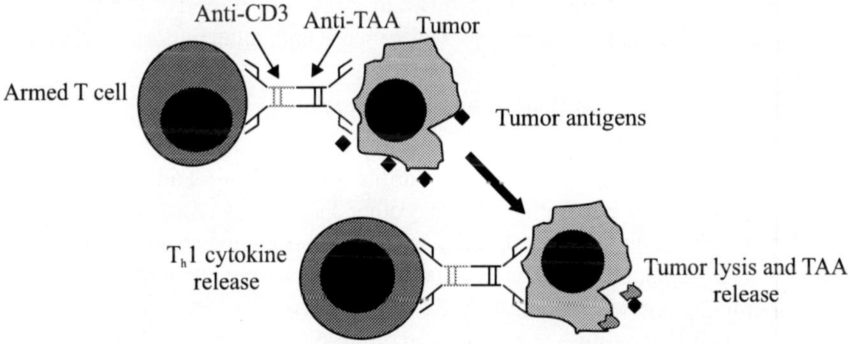

Fig. 5.16. Mode of action of heteroconjugate monoclonal antibody

Carcinoembryonic antigen (CEA) is a glycoprotein expressed on neoplasms and other adenocarcinomas derived gastrointestinal tract of endodermal origin. Being a surface antigen overexpressed by gastrointestinal tumor cells and high amount of it is released into circulation. However, normal tissues of the luminal surface of the gut also expressed it where mAbs cannot reach. mAbs developed against CEA have been used in radioimmunotherapy, antibody dependent enzyme pro-drug therapy (ADEPT) and in radioimmunoguided surgery (RIGS).

Tumor necrosis factor related apoptosis-inducing ligand (TRAIL) is a member of the TNF ligand superfamily responsible for inducing apoptosis of tumor cells with hardly any effect on most normal cells. mAb agonists of TRAIL-R1 or TRAIL-R2 of rabbit or marine origin have been used in humans, and have shown anti-tumor activity.

HGS-ETR1 **(mapatumumab)** is a high affinity, fully human agonistic mAb with specificity for TRAIL-R1, induces cell death in tumor cells by activating both intrinsic and extrinsic death signaling pathways. The lymphotoxin-β receptor, the third TNF family receptor, has been used as another target in mAb therapy. RAV12 is a chimeric mAb (IgG1k) with high affinity directed against an N-linked glycotope (RAG12) that is expressed on the vast majority of colon, gastric and pancreatic carcinomas. The mechanism of action of mAb involves induction of oncolysis,a process of cell death by necrosis involving cell swelling.

5.5.7.4 Bispecific monoclonal antibodies in cancer immunotherapy

Among the antibody-based cancer immunotherapies, bispecific antibody (biAb) therapy features predominantly under next-generation therapies. biAbs can be categorized into *trans*-acting and *cis*-acting depending on whether they bridge two targets on the same or on different cells. Vast majority of biAbs used in cancer therapeutic are *trans*-acting. For example, CD47 × CD20 and CD47 × CD19 biAbs were developed to confine CD47/SIRPα axis blockade to malignant and normal B cells.

At present T-cell engaging biAbs (T-biAbs) are the dominating therapies being practiced for the treatment of hematological cancers and solid tumors of various tissues. **Blinatumomab** (Blincyto® by Amgen) is currently the only T-biAb therapy that has been approved by US-FDA in 2014 and European Union EMA in 2015 for the treatment of hematological cancers and solid tumors of various tissues.

1. **T-biAbs for the treatment of hematological malignancies**

   T-biAbs can mediate a potent and selective cytotoxic response by recruiting and activating T cells with one Fab arm of the antibody and targeting the tumor cell surface receptor with the other Fab arm. Majority of T-biAbs approved till date for clinical trials use anti-CD3 specific Fab arm, especially directed against CD3ε as T cell engaging arm. CD3 engagement by T-biAbs generates cytotoxic response by establishing synapse between T cell and tumor cell that mimics the natural immunological synapse of T cell with antigen presenting cell through the interaction of class I and II MHC with T cell receptor (TCR). US-FDA and EMA approved T-biAb is blinatumomab, which has anti-CD3 specific one Fab arm and the other Fab arm is specific for CD19 for the treatment of adult and children suffering from Pre-B cell acute lymphoblastic leukemia (pre-B-ALL).

   Recently, two more pre-B-ALL therapies have been approved by US-FDA and EMA, namely, CD-19 targeting chimeric antigen receptor T cell (CAR–T) therapy Tisagenlecleucel (Kymriah® by Novartis for pediatric pre-B-ALL and CD22-targetingantibody-drug conjugate (ADC) inotuzumab ozogamycin (Besponsa® by Pfizer for adult pre-B-ALL. Conceptually, similar to T-biAbs, CAR-Ts, tisagenlecleucel and axicabtagene ciloleucel (Yescarta® by Gilead have received approval from US-FDA and EMA for the treatment of pediatric pre-B-ALL (tisagenlecleucel) and adult B cell non-Hodgkin's lymphoma (B-NHL) (tisagenlecleucel and axicabtagene ciloleucel). In addition to CD19 and CC20 T-biAbs, other clinical trials are in progress against BCMA for multiple myeloma (MM), CD123 for acute myeloid leukemia (AML), chronic myeloid leukemia (CML), CD33 for AML; and CD38 for MM.

2. **T-biAbs for the treatment of solid tumor malignancies**

   Most of the T-biAbs therapies against solid tumor malignancies are in phase I and II trials and in some have met with failure due to tumor microenvironment induced immunosuppressive effects. To overcome this suppressive effect alternative approaches have been followed using blocking antibodies against immunosuppressive components of tumor microenvironment. Targets that are pursued for T-biAbs therapy against solid tumor malignancies are HER2 in breast and gastric cancers; PSMA in prostate cancer; glypican 3 (GPC3) in liver, lung, and other cancers; ROR1, which is expressed in both hematological and solid tumor malignancies; p95HER2 in breast cancer; mucin 16 (MUC 16) in ovarian cancer.

3. **Oncolytic viruses for in situ expression of T-biAbs**

   Since inflamed tumor microenvironment is more capable of blocking the immune response and T-biAbs action on solid tumors, oncolytic viruses (OVs) have come to rescue to overcome this problem. In 2015, US-FDA and EMA approved OV therapy for the immunosuppressed solid tumor treatment. Talimogene laherparepvec (Imlygic® by Amgen), which is a live attenuated herpes simplex virus 1 (HSV-1) with a human GM-CSF transgene was administered to drug-resistant melanoma patients intratumoral administration. OVs have been designed and engineered to selectively lyse the tumor cells and stimulate systemic immune response without harming the normal cells and tissues by equipping them with an expression cassette encoding a therapeutic transgene, such as functional T-biAbs. OVs help in transduction of tumor cells by delivering T-biAb gene into the cytoplasm of tumor cells. Adenovirus and measles virus have been engineered to deliver transgene into tumor cells. Introduction of both T-biAb and CAR transgene into T cells for an EGFRvIII-targeting CAR T cells expressing CD3 × EGFR T-biAb in mouse model of glioblastoma multiforme (GBM) is an attractive approach for confining T-biAb to the tumor cell microenvironment.

5.5.7.5 *Antibody and complement mediated lysis or complement-dependent cytotoxicity (CDC) of bone marrow tumor cells in vitro*

It is used during autologous bone marrow transplantation carried out in B cell lymphoma patients. In this procedure, bone marrow from the B cell lymphoma patient is removed, and the patient is subjected to whole body radiation and chemotherapy, which results in destruction of normal marrow cells and tumor cells. The bone marrow removed from the patient is subjected to treatment with antibodies directed against B lymphocyte specific antigens, which are specifically expressed on B cell lymphomas. Antibody bound lymphoma cells are subjected to complement-mediated lysis by adding the complements. The treated marrow, having been depleted of B cell lymphoma cells, is transplanted back into the patient who restores the hematopoietic system, which was destroyed by radiation and chemotherapy.

CD46, CD55 and CD59 are overexpressed in cancer cells to evade complement mediated lysis. To overcome this blockade, in B-NHL (non-Hodgkin's lymphoma), *cis*-acting CD55 × CD20 and CD59 × CD20 biAbs were used to enhance CDC.

5.5.7.6 Antibody-directed enzyme prpo-drug therapy (ADEPT)

Antibody-directed enzyme pro-drug therapy (ADEPT) is a two-step approach to cancer therapy in which, first a tumor-specific mAb conjugated to enzyme is administered to a cancer patient that concentrates within tumor mass and will not be in systemic circulation over time. Once the tumor to non-tumor ratio reaches high level, an anticancer pro-drug is administered, which is converted to active drug at the tumor site by the mAB conjugated enzyme. Since the therapy is target oriented, soon after the enzyme converts pro-drug into drug, the drug enters specifically the cancer cell and causes cell death due to cytotoxicity, thereby preventing systemic toxicity of the drug.

5.5.8 Cytokines in Tumor Therapy

At present high grade, pure cytokines are made available through recombinant DNA technology and they are in sufficient quantity, hence, treatment of various tumors through cytokine mediated therapy has become feasible recently. The reason for using cytokines is because it can enhance one or more components of cell-mediated immune response. The transfection of tumor cells with cytokine gene makes them more susceptible for immune attack. Among the cytokines that have been evaluated in cancer immunotherapy are interferons α, β and γ, IL-1, IL-2, IL-4, IL-5 and IL-12, GM-CSF and TNFα.

Cytokine immunotherapy has its own drawbacks, such as systemic administration of some cytokines has serious side effects. Although, several experimental and clinical trials of cytokine therapy are discussed here it is important to note that this therapeutic approach is in its early stage and not approved for general practice.

Interleukin-2 (IL-2) in combination with adoptive cellular immune therapy or alone used in cancer therapy has the potential to increase T lymphocytes, NK cells in the blood and LAK cell activity, as well as increased levels of TNF, IL-1 and IFN-γ activity in the serum. In high doses IL-2 is toxic because it induces the production of other cytokines by T cells, which cause deleterious effects such as pulmonary edema, fever and often shock. This therapeutic approach has been approved by United States Food and Drug Administration for the treatment of advanced melanomas and renal cell carcinomas and has shown regression of tumors in 10 to 15% patients.

Tumor necrosis factor alpha (TNFα) and TNFβ, both exhibit anti-tumor activity by inducing hemorrhagic necrosis of tumors. TNFα inflicts damage to vascular endothelial cells in the vicinity of tumors and inhibits tumor-induced angiogenesis, thereby starving the tumor of nutrition, blood-flow and oxygen leading to death of tumor cells. TNFα therapy has its own limitations because of its short half-life, repeated injections are necessary, which leads to many side effects like fever, blood pressure and decreased WBC count. Only the drawback with this treatment is TNFα is highly toxic and causes many undesirable side effects. Recommended dose for human treatment is 0.04 mg/kg body weight.

Interferon-α (IFN-α) is a type I interferon, largely produced by leukocytes, enhances the class I MHC expression on various cell types and increases the NK cell-mediated lysis. Clinical trials of humans showed that daily administration of IFNα causes complete regression of tumor in some patients with myelomas, leukemias, and lymphomas (hematopoietic malignancies) and solid tumors such as melanomas, Kaposi's sarcoma, renal tumor, and breast cancer.

IFN-α, β and γ are known to increase Class I MHC expression on tumor cells hence make them prone to CTL-mediated cell killing. Increased expression of class II MHC on macrophages is known to occur due to the influence of IFN-γ, which facilitates expression for processed antigens of tumors, thereby increasing T_H cell response against tumors. Tumor cells are known to express decreased levels of class I MHC and interferons restore MHC expression by tumor cells.

IFN-γ activates macrophages and NK cells and upregulates MHC expression, which would facilitate anti-tumor immunity. Currently, intraperitoneal administration of IFN-γ for the treatment of ovarian cancer is being evaluated.

Growth factor of hematopoietic tissue, such as *granulocyte-macrophage colony stimulating factor* (GM-CSF) and *granulocyte colony stimulating factor* (G-CSF) are being exploited for cancer treatment. Generally, post-chemotherapy or autologous bone marrow transplantation, the patient suffers from neutropenia (decreased neutrophil population). Immune response against tumor can be enhanced by administering GM-CSF or G-CSF, which stimulates maturation of granulocyte precursor thereby indirectly enhancing anti-tumor activity.

5.5.8.1 Enhancement of APC activity through cytokines for immune therapy of cancer

Dendritic cells derived from mouse cultured in vitro were provided GM-CSF and incubated with liver tumor cells activate both T_H-cells and CTLs specific for the tumor antigens. These cells were injected back into mice were shown to display tumor immunity against liver tumor.

A more effective approach on similar lines has been tried, where tumor cells are transfected with gene encoding GM-CSF. These transfected cells are injected back into the same patient from whom the tumor cells were obtained. Genetically engineered cells start secreting GM-CSF, which enhances the differentiation of APCs, namely, dendritic cells. Dendritic cells start accumulating around the tumor cells, where tumor antigens are presented to T_H-cells and CTLs by dendritic cells.

Clinical trials are underway in melanoma patients, whose melanoma cells are transfected with GM-CSF.

Another approach is to expand peripheral blood dendritic cell population in culture in the presence of GM-CSF, TNF-α and IL-4. Highly proliferated dendritic cells are pulsed with tumor fragments and introduced back into the patients. These dendritic cells now activate T_H-cells and T-cytotoxic cells specific for tumor antigens.

5.6 NANOPARTICLES AS THERAPEUTICS FOR CANCER TREATMENT

Nanoparticles have been used as effective vehicles for the transport and delivery of poorly soluble chemotherapeutic drugs like paclitaxel. For the treatment of refractory breast cancer, protein-bound paclitaxel (**Abraxane**) or nab-paclitaxel was approved by the US FDA in January 2005, where paclitaxel bound to human albumin as a vehicle is used and not the Cremophore vehicle used in Taxol, another counterpart of paclitaxel. By externally applied magnetic field, magnetic nanoparticles bound to chemotherapeutic agents can be concentrated at tumor sites.

Importantly, multiple therapeutic functions can be combined into one in nanoparticles to target them to specific tissues or to reach particular sub-cellular compartment or target malignant cells in circulation by coating or binding the nanoparticles with specific proteins or receptors for targeted delivery. Circulating malignant cells can also be targeted by nanoparticles through antibody dependent enzyme pro-drug therapy ADEPT or targeting the ligand through the administration of immunotherapy, which otherwise would have been difficult with conventional approach.

Nanoparticle size, surface charge, mechanical properties, and chemistry, as well as the route of administration, play a major role in determining the localization of nanoparticles in specific organs. Because of the blood-brain barrier (BBB), treatment of brain tumor is considered to be the most challenging since only lipophilic substances can cross the BBB. Nanoparticle uptake in other organs is in the higher nanoscale range, whereas particle size of under 15 nm are allowed to pass across the BBB. Modification of the nanoparticle surface with lipophilic constituents and reduction in the surface charges facilitates BBB passage. Nanoparticles bound by apolipoprotein E (ApoE) conjugated to engineered monoclonal antibodies have been successfully transported across BBB in mouse model may turn out fruitful towards treatment of brain tumors due to increased uptake of drugs into the brain parenchyma.

Iron oxide nanoparticles coated with dextran leads to increased accumulation in lymph nodes, which can be exploited for the treatment of B cell lymphomas by conjugating chemotherapeutic drugs with nanoparticles. In general, nanoparticles charged negatively are taken up by the cells at faster rates than positively charged or uncharged particles. Nanoparticles coated with polyethylene glycol (PEG) 'stealth polymers' inhibit the uptake of nanoparticles by leukocytes, thereby reducing accumulation in the lymph nodes.

Lipids are amphiphilic in nature, therefore organize themselves into bilayered vesicles or liposomes, micelles or lipoplexes (amorphous particles). By using nanoparticles as carriers of these lipid-based vehicles, which can be surface modified for the targeted delivery of both water-soluble and insoluble therapeutics to the cells. Properties of the nanoparticles such as size, carrying capacity and targeting capabilities can also be modified by coupling the nanoliposomes with appropriate targeting ligand. The targeting ligand could be integrin-binding peptides which would facilitate accumulation of liposomes in the tumor vasculature during angiogenesis and can deliver a therapeutic payload of chemotherapeutic drugs. Release of the chemotherapeutic drugs could be controlled by pH-sensitive and temperature-sensitive formulations. Since liposomes are cleared fast through reticuloendothelial system (RES), they are coated with polyethylene glycol (PEG), which increases their retention time. PEG also helps as binding agent for drugs or antibody conjugation with liposomes.

5.6.1 Liposome Based Antibody Targeting

PEG coated liposomes could serve as antibody carriers to deliver antibody to specific target. The antibody is attached to the liposome through the terminus of PEG, such liposomes are called immunoliposomes. Ten to thirty antibody molecules are attached per liposome, which is found to be effective concentration to deliver the payload. Tumors expressing EGFR are treated with anti-EGFR liposomes carrying toxic drug (paclitaxel) has resulted in regression of EGFR positive tumors.

Folate receptor targeting liposomes have also been designed because most of the tumors are known to express folate receptor.

Among other important ligands that can be targeted using liposomes is transferrin receptor-1 (TFR1), which is overexpressed in many tumors.

Gold nanoparticles like gold shells, spheres and rods have been used for thermoablative therapies using near-infrared light, which releases the thermal energy in the form of heat that facilitates the coagulation of the tumor vasculature. Multiple ligands are attached to gold nanoparticles which serve as scaffolds.

A neovasculature-specific receptor integrin $\alpha v\beta 3$ is coated on lipid-based nanoparticles and this integrin receptor is not only specific to newly growing vessels but also facilitates internalization of viruses and small particles, which can be exploited for gene delivery.

Regression of primary and metastatic tumors can be brought about by coupling a mutant form of the Raf gene to the nanoparticles and it was used for inhibiting the Raf pathway critical for angiogenesis in vivo.

5.6.2 Synthetic Polymeric Nanoparticles for Vaccine Delivery

Poly-lactic acid (PLA), poly-glycolic acid (PGA), poly-lactide-co-glycolide (PLGA) are the most widely used polymers for nanoparticles coating. Polymeric nanoparticles have been found to be taken up by the mucosal tissue and these nanoparticles also can cross GI tract and the nasal mucosa and subsequently deliver the antigen into the bloodstream.

5.6.3 Chitosan Based Nanoparticles for DNA Delivery

Chitosan loaded with naked DNA as vaccine against tumor cell lines has been tried and it has yielded favorable results. Plasmid DNA carrying p53 gene was delivered to the lung cancer cells resulted in restoration of wild-type p53 function.

5.6.4 Targeting Several Steps of Metastasis at Once by Nanoparticles

Metastasis of tumor cells from a primary tumor site to a secondary site involves several steps. Recently "gene signatures" associated with primary tumor pertaining to risk of metastasis have been identified. Four gene signatures in human lung cancer metastasis have been identified, like EGFR ligand epiregulin, COX2, and MMP1 and MMP2. In mice, these genes have been proved to be responsible for tumor growth, angiogenesis, migration, intravasation, and extravasation. In the experimental approach, short hairpin RNA interference was used to target four genes simultaneously for reduced expression. Inhibition of all four genes suppressed the tumor growth and lung metastasis. Applying the same concept in the context of cancer therapeutics, a combination of the existing drugs like cetuximab (an anti-EGFR antibody), celecoxib (a COX inhibitor), and GM6001 (an MMP inhibitor) were able to target the protein products of the four genes and suppressed the tumor growth and metastasis. From the future cancer therapeutic perspective, these results hold great potential because if a cancer is caught at an early stage and metastasis is blocked, there is a hope of managing the cancer and survival rate in individual can be increased.

Exercise

1. Name the chemotherapeutic drugs that have been used till date for the treatment of cancer and explain their mechanism of action.
2. Plant derived drugs can be used for the treatment of cancer. Give details of plant derived drugs till date being used for cancer treatment.
3. External beam radiation therapy is being used for the treatment of various types of cancers, explain how it is being used for treatment of cancer.

   OR

   Internal beam radiation therapy is being used for treatment of various types of cancers, explain how it is being used for the treatment of cancer?
4. Strategies of targeting various molecular targets in cancer as a means of therapeutics.
5. How are the following therapeutic strategies employed for the treatment of cancer?

(a) Synthetic lethal strategy as a target of DNA repair pathway (schematic diagram)
(b) Inhibitors of DNA methylation
(c) Inhibitors of histone deacetylases
(d) Telomerase inhibitors
(e) Anti-EGFR drug
(f) Strategies against Raf
(g) Imatinib
(h) Cyclin dependent kinase inhibitors
(i) Inhibitors of mitotic spindle
(j) Strategies that aim to correct p53 mutation (schematic diagram)
(k) Strategies that aim to activate endogenous p53
(l) Strategies that aim to suppress endogenous p53
(m) Direct and indirect activation of caspases
(n) Regulation of Bcl-2 family proteins (schematic diagram)
(o) Targeting TRAIL and its receptor
(p) Inhibitors of Wnt pathway or Hh pathway (schematic presentation)
(q) Leukemia differentiation therapies
(r) Metalloproteinase inhibitors and metastasis suppressor
(s) Anti-angiogenic therapy and vascular targeting

6. Explain the following strategies of immune therapies against cancer:
   (a) Whole cell vaccines
   (b) Adoptive immune therapy
   (c) Peptide vaccines
   (d) Inhibition of inflammation
   (e) Vaccination against cancer
7. What is meant by passive therapy for cancer? How is it done?
8. Write in detail cancer therapy with anti-tumor antibodies.
9. How does cytokine therapy work for cancer treatment? Explain.
10. What is meant by nanomedicine? How is it used in cancer therapeutics?
11. Explain the application of nanoparticles in the treatment of cancer.
12. How liposome-based cancer therapy is carried out? With a suitable example explain the process.

Glossary

Abasic: Referring to the nucleotide that has lost its purine or pryrimidine base, *See also* **apurinic; apyrimidinic.**

Ablate: To eliminate.

Acellular: Lacking or deprived of cells.

Acetylation: Covalent attachment of acetyl group to a second molecule such as protein.

Adduct: The novel molecular structure arising after covalent linkage of a mutagen with one or another portion of a DNA molecule.

Adenocarcinoma: Tumor derived from secretary epithelial cells.

Adenoma (adj., -adenomatous): Any of the series of pre-malignant, noninvasive growths in various epithelial tissues, many of which have the potential to progress further to carcinomas. *See also* **polyp.**

Adipocytes: Specialized cells of the mesenchymal lineage, closely related to fibroblasts that create fat and store it in large globules in the cytoplasm; the dominant cell types in fatty (adipose) tissue.

Adjuvant: A substance not being antigenic itself is a strong stimulant of immune response. A substance used in combination with a therapy to enhance the efficacy.

Adoptive transfer: Procedure in which immune cells are transferred from one donor to a recipient of the same species.

Agonist: Activating agent: opposite of antagonist.

Alkylating: Capable of attaching an alkyl group or similarly structured chemical group to a substrate such as a DNA base.

Allele: One alternative among different versions of a gene that may be defined by the phenotype that it creates, by the protein that it specifies, or by its nucleotide sequence.

Amphiphillic or amphipathic: A molecule containing distinct hydrophilic and hydrophobic groups.

Amplification: Genetic mechanism by which the copy number of a gene is increased above its normal level in a diploid genome or existence of many copies of the same gene in a diploid cell.

Anaplastic: Referring to the tumor, lacking the cellular architecture differentiated characteristic of a tissue origin.

Anchorage dependence: Requirement of normal cells for attachment to a solid surface before they grow or multiply.

Anchorage independence: Ability of a cell to proliferate without attaching to the solid support.

Aneuploid: A karyotype that deviates from the diploid number because of increase or decrease in number of certain chromosomes.

Angiogenesis: A process by which new blood vessels are formed.

Angiogenic factor: Type of growth factor that facilitates growth of blood vessels.

Angiosarcoma: Tumor of the cells that are precursors to endothelial cells.

Anoxia: A state of oxygenless condition.

Antibody: A soluble protein produced against antigens by plasma cells of the immune system. *See also* **immunoglobulin**

Antigen: A molecule that can trigger an immune response, bind to antibody produced against it, presented by class I and II MHC and bind to T cell receptor.

Antigen-presenting cells: A class of immune cells often called professional antigen presenting cells like dendritic cells, macrophage, and B cells. They present antigen on class II MHC on their surface to T cell receptor.

Apoptosis: Programmed cell death induced by various factors in a cell when the cell shows severe abnormality in genetic milieu or biochemical pathways.

Apoptosome: A multiprotein complex consisting of cytochrome c complexed with apoptosome activation factor (Apaf-1) that facilitates apoptosis.

Apurinic: Refers to the product of depurination, in which glycosidic bond linking a deoxyribose to a purine base is broken, leaving behind only the deoxyribose in the DNA.

Aromatic: Refers to an organic molecule that contains one or more benzene rings.

Ascites: The fluid that accumulates in the peritoneal cavity of some cancer patients, often containing malignant cells.

Astrocytoma: Tumor of the astrocytes, neuronal support cells in the brain.

Ataxia: Loss of muscle coordination.

Autocrine: A hormone or protein factor acting on the cell that produces it.

Autologous: Refers to biological material that belongs to one's own body.

Base excision repair: A form of DNA repair that initially involves cleavage of glycosidic bond between base and deoxyribose by a repair enzyme leaving behind abasic nucleotide.

Basement membrane: A specialized extracellular matrix that forms a sheet separating epithelial from stromal cells, sometimes called **basal limina.**

Benign: Abnormal growth of cells confined to a specific site in a tissue surrounded by a connective tissue capsule showing no evidence of migration into neighboring area.

Bispecific: Able to specifically recognize two objects simultaneously.

Body-mass index: Weight in kilograms divided by the square of the height in meters.

Breakpoint: Location on the chromosome where the chromosome breaks or fuses with other chromosome during translocation.

Bronchial: Referring to the major airway of the lung.

Buccal: Referring to the tissue of the oral cavity.

Carcinogen: An agent that contributes to the cancer development.

Carcinogenic: An agent capable of causing cancer.

Carcinoma: Cancer arising from epithelial cells.

Caspase: A cystein-aspartyl-specific protease.

CD4: A receptor specific T-helper cells (T_H cell) expressed on its membrane.

CD8: A receptor specific T-cytotoxic cells (T_C cell) expressed on its membrane.

CD20: An antigen specific to B cells expressed on its membrane and over-expressed in B cell lymphomas.

Cell cycle: Progress of cell division in a cyclical manner with changes in chromosomal morphology and biochemical events as it progresses culminating in cell division.

Cell cycle clock: A network of signaling proteins that regulate the cell cycle culminating in cell division.

Cell lines: The cells derived from a tissue adapted grow endlessly in culture medium.

Cellular (cell-mediated) immune response: Involvement of specific cell types of the immune system to provide defence, like T-helper cells, cytotoxic T cells, NK cells and macrophages.

Checkpoint: Control point that ensures that the next step in the cell cycle does not proceed until a series of preconditions have been fulfilled including the completion of DNA repair.

Chimera (Chimeric): Organisms or combinations in which different cells or molecules derived from genetically distinct parents or chemical constitution are brought together

Referring to a protein product of a re-engineered gene in which two portions of the protein derive from two distinct sources.

Chromatid: A half chromosome that exists after S phase and before M phase; paired chromatids are separated at M phase, whereupon each becomes a chromosome.

Chromatin: Complex of DNA with protein that constitutes a chromosome.

Clone: Copy of a gene that has been isolated from recombinant DNA technology and amplified into a large number of identical copies.
Population of cells all of which descend from a common progenitor cell.

Co-carcinogen: An agent or substance that is as such not being carcinogenic on its own, collaborates with another agent to enable carcinogenesis to proceed.

Colonization: Proliferation of cells within a micrometastasis that leads to the establishment of a macroscopic metastasis.

Colony: A cluster of cells usually of clonal origin.

Colorectal: Referring to the lower gastrointestinal tract including the colon and rectum.

Complement: A group of collaborating plasma proteins that undergoes activation in a cascading manner and comes together to form a complex with antigen-antibody complex on the cell membrane and causes cell lysis by creating pores on the cell membrane.

Complete carcinogen: An agent that can act as both initiator and promoter of tumor growth and progression.

Contact inhibition: A behavior exhibited by the cells propagated in tissue culture as monolayer.

Copy choice: A molecular genetic mechanism whereby a growing DNA strand can select the template for its further elongation from among alternative complementary DNA strands.

Crisis: A state arising when cells lose telomeres of certain length, resulting in end-to-end fusion of chromosomes, karyotypic chaos leading to widespread cell death and apoptosis.

Crypt: Deep cavity in the wall of small or large intestine in which enterocyte stem cell proliferation and initial differentiation occur.

Cyclin: A protein that associates with a cyclin-dependent kinase and serves as a regulatory subunit of this kinase by activating its catalytic activity and directing it to appropriate substrates.

Cyclin-dependent kinase: Type of serine-threonine kinase deployed by the cell cycle machinery that depends on an associated cyclin protein for proper functioning.

Cytokines: Growth factors that stimulate one or several of the cell types of the hematopoietic system. Regulatory factors of the immune system that regulate immune cell reactions.

Cytoskeleton: Network of proteins in the cell, largely in the cytoplasm that provide structural rigidity to the cell and helps in cell division as well as in cell motility

Cytosol: The cytoplasm of the cell containing soluble materials present in the free form.

Deamination: Loss of an amine group from a larger molecule such as a DNA base.

Dedifferentiation: Reversion of differentiated cell to the phenotype of a less differentiated cell of embryonic condition.

Dendritic cells: An immune cell capable of phagocytosis of infectious agents and cell fragments and then present oligopeptides derived from these phagocytosed particles to T-helper cell on Class II MHC.

Density dependent growth: *See* Contact inhibition.

Depurination: Breaking of glycosidic bond that links purine bases to the deoxyribose of DNA.

Depyrimidination: Breaking of glycosidic bond that links pyrimidine bases to the deoxyribose of DNA.

Dermal: Referring to thick layer of stromal cells, largely fibroblasts beneath the epidermis of the skin.

Dicentric: Refers to chromatids or chromosome having two distinct centromeres.

Differentiation: A process whereby a cell acquires a specialized phenotype particular to a tissue.

Dimer: Molecular complex composed of two subunits.

Diploid: Refers to the genome of a cell in which all chromosomes are present in pairs, one of each pair is inherited from a father and the other from a mother.

Disseminated: Spread or seeded widely.

Dominant: Referring to one of several alternative genes that can be specified by a genetic locus; when the locus is heterozygous and carries information specifying two distinct traits, the dominant trait will express.

Dominant interfering: *See* dominant negative.

Dominant negative: Referring to a mutant allele of a gene that, when co-exists with wild type allele will co-express with wild type allele of the gene and interfere with the functioning of wild-type allele.

Double minute: A chromosomal segment the becomes separated from the chromosome in which normally resides and is able to perpetuate itself as an extrachromosomal particle unlinked to a centromere.

Dysplasia (adj., Dysplastic): Premalignant tissue consisting of abnormal appearing cells constituting tissue architecture that deviates from normal.

Ectodomain: Portion of the cell surface protein that protrudes from the plasma membrane into the exterior.

Effector: An agent such as protein that carries out actual work of a biological process rather than regulating it.

Electrophile: Referring to a molecule that seeks out and reacts with electron-rich substrates.

Endocrine: Referring to a gland that secretes fluids into a general circulation without using ducts.

Endoderm: Innermost layer of the cells in a developing embryo.

Endogenous: Originating from within a cell.

Endothelial cells: Mesenchymal cells that form the walls of blood capillaries and lymph ducts.

Enterocyte: Epithelial cells lining luminal wall of the gastrointestinal tract.

Epithelial-mesenchymal transition: Acquisition by epithelial cells the phenotypic characteristic of mesenchymal cells.

Epithelium: A layer of cells that forms the lining of a cavity or duct, including the epithelium that forms the upper layer of skin.

Erythroblastosis: Malignancy of the precursors of red blood cells.

Ex vivo: Occurring outside of a living body or organism.

Exocyclic: Referring to the chemical group that is attached or protrudes from the aromatic ring.

Extracellular matrix: Meshwork of secreted proteins, largely glycoproteins and proteoglycans that surround most cells in a tissue and create structure in the intercellular space.

Familial: Referring to trait that is inheritable and therefore found in clusters in certain families.

Fibrin: Protein formed by the cleavage of plasma fibrinogen and assembles in the form of fibers binding the platelets together in clots.

Fibrinogen: *See* Fibrin

Fibroblast: A type of mesenchymal cells found commonly in connective tissue and the stromal compartment of epithelial tissue and is characterized by its secretion of collagen.

Fibrocyte: A relatively undifferentiated circulating cell of bone marrow origin that express collagen, adheres tightly to substrates when cultures in vitro and appears as precursor of fibroblasts.

Fibrosis: Development of dense fibrous stroma within a tissue particularly after inflammatory response, replaces normal epithelium resulting in loss of function of the tissue.

Focus (pl., **foci**): A cluster of transformed cells surrounded by normal cells.

Gate keeper: The gene that operates to hinder cell division or further cell differentiation, in this way prevents the appearance of neoplastic cells.

Gene amplification: Increase in the number of copies of a gene normally present in the diploid genome.

Genetic polymorphism: A variant sequence genome of an organism that has no effect on phenotype and genetically transmitted in Mendelian fashion.

Genotoxic: Referring to an agent that is capable of damaging the genome, i.e., mutagenic.

Germ line: The cells within a multicellular organism that are responsible for carrying and transmitting genes from one individual to its offspring.

Glioblastoma: Tumor of the glial cells of the brain.

Glioma: *See* Glioblastoma

Glycoprotein: A protein that has undergone post-translational modification and conjugated to carbohydrate moiety.

Gray (Gy): Unit of radiation exposure equal to the absorption of one joule of energy per kilogram of exposed tissue.

Growth factor: Protein that is able to stimulate growth/proliferation of cells by binding to specific cell surface receptors.

Half-life: Time during which half of a population of metabolically unstable molecules decays or is eliminated or the time required for half of a physiologic signal to decrease.

Haploinsufficiency: State in which the presence of only a single functional copy of a gene yields a mutant or partially mutant phenotype.

Hemangioblastoma: Tumor of the precursor of the endothelial cells.

Hemizygosity: Presence of only one copy of the autosomal gene per cell.

Hepatocellular carcinoma: *See* Hepatoma

Hepatocyte: Epithelial cells of the liver that constitutes bulk of the liver and is responsible for all of the metabolic activity of the liver.

Hepatoma: Tumor of the liver epithelial cells, also known as **hepatocellular carcinoma.**

Herceptin: Chimeric anti-HER2/Neu monoclonal antibody bearing murine antigen combining (variable) Fab domain and human constant region (Fc) domain, also called **trastuzumab.**

Heterochromatin: Chromatin that contains transcriptionally inactive tightly coiled, compact region, that stains darkly.

Heterodimer: Molecular complex composed of two distinct subunits.

Heterozygous: Referring to the configuration of genetic locus in which two copies of the associated gene carry different version (alleles) of genes responsible for two different traits.

High-grade: Referring to a tumor that has progressed through many steps of multi-step tumorigenesis and become highly malignant.

Hydrocarbon: A molecule composed of hydrogen and carbon atoms.

Hyperoxia: State of oxygen tension that is elevated above physiologic levels.

Hyperphosphorylated: Referring to elevated phosphorylation of protein.

Hyperplasia (adj., hyperplastic): Accumulation of excessive number of normal-appearing cells within a tissue.

Hypophosphorylated: Referring to relatively weak phosphorylation of protein.

Hypoxia: State of lower than normal oxygen tension.

Idiotype: Fab region of the antibody molecule with specific amino acid sequence.

Immortality: Proliferative ability of the cells without mortality or dying.

Immortalization: The cell that gains the ability of indefinite proliferation.

Immunoglobulins: Globular glycoprotein molecule capable of binding to antigen produced by plasma cells of the immune system.

Immunotoxin: Antibody conjugated to toxin molecule usually derived from bacteria.

In situ: Occurring in the site of origin.

In vitro: Occurring in a tissue culture dish or in a glass container.

In vivo: Occurring in a living organism.

Initiation: The first step in the multistep process of tumorigenesis, i.e., first change observed in a cell be means of a mutation.

Initiator: Agent that triggers the mutation in the multistep process of tumorigenesis.

Insertional mutagenesis: Process whereby a gene becomes mutated through the insertion or integration of another genetic segment (element) in the chromosomal DNA, such as, insertion of viral genome in the DNA.

Integration: Insertion of fragment of foreign DNA (genome of virus) into chromosomal DNA so that it becomes the part and parcel of host genome in which it is inserted.

Internalization: Process by which proteins and other molecules are imported into the cell cytoplasm.

Interstitial deletion: Refers to loss of chromosomal segment in the midst of the chromatid.

Invasion: Migration of cancer cells from the primary tumor to the neighboring area of normal tissue.

Kinase: Enzyme that covalently attaches phosphate groups to substrate molecules, often proteins.

Leiomyoma: Benign tumor of the mesenchymal cells forming the wall of the uterus.

Leukemia: Malignancy of any variety of hematopoietic cells.

Leukosis: Leukemia like disease of chicken.

Ligand: Molecule that binds specifically to a receptor and activates its signaling power.

Lineage: Linear succession of cells extending from an ancestral cell to its descendents.

Locus: Region of the chromosome that can be studied genetically and is presumed to be associated with a specific gene.

Low-grade: Referring to a tumor that has progressed minimally and is still relatively benign.

Lumen: The bore of a hollow, tube-like structure.

Luminal: Referring to the cells that line and face the lumen of a tube-like structure.

Lymphocytes: Class of immune cells that mediate humoral and cell-mediated immune response, encompassing B cells, T cells and NK cells.

Lymphoma: Solid tumor of the lymphoid cells.

Malignant: The growth of tumor cells that shows invasive and possibly metastatic ability.

Medulloblastoma: Tumor of the neurons of the cerebellum.

Melanocyte: Cells of the neural crest origin that produces pigment in the skin and iris.

Melanoma: Tumor arising from the melanocytes.

Menarche: Time in the life of women when the menstrual cycle begins.

Mesenchymal: Referring to the tissue composed of the cells of the mesodermal origin.

Mesenchymal-epithelial transition: The reversal of the epithelial-mesenchymal transition (*see also* epithelial-mesenchymal transition).

Metalloproteinase: A protease that contains a metal atom, usually zinc, in its catalytic site.

Metaplasia: Replacement in tissue of cells of one differentiation lineage by cells of another lineage.

Metastasis: Malignant growth forming at one site in the body, the cells of which derive from a malignant tumor located elsewhere in the body.

Micrometastasis: A metastasis composed of a single cell derived from malignant tumor or a small clump of cells derived from malignant tumor.

Missense mutation: The change of a single base pair causes the substitution of a different amino acid in the resulting protein.

Murine: Referring to the rodent group that includes mice.

Mutagen (adj., mutagenic): An agent that induces mutation.

Mutation: Change in the genotype of a species that involves alteration in nucleotide sequence of DNA segment leading to change in trait.

Myelogenous: Originating in the bone marrow. (*See also* **myeloid**)

Myeloid: Referring to lineage of hematopoietic tissue of bone marrow origin.

Myeloma: Malignancy of antibody producing cells of the bone marrow.

Necrosis: Process of cell death involving the breakdown of a cell and its constituents through steps that are distinct from apoptosis.

Neoplasia (adj., neoplastic): Cells showing abnormal growth or proliferation.

Neural crest: Adjacent region to neural tube in the early embryonic development of neurula stage of vertebrate embryos as the neural tube is being formed.

Neuroblastoma: Tumor originating from precursor neural cells of peripheral nervous system and adrenal medulla.

Neuroectodermal: Referring to the component of the nervous system derived from early embryonic ectoderm through the process of invagination of ectoderm.

Neurofibroma: Benign tumor of the cells forming the sheath around the axon.

Neurofibrosarcoma: Malignant tumor of the cells forming the sheath around the axon.

Nonhomologous end joining (NHEJ): Type of DNA repair consisting of joining of double stranded DNA ends is not directed by sequence in a sister chromatid or homologous chromosome.

Nonsense codon: Triplet codon in the genetic code that specifies termination of growing amino acid chain (peptide chain).

Nonsense mutation: Mutation causing premature termination of a growing protein chain.

Non-small-cell lung carcinoma: Several types of lung cancers with the exception of small cell lung carcinoma.

Normoxia: Normal oxygen concentration experienced by cells in a specific tissue environment.

Nucleophilic: Referring to molecule that seeks out and reacts with electron poor substrates.

Nucleotide-excision repair: A type of DNA repair with which the initial step involves the excision of DNA bases together with associated nucleotides.

Oncofoetal: Referring to a antigen that is normally expressed during embryonic tissue during early stage of development and is also expressed by some tumor cells.

Oncogene (adj., Oncogenic): A gene that can transform cells or a cancer-inducing gene.

Oncoprotein: A protein product of an oncogene.

Osteosarcoma: Cancer of the bone tissue.

Overexpression: Expression of RNA or protein at higher than normal level.

Papilloma: A benign adenomatous proliferation of epithelial cells of skin.

Papova viruses: The class of viruses that includes SV40, polyoma virus, and pailloma viruses.

Paracrine: Referring to the signaling path of a hormone or factor released by one cell and acts on other cells.

Pericytes: Cells closely related to smooth muscle cells that surround blood capillaries and support the capillary wall together with endothelial cells.

Pheochromocytoma: Tumor of the neuroectodermal cells of adrenal medulla.

Phosphotase: An enzyme that removes phosphates from phosphorylated substrates.

Phosphorylation: Covalent attachment of a phosphate group to a substrate.

Plasminogen: The inactive pro-enzyme converted to active plasmin protease through proteolytic cleavage.

Pocket protein: The term referring to pRb (retinoblastoma protein) and two of its cousins p107 and p130.

Point mutation: Substitution of a single base for another in a DNA sequence.

Polyclonal: Describing a population of cells so that their origin can be traced to two or more ancestral cells.

Polycyclic: Referring to molecules with more than one benzene ring structure.

Polycyclic aromatic hydrocarbons: A hydrocarbon having more than one benzene ring.

Primary cells: Cells that have been recently removed from living tissue and put into culture and have not been propagated.

Primary tumor: Tumor growing at the anatomical site where tumor progression began to yield a mass of cells.

Procarcinogen: A chemical compound which is nonreactive chemically can be converted into highly reactive carcinogen through metabolic process.

Proto-oncogene: A normal cellular gene, upon mutation by chemicals or virus transforms itself into oncogene.

Rad: Unit of radiation corresponding to 0.01 joule of absorbed radiation or 0.01 grey.

Radiotherapy: Treatment of disease like cancer by X-ray radiation or gamma radiation.

Refractory: Unresponsive to some type of signal or therapeutic agent.

Relapse: Recurrence of a disease, i.e., reappearance of a tumor.

Remission: Retreat or disappearance of a disease.

Restriction point: A decision-making point in the cell cycle in G1 phase before the cell enters division cycle

Retinoblastoma: Tumor of the retinal cells.

Retrovirus: A class of virus having RNA as its genetic material.

Reverse transcriptase: The enzyme capable of making complementary DNA be reading or copying the nucleotide sequence of RNA molecule which acts as a template.

Rituxan: Chimeric anti-CD 20 monoclonal antibody bearing murine antigen combining (variable) Fab domain and human constant region (Fc) domain, also called **Rituximab.**

Sarcoma: Tumor derived from mesenchymal cells, usually those constituting connective tissue cells, muscle cells, fibroblasts, osteoblasts, and chondrocytes.

Schwannoma: Tumor of the Schwann cells forming sheath around axonic neuron.

Small-cell lung carcinoma: Tumor of neurosecretory cells of lung.

Somatic mutation: Mutation that strikes the genome of cells other than germ-line cells or gametic cells or gonadal cells.

Sporadic: The disease that occurs randomly or suddenly in a large population without any predisposition

Squamous: Referring to epithelial cells that line a duct but not secretory in function.

Stem cell: Cell type within a tissue that is capable of self-renewal and is also capable generating daughter cells that undergo differentiation to form specialized cells.

Stroma: Mesenchymal component of epithelial and hematopoietic tissues and tumors.

Subcutaneous: Beneath the skin.

T-loop: Configuration of the telomeric DNA that involves the insertion of its 3′ overhanging strand into its double stranded region.

Telomerase: An enzyme specialized to extend the telomeric DNA having RNA as template in the core of the enzyme with reverse transcriptase action.

Telomere: End part of the eukaryotic chromosome (chromatid) that protects the chromosome from sticking to each other having repetitive sequence of nitrogenous bases.

Therapy: A treatment procedure.

Transformation: Process of converting normal cell into to a cell having cancer characteristics.

Transit-amplifying cells: Relatively undifferentiated cells generated from stem cells and are capable of exponential proliferation for a limited number of generation before differentiating themselves into specialized cells.

Translocation: Rearrangement of chromosome by breaking off a chromatid and fusing it with another chromosome that does not belong to homologous pair resulting in alteration of chromosome morphology and genetic sequence.

Tumor progression: Process of multistep evolution of a normal cell into a tumor cell.

Tumor rejection: Process by which an organism prevents formation of tumor.

Tumor suppressor gene: A gene whose partial or complete inactivation leads to an increased likelihood of cancer development.

Tumoricidal: Able to kill/destroy tumor cells.

Tumorigenic: Ability to form tumors when introduced into other animal hosts.

Ubiquitylation: Process by which one or more ubiquitin molecules attach to a protein substrate, which often results in destruction of protein.

Ultimate carcinogen: A chemical compound that is able to directly contribute to the induction of cancer without prior modification or metabolism by directly interacting with DNA and bring about mutation.

Vimentin: An intermediate filament protein of the cytoskeleton of mesenchymal cells such as fibroblasts.

Wild type: The allele of the gene that is commonly present in all the cells in an individual species.

Zymogen: Inactive form of enzyme stored in the cell cytoplasm in the form of granule.

Index

[A]

[B]

[C]

[D]

[E]

[F]

[G]

[H]

[I]

[K]

[N]

[O]

[P]

[Q]

[R]

[S]

[T]

[U]